Household Safety Sourcebook

Hypertension Sourcebook

Immune System Disorders Sourcebook

Infant & Toddler Health Sourcebook

Infectious Diseases Sourcebook

Injury & Trauma Sourcebook

Kidney & Urinary Tract Diseases & Disorders Sourcebook

Learning Disabilities Sourcebook, 2nd Edition

Leukemia Sourcebook

Liver Disorders Sourcebook

Lung Disorders Sourcebook

Medical Tests Sourcebook, 2nd Edition

Men's Health Concerns Sourcebook, 2nd Edition

Mental Health Disorders Sourcebook, 3rd Edition

Mental Retardation Sourcebook

Movement Disorders Sourcebook

Muscular Dystrophy Sourcebook

Obesity Sourcebook

Osteoporosis Sourcebook

Pain Sourcebook, 2nd Edition

Pediatric Cancer Sourcebook

Physical & Mental Issues in Aging Sourcebook

Podiatry Sourcebook

Pregnancy & Birth Sourcebook, 2nd Edition

Prostate Cancer

Public Health Sourcebook

Reconstructive & Cosmetic Surgery Sourcebook

Rehabilitation Sourcebook

Respiratory Diseases & Disorders Sourcebook

Sexually Transmitted Diseases Sourcebook, 2nd Edition

Skin Disorders Sourcebook

Sleep Disorders Sourcebook, 2nd Edition

Smoking Concerns Sourcebook

Sports Injuries Sourcebook, 2nd Edition

Stress-Related Disorders Sourcebook

Stroke Sourcebook

Substance Abuse Sourcebook

Surgery Sourcebook

Thyroid Sourcebook

Transplantation Sourcebook

Traveler's Health Sourcebook

Vegetarian Sourcebook

Women's Health Concerns Sourcebook, 2nd Edition

Workplace Health & Safety Sourcebook

Worldwide Health Sourcebook

Teen Health Series

Alcohol Information for Teens

Asthma Information for Teens

Cancer Information for Teens

Diet Information for Teens

Drug Information for Teens

Eating Disorders Information for Teens

Fitness Information for Teens

Mental Health Information for Teens

Sexual Health Information for Teens

Skin Health Information for Teens

Sports Injuries Information for Teens

Suicide Information for Teens

Health Reference Series

Second Edition

Immune System Disorders SOURCEBOOK

Basic Consumer Health Information about Disorders of the Immune System, Including Immune System Function and Response, Diagnosis of Immune Disorders, Information about Inherited Immune Disease, Acquired Immune Disease, and Autoimmune Diseases, Including Primary Immune Deficiency, Acquired Immunodeficiency Syndrome (AIDS), Lupus, Multiple Sclerosis, Type 1 Diabetes, Rheumatoid Arthritis, and Graves Disease

Along with Treatments, Tips for Coping with Immune Disorders, a Glossary, and a Directory of Additional Resources

Edited by
Joyce Brennfleck Shannon

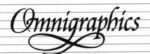

Omnigraphics

615 Griswold Street • Detroit, MI 48226

Bibliographic Note

Because this page cannot legibly accommodate all the copyright notices, the Bibliographic Note portion of the Preface constitutes an extension of the copyright notice.

Edited by Joyce Brennfleck Shannon

Health Reference Series

Karen Bellenir, *Managing Editor*
David A. Cooke, M.D., *Medical Consultant*
Elizabeth Barbour, *Research and Permissions Coordinator*
Cherry Stockdale, *Permissions Assistant*
Dawn Matthews, *Verification Assistant*
Laura Pleva Nielsen, *Index Editor*
EdIndex, Services for Publishers, *Indexers*

* * *

Omnigraphics, Inc.

Matthew P. Barbour, *Senior Vice President*
Kay Gill, *Vice President—Directories*
Kevin Hayes, *Operations Manager*
Leif Gruenberg, *Development Manager*
David P. Bianco, *Marketing Director*

* * *

Peter E. Ruffner, *Publisher*

Frederick G. Ruffner, Jr., *Chairman*

Copyright © 2005 Omnigraphics, Inc.

ISBN 0-7808-0748-0

Library of Congress Cataloging-in-Publication Data

Immune system disorders sourcebook : basic consumer healthinformation about disorders of the immune system, including immune system function and response, diagnosis of immune disorders, information about inherited immune disease, acquired immune disease, and autoimmune diseases, including primary immune deficiency, acquired immunodeficiency syndrome (AIDS), lupus, multiple sclerosis, type 1 diabetes, rheumatoid arthritis, and Graves disease; along with treatments, tips for coping with immune disorders, a glossary, and a directory of additional resources / edited by Joyce Brennfleck Shannon.-- 2nd ed.
    p. cm. -- (Health reference series)
    Summary: "Provides basic consumer health information about immune system function,diseases,treatments,and management of related disorders. Includes index, glossary of related terms, and other resources"--Provided by publisher.
    Includes bibliographical references and index.
    ISBN 0-7808-0748-0 (hardcover : alk. paper)
    1. Immunologic diseases--Popular works. I. Shannon, Joyce Brennfleck. II. Health reference series (Unnumbered).
    RC582.I4626 2005
    616.07'9--dc22
                                                                2005014226

The information in this publication was compiled from the sources cited and from other sources considered reliable. While every possible effort has been made to ensure reliability, the publisher will not assume liability for damages caused by inaccuracies in the data, and makes no warranty, express or implied, on the accuracy of the information contained herein.

This book is printed on acid-free paper meeting the ANSI Z39.48 Standard. The infinity symbol that appears above indicates that the paper in this book meets that standard.

Printed in the United States

Table of Contents

Visit www.healthreferenceseries.com to view *A Contents Guide to the Health Reference Series*, a listing of more than 10,000 topics and the volumes in which they are covered.

Part III: Inherited Immune Deficiency Diseases

Part VI: Other Altered Immune Responses

Part VII: Treatments for Immune Deficiencies and Diseases

Preface

About This Book

The body's immune system usually works efficiently to ward off disease, but things can go wrong. Sometimes dysfunctions result from inherited conditions. Sometimes they are caused when bacteria or viruses, such as the human immunodeficiency virus (HIV), slip past normal immune system defenses. Sometimes, for reasons poorly understood, the immune system begins to attack normal body cells; this can result in an autoimmune disease. Autoimmune diseases afflict approximately five percent of the U.S. population, and more than one in every 500 U.S. citizens is born with an inherited immune system disorder.

Immune System Disorders Sourcebook provides information about immune system function and related disorders. Readers will learn about inherited, acquired, and autoimmune diseases, including primary immune deficiency, acquired immunodeficiency syndrome (AIDS), lupus, multiple sclerosis, type 1 diabetes, rheumatoid arthritis, and Graves disease. Information about symptoms and treatments is included along with tips for coping with an immune disorder, suggestions for caregivers, glossaries of terms and diseases, and a directory of additional resources.

How to Use This Book

This book is divided into parts and chapters. Parts focus on broad areas of interest. Chapters are devoted to single topics within a part.

Part I: Immune System Overview describes how the immune system works and explains both natural and acquired immunity. It summarizes the types of disorders that affect the immune system and describes factors that influence its function. Research initiatives to help better understand the immune system and learn how it can be manipulated to produce health benefits are also described.

Part II: Diagnosis of Immune System Disorders provides information for people concerned about the diagnostic challenges involved in identifying immune disorders. Facts about the tests most commonly used, including blood, gene, and allergy tests, are provided.

Part III: Inherited Immune Deficiency Diseases explains the symptoms, diagnosis, and treatment of diseases that result when genetic defects cause essential parts of the immune system to be missing or to malfunction. Inherited immune deficiency diseases include primary immune deficiency (PID), ataxia-telangiectasia, selective IgA deficiency, and severe combined immunodeficiency (SCID), which is more commonly known as "bubble boy disease."

Part IV: Acquired Immune Deficiency Diseases describes immune system diseases that are not present at birth but that are acquired later. These can result from exposure to the human immunodeficiency virus (HIV), the body's response to a transplant, or the inability to tolerate a substance in the environment.

Part V: Autoimmune Diseases explains the symptoms, diagnosis, and treatment of diseases caused when immune cells mistake the body's own cells as invaders and attack them. Individual chapters cover diseases alphabetically from Addison disease to vitiligo.

Part VI: Other Altered Immune Responses describes immune system reactions to environmental triggers and medical treatments. Topics include allergies and asthma, serum sickness, blood transfusion reaction, transplant rejection, and anaphylaxis.

Part VII: Treatments for Immune Deficiencies and Diseases contains information about drug and gene therapies, plasmapheresis, and stem cell transplantation. Treatments used for specific immune diseases are also described.

Part VIII: Coping with Immune Disease provides tips for individuals and families living with an autoimmune or immune system disease, including facts for caregivers, immunization recommendations, and suggestions for students and travelers with immune system disorders.

Part IX: Additional Help and Information offers glossaries of immune system terms and autoimmune diseases and a directory of resources.

Bibliographic Note

This volume contains documents and excerpts from publications issued by the following U.S. government agencies: Centers for Disease Control and Prevention (CDC); National Heart, Lung, and Blood Institute (NHLBI); National Human Genome Research Institute (NHGRI); National Institute on Alcohol Abuse and Alcoholism (NIAAA); National Institute of Allergy and Infectious Diseases (NIAID); National Institute of Arthritis and Musculoskeletal and Skin Diseases (NIAMS); National Institute of Child Health and Human Development (NICHD); National Institute of Diabetes and Digestive and Kidney Diseases (NIDDK); National Institute of Mental Health (NIMH); National Institute of Neurological Disorders and Stroke (NINDS); National Institutes of Health Clinical Center; National Women's Health Information Center (NWHIC); and the U.S. Food and Drug Administration (FDA).

In addition, this volume contains copyrighted documents from the following organizations and individuals: A.D.A.M., Inc.; American Academy of Family Physicians (AAFP); American Association for Clinical Chemistry; American Autoimmune Related Diseases Association; American Liver Foundation; American Society of Health-System Pharmacists; Arthritis Foundation; Ataxia-Telangiectasia Children's Project, Inc.; Immune Deficiency Foundation; International Pemphigus Foundation; Jeffrey Modell Foundation; Muscular Dystrophy Association-USA; Myositis Association; National Academies of Science; National Graves' Disease Foundation (NGDF); National Jewish Medical and Research Center; Nemours Center for Children's Health Media; Scleroderma Foundation; Spondylitis Association of America; University of Cincinnati Center for Environmental Genetics; and University of Washington.

Full citation information is provided on the first page of each chapter. Every effort has been made to secure all necessary rights to reprint the copyrighted material. If any omissions have been made, please contact Omnigraphics to make corrections for future editions.

Acknowledgements

In addition to the listed organizations, agencies, and individuals who have contributed to this *Sourcebook*, special thanks go to managing editor Karen Bellenir, research and permissions coordinator Liz Barbour, medical consultant Dr. David Cooke, verification assistant Dawn Matthews, and document engineer Bruce Bellenir for their help and support.

About the Health Reference Series

The *Health Reference Series* is designed to provide basic medical information for patients, families, caregivers, and the general public. Each volume takes a particular topic and provides comprehensive coverage. This is especially important for people who may be dealing with a newly diagnosed disease or a chronic disorder in themselves or in a family member. People looking for preventive guidance, information about disease warning signs, medical statistics, and risk factors for health problems will also find answers to their questions in the *Health Reference Series*. The *Series*, however, is not intended to serve as a tool for diagnosing illness, in prescribing treatments, or as a substitute for the physician/patient relationship. All people concerned about medical symptoms or the possibility of disease are encouraged to seek professional care from an appropriate health care provider.

Locating Information within the Health Reference Series

The *Health Reference Series* contains a wealth of information about a wide variety of medical topics. Ensuring easy access to all the fact sheets, research reports, in-depth discussions, and other material contained within the individual books of the *Series* remains one of our highest priorities. As the *Series* continues to grow in size and scope, however, locating the precise information needed by a reader may become more challenging.

A Contents Guide to the Health Reference Series was developed to direct readers to the specific volumes that address their concerns. It presents an extensive list of diseases, treatments, and other topics of general interest compiled from the Tables of Contents and major index headings. To access *A Contents Guide to the Health Reference Series*, visit www.healthreferenceseries.com.

Medical Consultant

Medical consultation services are provided to the *Health Reference Series* editors by David A. Cooke, M.D. Dr. Cooke is a graduate of Brandeis University, and he received his M.D. degree from the University of Michigan. He completed residency training at the University of Wisconsin Hospital and Clinics. He is board-certified in Internal Medicine. Dr. Cooke currently works as part of the University of Michigan Health System and practices in Brighton, MI. In his free time, he enjoys writing, science fiction, and spending time with his family.

Our Advisory Board

We would like to thank the following board members for providing guidance to the development of this *Series*:

- Dr. Lynda Baker, Associate Professor of Library and Information Science, Wayne State University, Detroit, MI

- Nancy Bulgarelli, William Beaumont Hospital Library, Royal Oak, MI

- Karen Imarisio, Bloomfield Township Public Library, Bloomfield Township, MI

- Karen Morgan, Mardigian Library, University of Michigan-Dearborn, Dearborn, MI

- Rosemary Orlando, St. Clair Shores Public Library, St. Clair Shores, MI

Health Reference Series *Update Policy*

The inaugural book in the *Health Reference Series* was the first edition of *Cancer Sourcebook* published in 1989. Since then, the *Series* has been enthusiastically received by librarians and in the medical community. In order to maintain the standard of providing high-quality health information for the layperson the editorial staff at Omnigraphics felt it was necessary to implement a policy of updating volumes when warranted.

Medical researchers have been making tremendous strides, and it is the purpose of the *Health Reference Series* to stay current with the most recent advances. Each decision to update a volume is made on an individual basis. Some of the considerations include how much new information is available and the feedback we receive from people who use the books. If there is a topic you would like to see added to the update list, or an area of medical concern you feel has not been adequately addressed, please write to:

Editor
Health Reference Series
Omnigraphics, Inc.
615 Griswold Street
Detroit, MI 48226
E-mail: editorial@omnigraphics.com

Part One

Immune System Overview

Chapter 1

Understanding the Immune System: How It Works

The immune system is a network of cells, tissues, and organs that work together to defend the body against attacks by foreign invaders. These are primarily microbes (germs)—tiny, infection-causing organisms such as bacteria, viruses, parasites, and fungi. Because the human body provides an ideal environment for many microbes, they try to break in. It is the immune system's job to keep them out, or failing that, to seek out and destroy them. When the immune system hits the wrong target or is crippled, it can unleash a torrent of diseases, including allergy, arthritis, or acquired immunodeficiency syndrome (AIDS).

The immune system is amazingly complex. It can recognize and remember millions of different enemies, and it can produce secretions and cells to match up with and wipe out each one of them. The secret to its success is an elaborate and dynamic communications network. Millions and millions of cells, organized into sets and subsets, gather like clouds of bees swarming around a hive and pass information back and forth. Once immune cells receive the alarm, they undergo tactical changes and begin to produce powerful chemicals. These substances allow the cells to regulate their own growth and behavior, enlist their fellows, and direct new recruits to trouble spots.

Excerpted from "Understanding the Immune System: How It Works," National Institute of Allergy and Infectious Diseases (NIAID), NIH Publication No. 03–5423, September 2003.

Self and Non-Self

The key to a healthy immune system is its remarkable ability to distinguish between the body's own cells (self), and foreign cells (non-self). The body's immune defenses normally coexist peacefully with cells that carry distinctive self marker molecules. But when immune defenders encounter cells or organisms carrying markers that are foreign, they quickly launch an attack.

Anything that can trigger this immune response is called an antigen. An antigen can be a microbe such as a virus, or even a part of a microbe. Tissues or cells from another person (except an identical twin) also carry foreign markers and act as antigens. This explains why tissue transplants may be rejected.

In abnormal situations, the immune system can mistake cells as foreign and launch an attack against the body's own cells or tissues. The result is called an autoimmune disease. Some forms of arthritis and diabetes are autoimmune diseases. In other cases, the immune system responds to a seemingly harmless foreign substance such as ragweed pollen. The result is allergy, and this kind of antigen is called an allergen.

The Structure of the Immune System

The organs of the immune system are positioned throughout the body. They are called lymphoid organs because they are home to lymphocytes, small white blood cells that are the key players in the immune system.

Bone marrow, the soft tissue in the hollow center of bones, is the ultimate source of all blood cells, including white blood cells destined to become immune cells.

The thymus is an organ that lies behind the breastbone; lymphocytes known as T lymphocytes, or just T cells, mature in the thymus.

The spleen is a flattened organ at the upper left of the abdomen. Like the lymph nodes, the spleen contains specialized compartments where immune cells gather and work, and serves as a meeting ground where immune defenses confront antigens.

Clumps of lymphoid tissue are found in many parts of the body, especially in the linings of the digestive tract and the airways and lungs—territories that serve as gateways to the body. These tissues include the tonsils, adenoids, and appendix.

Lymphatic vessels carry lymph, a clear fluid that bathes the body's tissues. Lymphocytes can travel throughout the body using the blood vessels. The cells can also travel through a system of lymphatic vessels that closely parallels the body's veins and arteries. Cells and

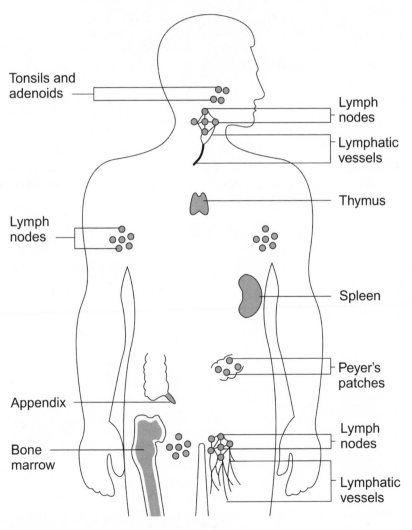

Figure 1.1. *Organs of the Immune System*

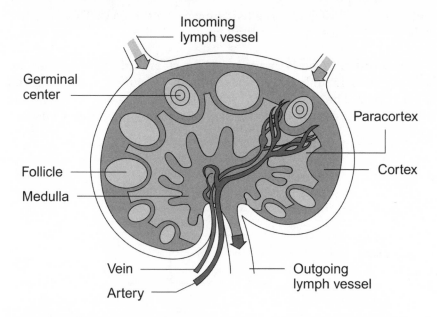

Figure 1.2. The lymph node contains numerous specialized structures. T cells concentrate in the paracortex, B cells in and around the germinal centers, and plasma cells in the medulla.

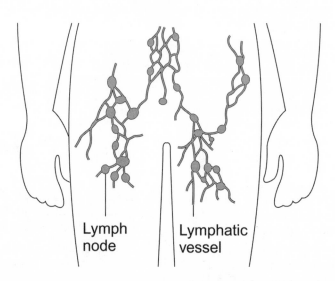

Figure 1.3. Immune cells and foreign particles enter the lymph nodes via incoming lymphatic vessels or the lymph nodes' tiny blood vessels.

fluids are exchanged between blood and lymphatic vessels, enabling the lymphatic system to monitor the body for invading microbes.

Lymph nodes—small, bean-shaped nodes—are laced along the lymphatic vessels, with clusters in the neck, armpits, abdomen, and groin. Each lymph node contains specialized compartments where immune cells congregate, and where they can encounter antigens.

All lymphocytes exit lymph nodes through outgoing lymphatic vessels. Once in the bloodstream, they are transported to tissues throughout the body. They patrol everywhere for foreign antigens, then gradually drift back into the lymphatic system, to begin the cycle all over again.

Immune Cells and Their Products

The immune system stockpiles a huge arsenal of cells, not only lymphocytes, but also cell-devouring phagocytes and their relatives. Some immune cells take on all comers, while others are trained on highly specific targets. To work effectively, most immune cells need the cooperation of their comrades. Sometimes immune cells communicate by direct physical contact, sometimes by releasing chemical messengers.

The immune system stores just a few of each kind of the different cells needed to recognize millions of possible enemies. When an antigen appears, those few matching cells multiply into a full-scale army. After their job is done, they fade away, leaving sentries behind to watch for future attacks.

All immune cells begin as immature stem cells in the bone marrow. They respond to different cytokines and other signals to grow into specific immune cell types, such as T cells, B cells, or phagocytes. Because stem cells have not yet committed to a particular future, they are an interesting possibility for treating some immune system disorders. Researchers are investigating if a person's own stem cells can be used to regenerate damaged immune responses in autoimmune diseases and immune deficiency diseases.

B Lymphocytes

B cells and T cells are the main types of lymphocytes. B cells work chiefly by secreting substances called antibodies into the body's fluids. Antibodies ambush antigens circulating the bloodstream. However, they are powerless to penetrate cells. The job of attacking target cells—either cells that have been infected by viruses or cells that have been distorted by cancer—is left to T cells or other immune cells.

Each B cell is programmed to make one specific antibody. For example, one B cell will make an antibody that blocks a virus that causes the common cold, while another produces an antibody that attacks a bacterium that causes pneumonia.

When a B cell encounters its triggering antigen, it gives rise to many large cells known as plasma cells. Every plasma cell is essentially a factory for producing an antibody. Each of the plasma cells descended from a given B cell manufactures millions of identical antibody molecules and pours them into the bloodstream.

An antigen matches an antibody much as a key matches a lock. Some match exactly; others fit more like a skeleton key. But whenever antigen and antibody interlock, the antibody marks the antigen for destruction.

Antibodies belong to a family of large molecules known as immunoglobulins. Different types play different roles in the immune defense strategy.

- Immunoglobulin (Ig) G, or IgG, works efficiently to coat microbes, speeding their uptake by other cells in the immune system.

- IgM is very effective at killing bacteria.

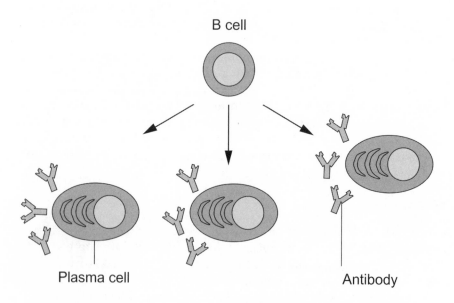

B cell

Plasma cell

Antibody

Figure 1.4. *B cells mature into plasma cells that produce antibodies.*

8

- IgA concentrates in body fluids—tears, saliva, the secretions of the respiratory tract, and the digestive tract—guarding the entrances to the body.

- IgE, whose natural job probably is to protect against parasitic infections, is the villain responsible for the symptoms of allergy.

- IgD remains attached to B cells and plays a key role in initiating early B cell response.

T Cells

Unlike B cells, T cells do not recognize free-floating antigens. Rather, their surfaces contain specialized antibody-like receptors that see fragments of antigens on the surfaces of infected or cancerous cells. T cells contribute to immune defenses in two major ways: some direct and regulate immune responses; others directly attack infected or cancerous cells.

Helper T cells, or Th cells, coordinate immune responses by communicating with other cells. Some stimulate nearby B cells to produce antibodies, others call in microbe gobbling cells called phagocytes, still others activate other T cells.

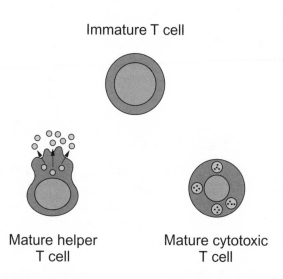

Immature T cell

Mature helper
T cell

Mature cytotoxic
T cell

Figure 1.5. *Types of T Cells*

Killer T cells—also called cytotoxic T lymphocytes (CTLs)—perform a different function. These cells directly attack other cells carrying certain foreign or abnormal molecules on their surfaces. CTLs are especially useful for attacking viruses because viruses often hide from other parts of the immune system while they grow inside infected cells. CTLs recognize small fragments of these viruses peeking out from the cell membrane and launch an attack to kill the cell.

In most cases, T cells only recognize an antigen if it is carried on the surface of a cell by one of the body's own major histocompatibility complex (MHC) molecules. MHC molecules are proteins recognized by T cells when distinguishing between self and non-self. A self MHC molecule provides a recognizable scaffolding to present a foreign antigen to the T cell.

Although MHC molecules are required for T cell responses against foreign invaders, they also pose a difficulty during organ transplantations. Virtually every cell in the body is covered with MHC proteins, but each person has a different set of these proteins on his or her cells. If a T cell recognizes a foreign MHC molecule on another cell, it will destroy the cell. Therefore, doctors must match organ recipients with donors who have the closest MHC makeup. Otherwise the recipient's T cells will likely attack the transplanted organ, leading to graft rejection.

Natural killer (NK) cells are another kind of lethal white cell, or lymphocyte. Like killer T cells, NK cells are armed with granules filled with potent chemicals. But while killer T cells look for antigen fragments bound to self-MHC molecules, NK cells recognize cells lacking self-MHC molecules. Thus NK cells have the potential to attack many types of foreign cells.

Both kinds of killer cells slay on contact. The deadly assassins bind to their targets, aim their weapons, and then deliver a lethal burst of chemicals.

Phagocytes and Their Relatives

Phagocytes are large white cells that can swallow and digest microbes and other foreign particles. Monocytes are phagocytes that circulate in the blood. When monocytes migrate into tissues, they develop into macrophages. Specialized types of macrophages can be found in many organs, including lungs, kidneys, brain, and liver.

Macrophages play many roles. As scavengers, they rid the body of worn-out cells and other debris. They display bits of foreign antigen

10

in a way that draws the attention of matching lymphocytes. And they churn out an amazing variety of powerful chemical signals, known as monokine, which are vital to the immune responses.

Granulocytes are another kind of immune cell. They contain granules filled with potent chemicals, which allow the granulocytes to destroy microorganisms. Some of these chemicals, such as histamine, also contribute to inflammation and allergy.

One type of granulocyte, the neutrophil, is also a phagocyte; it uses its prepackaged chemicals to break down the microbes it ingests. Eosinophils and basophils are granulocytes that spray their chemicals onto harmful cells or microbes nearby.

The mast cell is a twin of the basophil, except that it is not a blood cell. Rather, it is found in the lungs, skin, tongue, and linings of the nose and intestinal tract, where it is responsible for the symptoms of allergy.

A related structure, the blood platelet, is a cell fragment. Platelets, too, contain granules. In addition to promoting blood clotting and wound repair, platelets activate some of the immune defenses.

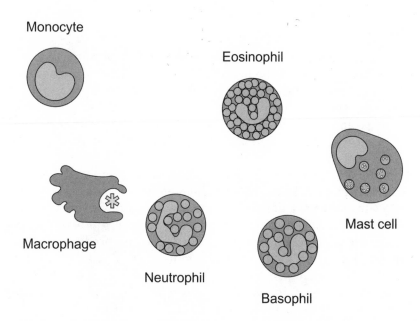

Figure 1.6. *Phagocytes, granulocytes, and mast cells, all with different methods of attack, demonstrate the immune system's versatility.*

Cytokines

Components of the immune system communicate with one another by exchanging chemical messengers called cytokines. These proteins are secreted by cells and act on other cells to coordinate an appropriate immune response. Cytokines include a diverse assortment of interleukins, interferons, and growth factors. Some cytokines are chemical switches that turn certain immune cell types on and off.

One cytokine, interleukin 2 (IL-2), triggers the immune system to produce T cells. IL-2's immunity-boosting properties have traditionally made it a promising treatment for several illnesses. Clinical studies are ongoing to test its benefits in other diseases such as cancer, hepatitis C, human immunodeficiency virus (HIV) infection, and AIDS. Other cytokines also are being studied for their potential clinical benefit.

Other cytokines chemically attract specific cell types. These so-called chemokines are released by cells at a site of injury or infection and call other immune cells to the region to help repair the damage or fight off the invader. Chemokines often play a key role in inflammation and are a promising target for new drugs to help regulate immune responses.

Complement

The complement system is made up of about 25 proteins that work together to complement the action of antibodies in destroying bacteria. It also helps to rid the body of antibody-coated antigens (antigen-antibody complexes). Complement proteins, which cause blood vessels to become dilated and then leaky, contribute to the redness, warmth, swelling, pain, and loss of function that characterize an inflammatory response.

Complement proteins circulate in the blood in an inactive form. When the first protein in the complement series is activated—typically by antibody that has locked onto an antigen—it sets in motion a domino effect. Each component takes its turn in a precise chain of steps known as the complement cascade. The end product is a cylinder inserted into and puncturing a hole in the cell's wall. With fluids and molecules flowing in and out, the cell swells and bursts. Other components of the complement system make bacteria more susceptible to phagocytosis or beckon other cells to the area.

Chapter 2

Natural and Acquired Immunity

Understanding the Immune System: Immunity

Long ago, physicians realized that people who had recovered from the plague would never get it again—they had acquired immunity. This is because some of the body's activated T and B cells become memory cells. The next time an individual meets up with the same antigen, the immune system is set to demolish it. Immunity can be strong or weak, short-lived or long-lasting, depending on the type of antigen, the amount of antigen, and the route by which it enters the body. Immunity can also be influenced by inherited genes. When faced with the same antigen, some individuals will respond forcefully, others feebly, and some not at all.

An immune response can be sparked not only by infection but also by immunization with vaccines. Vaccines contain microorganisms— or parts of microorganisms—that have been treated so they can provoke an immune response, but not full-blown disease.

Immunity can also be transferred from one individual to another by injections of serum rich in antibodies against a particular microbe (antiserum). For example, immune serum is sometimes given to protect travelers to countries where hepatitis A is widespread. Such passive immunity typically lasts only a few weeks or months.

This chapter includes an excerpt from "Understanding the Immune System: How It Works," National Institute of Allergy and Infectious Diseases (NIAID), NIH Publication No. 03–5423, September 2003; and "Immune Response," © 2005 A.D.A.M., Inc. Reprinted with permission.

Infants are born with weak immune responses but are protected for the first few months of life by antibodies received from their mothers before birth. Babies who are nursed can also receive some antibodies from breast milk that help to protect their digestive tracts.

Immune Tolerance

Immune tolerance is the tendency of T or B lymphocytes to ignore the body's own tissues. Maintaining tolerance is important because it prevents the immune system from attacking its fellow cells. Scientists are hard at work trying to understand how the immune system knows when to respond or not respond.

Tolerance occurs in at least two ways. Central tolerance occurs during lymphocyte development. Very early in each immune cell's life, it is exposed to many of the self molecules in the body. If it encounters these molecules before it has fully matured, the encounter activates an internal self-destruct pathway and the immune cell dies. This process, called clonal deletion, helps ensure that self reactive T cells and B cells do not mature and attack healthy tissues.

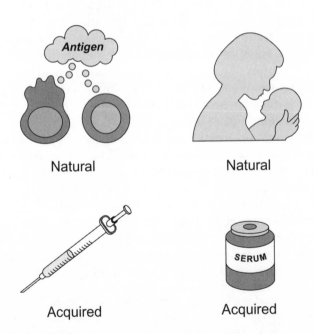

Figure 2.1. Sources of Natural and Acquired Immunity

Because maturing lymphocytes do not encounter every molecule in the body, they must also learn to ignore mature cells and tissues. In peripheral tolerance, circulating lymphocytes might recognize a self molecule, but cannot respond because some of the chemical signals required to activate the T or B cell are absent. So-called clonal anergy keeps potentially harmful lymphocytes switched off. Peripheral tolerance may also be imposed by a special class of regulatory T cells that inhibits helper or cytotoxic T-cell activation by self antigens.

Vaccines

Medical workers have long helped the body's immune system prepare for future attacks through vaccination. Vaccines consist of killed or modified microbes, components of microbes, or microbial DNA that trick the body into thinking an infection has occurred. An immunized person's immune system attacks the harmless vaccine and prepares for subsequent invasions. Vaccines remain one of the best ways to prevent infectious diseases and have an excellent safety record. Previously devastating diseases such as smallpox, polio, and whooping cough have been greatly controlled or eliminated through worldwide vaccination programs.

Immune Response

Alternative names: Innate immunity; humoral immunity; cellular immunity; immunity; inflammatory response; acquired (adaptive) immunity.

Definition: The immune response is the way the body recognizes and defends itself against microorganisms, viruses, and substances recognized as foreign and potentially harmful to the body.

The Immune System

The immune system protects the body from potentially harmful substances by recognizing and responding to so-called antigens. Antigens are large molecules (usually proteins) on the surface of cells, viruses, fungi, or bacteria. Some non-living substances such as toxins, chemicals, drugs, and foreign particles (such as a splinter) can be antigens. Substances that contain these antigens are recognized and destroyed by the immune system. Even your own body cells have proteins that are antigens these include a group of antigens called human leukocyte antigens (HLA). Your immune system learns to see these antigens as normal and does not usually react against them.

Innate Immunity and Inflammation

One's innate immunity are the barriers that keep harmful materials from entering your body and form the first line of defense in the immune response. Some of these barriers are: the skin, stomach acid, mucous (traps microorganisms and small particles), the cough reflex, and enzymes in tears and skin oils. If an antigen gets past the external barriers, it is attacked and destroyed by other parts of the immune system. Innate immunity also includes those things that make humans resistant to many of the diseases of animals.

The immune system includes certain types of white blood cells. It also includes chemicals and proteins in the blood (such as complement proteins and interferon). Some of these directly attack foreign substances in the body, and others work together to help the immune system cells.

The inflammatory response (inflammation) is part of innate immunity. It occurs when tissues are injured by bacteria, trauma, toxins, heat, or any other cause. Chemicals including histamine, bradykinin, serotonin, and others are released by damaged tissue. These chemicals cause blood vessels to leak fluid into the tissues, resulting in localized swelling. This helps isolate the foreign substance from further contact with body tissues.

The chemicals also attract white blood cells that eat microorganisms and dead or damaged cells. The process where these white blood cells surround, engulf, and destroy foreign substances is called phagocytosis, and the cells are collectively referred to as phagocytes. Phagocytes eventually die. Pus is formed from a collection of dead tissue, dead bacteria, and live and dead phagocytes.

Acquired Immunity

In comparison to innate immunity, acquired (adaptive) immunity develops when the body is exposed to various antigens and builds a defense that is specific to that antigen.

Lymphocytes, a special type of white blood cell, contain subgroups, B and T lymphocytes, that are key players in acquired immune responses. B lymphocytes (also called B cells) produce antibodies. Antibodies attach to a specific antigen and make it easier for the phagocytes to destroy the antigen. T lymphocytes (T cells) attack antigens directly, and provide control of the immune response. B cells and T cells develop that are specific for one antigen type. When you are exposed to a different antigen, different B cells and T cells are formed.

As lymphocytes develop, they normally learn to recognize the body's own tissues (self) as distinctive from tissues and particles not normally found in your body (non-self). Once B cells and T cells are formed, a few of those cells will multiply and provide memory for the immune system. This allows the immune system to respond faster and more efficiently the next time you are exposed to the same antigen, and in many cases will prevent you from getting sick. For example, adaptive immunity accounts for an individual who has had chickenpox being called immune to getting chickenpox again.

Passive Immunity

Passive immunity involves antibodies that are produced in someone's body other than your own. Infants have passive immunity because they are born with antibodies that are transferred through the placenta from the mother. These antibodies disappear between 6 and 12 months of age. Gamma globulin is another form of getting passive immunity that is given by a doctor. Its protection is also temporary.

Immune System Disorders and Allergies

Immune system disorders occur when the immune response is inappropriate, excessive, or lacking. Allergies involve an immune response to a substance that, in the majority of people, the body perceives as harmless. Transplant rejection involves the destruction of transplanted tissues or organs and is a major complication of organ transplantation. Blood transfusion reaction is a complication of blood administration. Autoimmune disorders (such as systemic lupus erythematosus and rheumatoid arthritis) occur when the immune system acts to destroy normal body tissues. Immunodeficiency disorders (such as inherited immunodeficiency and acquired immunodeficiency syndrome—AIDS) occur when there is a failure in all or part of the immune system.

Signs of Inflammation

- localized redness
- pain in the area
- swelling of the affected area

- warmth of the affected area
- pus (sometimes)

Note: In many cases, no observable symptoms develop. Additional symptoms may include:

- fever
- general discomfort, uneasiness, or ill feeling (malaise)
- muscle aches
- agitation or confusion

Tests

During an infection, a complete blood count (CBC) usually shows increased numbers of white blood cells. A blood differential count may reveal an elevated percentage of phagocytes, indicating that the body is responding to a need to fight infection. If a problem is suspected, other tests may be performed to determine complement levels and the levels of specific immunoglobulins (antibodies).

Therapies

Usually, the immune response is desired. In some cases, suppression of the immune system is necessary (for example, in the treatment of autoimmune disorders or allergies). This is usually accomplished by administering corticosteroids or other immunosuppressive medications.

Suppression of the immune system may be an undesired side effect of certain treatments or disorders.

Vaccination (immunization) is a way to trigger the immune response. Small doses of an antigen (such as dead or weakened live viruses) are given to activate immune system memory (activated B lymphocytes and sensitized T lymphocytes). Memory allows your body to react quickly and efficiently to future exposures. As noted, this means that if you are exposed to a microorganism, it will be destroyed before it can cause illness.

Passive immunization involves transfusion of antiserum, which contains antibodies that are formed by another person (or animal). It provides immediate protection against an antigen, but does not provide long-lasting protection. Gamma globulin and equine (horse) tetanus antitoxin are examples of passive immunization.

Complications

An efficient immune response protects against many diseases and disorders. Inefficient immune response allows diseases to develop. Inadequate, inappropriate, or excessive immune response causes immune system disorders.

Complications related to altered immune response include:

- disease development
- allergy/hypersensitivity
- anaphylaxis
- autoimmune disorders
- blood transfusion reaction
- immunodeficiency disorders
- serum sickness
- transplant rejection
- graft versus host disease

Chapter 3

Immune Response

Immune System Response to Infectious Diseases

How an infectious disease is treated depends on the microbe that caused it and sometimes on the age and medical condition of the person affected. Certain diseases are not treated at all, but are allowed to run their course, with the immune system doing its job alone. Some diseases, such as the common cold, are treated only to relieve the symptoms. Others, such as strep throat, are treated to destroy the offending microbe as well as to relieve symptoms—requiring a doctor's prescription for appropriate medicine.

Your immune system has an arsenal of ways to fight off invading microbes. Most begin with B and T cells and antibodies whose sole purpose is to keep your body healthy. Some of these cells sacrifice their lives to rid you of disease and restore your body to a healthy state. Some microbes normally present in your body also help destroy microbial invaders. For example, normal bacteria in your digestive system help destroy disease-causing microbes, such as listeria in that hot dog you had at lunch. Other important ways your body reacts to an infection include fever, coughing, and sneezing.

This chapter includes information excerpted from two National Institute of Allergy and Infectious Diseases (NIAID) documents. Text under the heading "Immune System Response to Infectious Diseases," is from "Microbes: In Sickness and in Health," NIH Pub. No. 01–4914, September 2001. Text under the heading "Mounting an Immune Response" is from "Understanding the Immune System: How It Works," NIH Publication No. 03–5423, September 2003.

Fever is one of your body's special ways of fighting an infection. Many microbes are very sensitive to temperature changes and cannot survive in temperatures higher than normal body heat, which is usually around 98.6 degrees Fahrenheit. For example, your body uses fever to destroy flu viruses.

Coughing and sneezing: Another piece in your immune system's reaction to invading infection-causing microbes is mucus production. Coughing and sneezing help mucus move those germs out of your body efficiently and quickly.

Other methods your body may use to fight off an infection include the following:

- Inflammation
- Vomiting
- Diarrhea
- Fatigue
- Cramping

Mounting an Immune Response

Infections are the most common cause of human disease. They range from the common cold to debilitating conditions like chronic hepatitis to life-threatening diseases such as acquired immunodeficiency syndrome (AIDS). Disease-causing microbes (pathogens) attempting to get into the body must first move past the body's external armor, usually the skin or cells lining the body's internal passageways.

The skin provides an imposing barrier to invading microbes. It is generally penetrable only through cuts or tiny abrasions. The digestive and respiratory tracts—both portals of entry for a number of microbes—also have their own levels of protection. Microbes entering the nose often cause the nasal surfaces to secrete more protective mucus, and attempts to enter the nose or lungs can trigger a sneeze or cough reflex to force microbial invaders out of the respiratory passageways. The stomach contains a strong acid that destroys many pathogens that are swallowed with food.

If microbes survive the body's front-line defenses, they still have to find a way through the walls of the digestive, respiratory, or urogenital passageways to the underlying cells. These passageways are lined with tightly packed epithelial cells covered in a layer of mucus, effectively blocking the transport of many organisms. Mucosal surfaces also secrete a special class of antibody called immunoglobulin

(Ig) A, which in many cases is the first type of antibody to encounter an invading microbe. Underneath the epithelial layer a number of cells, including macrophages, B cells, and T cells, lie in wait for any germ that might bypass the barriers at the surface.

Next, invaders must escape a series of general defenses, which are ready to attack, without regard for specific antigen markers. These include patrolling phagocytes, natural killer cells, and complement.

Microbes that cross the general barriers then confront specific weapons tailored just for them. Specific weapons, which include both antibodies and T cells, are equipped with singular receptor structures that allow them to recognize and interact with their designated targets.

Bacteria, Viruses, and Parasites

The most common disease-causing microbes are bacteria, viruses, and parasites. Each uses a different tactic to infect a person, and each is thwarted by a different part of the immune system.

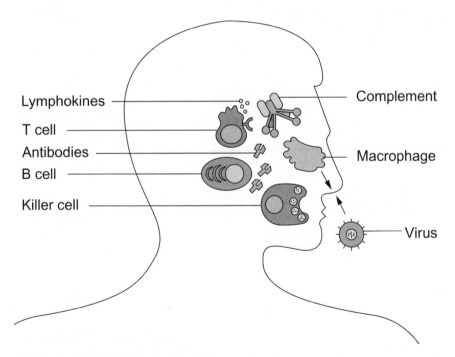

Figure 3.1. When challenged, the immune system has many weapons from which to choose.

Most bacteria live in the spaces between cells and are readily attacked by antibodies. When antibodies attach to a bacterium, they send signals to complement proteins and phagocytic cells to destroy the bound microbes. Some bacteria are eaten directly by phagocytes, which signal to certain T cells to join the attack.

All viruses, plus a few types of bacteria and parasites, must enter cells to survive, requiring a different approach. Infected cells use their major histocompatibility complex (MHC) molecules to put pieces of the invading microbes on the cell's surface, flagging down cytotoxic T lymphocytes to destroy the infected cell. Antibodies also can assist in the immune response, attaching to and clearing viruses before they have a chance to enter the cell.

Parasites live either inside or outside cells. Intracellular parasites such as the organism that causes malaria can trigger T cell responses. Extracellular parasites are often much larger than bacteria or viruses and require a much broader immune attack. Parasitic infections often trigger an inflammatory response when eosinophils, basophils, and other specialized granular cells rush to the scene and release their stores of toxic chemicals in an attempt to destroy the invader. Antibodies also play a role in this attack, attracting the granular cells to the site of infection.

Chapter 4

Vaccines and Immunity

How Vaccines Prevent Disease

Parents are constantly concerned about the health and safety of their children and they take many steps to protect them. These preventive measures range from childproof door latches to child safety seats. In the same respect, vaccines work to safeguard children from illnesses and death caused by infectious diseases. Vaccines protect children by helping prepare their bodies to fight often serious, and potentially deadly diseases.

Most vaccine-preventable diseases are caused by germs that are called viruses or bacteria. Vaccines to help prevent these diseases generally contain weakened or killed viruses or bacteria specific to the disease. Vaccines help your body recognize and fight these germs, and protect you each time you come in contact with someone who is sick with any of these diseases.

There are a series of steps that your body goes through in fighting vaccine-preventable diseases.

This chapter includes: "How Vaccines Prevent Disease," Centers for Disease Control and Prevention (CDC), July 2004; excerpts from "Understanding Vaccines: What They Are; How They Work," National Institute of Allergy and Infectious Diseases (NIAID), NIH Publication No. 03–4219, July 2003; and "News: Infant Immunizations Not Shown to Be Harmful to Children's Immune Systems," Copyright © 2002 National Academy of Sciences. All rights reserved. Reprinted with permission.

First: A vaccine is given by a shot (influenza vaccine may be given by a nasal spray).

Next: Over the next few weeks the body makes antibodies and memory cells against the weakened or dead germs in the vaccine.

Then: The antibodies can fight the real disease germs if the person is exposed to the germs and they invade the body. The antibodies will help destroy the germs and the person will not become ill.

Finally: Antibodies and memory cells stay on guard in the body for years after the vaccination to safeguard it from the real disease germs.

Most vaccines are given to babies and young children, but some are needed throughout your lifetime to make sure you stay protected. This protection is called immunity. Vaccines are an important and safe way to keep you healthy.

Why Are Vaccines Important?

Most newborn babies are immune to many diseases because they have antibodies passed from their mothers. However, this immunity only lasts a year or less. Further, most young children do not have maternal immunity from whooping cough, polio, hepatitis B, or *Haemophilus influenzae* type b.

Immunizing individual children also helps to protect the health of our community. People who cannot be vaccinated will be less likely to be exposed to disease germs that can be passed around by unvaccinated children. Immunization also prevents disease outbreaks.

If your child is not vaccinated and is exposed to a disease germ, the child's body may not be strong enough to fight the disease. Before vaccines, many children died of diseases vaccines prevent, like whooping cough, measles, and polio. Those germs still exist today, but children are now protected by vaccines so we do not see these diseases as often.

Understanding Vaccines: How They Work

Chances are you never had diphtheria. You probably do not know anyone who has suffered from this disease either. In fact, you may not know what diphtheria is. Similarly, diseases like whooping cough (pertussis), measles, mumps, and rubella may be unfamiliar to you. In the 19th and early 20th centuries, these illnesses struck hundreds of thousands of people in the United States each year, mostly children, and tens of thousands of people died. These diseases were frightening household words. Today, they are all but forgotten. That change happened largely because of vaccines.

Chances are you have been vaccinated against diphtheria. You even may have been exposed to the bacterium that causes it, but the vaccine prepared your body to fight off the disease so quickly that you were unaware of the infection.

Vaccines take advantage of your body's natural ability to learn how to eliminate almost any disease-causing germ, or microbe, that attacks it. Also, your body remembers how to protect itself from the microbes it has encountered before. Collectively, the parts of your body that recall and repel diseases are called the immune system. Without the immune system, the simplest illness—even the common cold—could quickly turn deadly.

On average, your immune system takes more than a week to learn how to fight off an unfamiliar microbe. Sometimes that is not soon enough. Stronger microbes can spread through your body faster than the immune system can fend them off. Your body often gains the upper hand after a few weeks, but in the meantime you are sick. Certain microbes are so powerful, or virulent, that they can overwhelm or escape your body's natural defenses. In those situations, vaccines can make all the difference.

Traditional vaccines contain either parts of microbes or whole microbes that have been killed or weakened so that they do not cause disease. When your immune system confronts these harmless versions of the germs, it quickly clears them from your body. In other words, vaccines fix the fight and at the same time teach your body important lessons about how to defeat its opponents.

What Do Cows Have to Do with Vaccines?

The word vaccine comes from the Latin word *vaccinus*, which means pertaining to cows. What do cows have to do with vaccines? The first vaccine was based on the relatively mild cowpox virus, which infected cows as well as people. This vaccine protected people against the related, but much more dangerous, smallpox virus.

More than 200 years ago, Edward Jenner, a country physician practicing in England, noticed that milkmaids rarely suffered from smallpox. The milkmaids often did get cowpox, a related but far less serious disease, and those who did never became ill with smallpox. In an experiment that laid the foundation for modern vaccines, Jenner took a few drops of fluid from a skin sore of a woman who had cowpox and injected the fluid into the arm of a healthy young boy who had never had cowpox or smallpox.

Six weeks later, Jenner injected the boy with fluid from a smallpox sore, but the boy remained free of smallpox. Dr. Jenner had discovered one of the fundamental principles of immunization. He had used a relatively harmless foreign substance to evoke an immune response that protected someone from an infectious disease. His discovery would ease the suffering of people around the world and eventually lead to the elimination of smallpox, a disease that killed a million people, mostly children, each year in Europe. By the beginning of the 20th century, vaccines were in use for diseases that had nothing to do with cows—rabies, diphtheria, typhoid fever, and plague—but the name stuck.

How Vaccines Mimic Infection

Vaccines teach your immune system by mimicking a natural infection. Yellow fever is no longer a problem in the United States, but the disease still occurs in other parts of the world, and the Centers for Disease Control and Prevention (CDC) recommend vaccination prior to traveling to those areas.

The yellow fever vaccine, first widely used in 1938, contains a weakened form of the virus that does not cause disease or reproduce very well. This vaccine is injected into your arm. Your macrophages cannot tell the vaccine viruses are duds. The macrophages gobble up the viruses as if they were dangerous and, in the lymph nodes, present yellow fever antigen to T and B cells.

The alarm is sounded, and your immune system swings into action. Yellow fever specific T cells rush out to meet the foe. B cells secrete yellow fever antibodies. The battle is over quickly. The weakened viruses in the vaccine cannot put up much of a fight. The mock infection is cleared, and you are left with a supply of memory T and B cells to protect you against yellow fever should a mosquito carrying the virus ever bite you.

Different Types of Vaccines

Live, attenuated vaccines: These vaccines contain a version of the living microbe that has been weakened in the lab so it cannot cause disease. This weakening of the organism is called attenuation.

Because a live, attenuated vaccine is the closest thing to an actual infection, these vaccines are good teachers of the immune system. They elicit strong cellular and antibody responses, and often confer lifelong immunity with only one or two doses. There is a remote possibility that the attenuated bacteria in the vaccine could revert to a virulent form and cause disease. For their own protection, people with compromised immune systems—such as people with cancer or people infected with human immunodeficiency virus (HIV)—usually are not given live vaccines.

Inactivated or killed vaccines: Scientists produce inactivated vaccines by killing the disease-causing microbe with chemicals, heat, or radiation. Such vaccines are more stable and safer than live vaccines—the dead microbes cannot mutate back to their disease-causing state. Most inactivated vaccines stimulate a weaker immune system response than do live vaccines. So it would likely take several additional doses, so-called booster shots, to maintain a person's immunity.

Subunit vaccines: Subunit vaccines dispense with the entire microbe and use just the important parts of it—the antigens that best stimulate the immune system. In some cases, these vaccines use epitopes—the very specific parts of the antigen that antibodies or T cells recognize and bind to. Because subunit vaccines contain only the essential antigens and not all the other molecules that make up the microbe, the chances of adverse reactions to the vaccine are lower.

Toxoid vaccines: If a bacterium secretes a toxin, or harmful chemical, a toxoid vaccine might work against it. These vaccines are used when a bacterial toxin is the main cause of illness. Scientists have found they can inactivate toxins by treating them with formalin, a solution of formaldehyde and sterilized water. Such detoxified toxins, called toxoids, are safe for use in vaccines.

When the immune system receives a vaccine containing a harmless toxoid, it learns how to fight off the natural toxin. The immune system produces antibodies that lock onto and block the toxin.

Conjugate vaccines: If a bacterium has an outer coating of sugar molecules called polysaccharides, researchers try to make a conjugate vaccine. Polysaccharide coatings disguise a bacterium's antigens so that the immature immune systems of infants and younger children cannot recognize or respond to them. Conjugate vaccines, a special type of subunit vaccine, get around this problem.

When making a conjugate vaccine, scientists link antigens or toxoids from a microbe that an infant's immune system can recognize to the polysaccharides. The linkage helps the immature immune system react to polysaccharide coatings and defend against the disease-causing bacterium. The vaccine that protects against *Haemophilus influenzae* type b (Hib) is a conjugate vaccine.

Experimental deoxyribonucleic acid (DNA) vaccines: Still in the experimental stages, these vaccines show great promise, and several types are being tested in humans. DNA vaccines take immunization to a new technological level. These vaccines dispense with both the whole organism and its parts and get right down to the essentials—the microbe's genetic material. In particular, DNA vaccines use the genes that code for those all-important antigens.

Researchers have found that when the genes for a microbe's antigens are introduced into the body, some cells will take up that DNA. The body's own cells become vaccine-making factories, creating the antigens necessary to simulate the immune system. The DNA vaccine could not cause the disease because it would not contain the bacterium, just copies of a few of its genes. In addition, DNA vaccines are relatively easy and inexpensive to design and produce.

Naked DNA vaccines inject the DNA directly into the body. These vaccines are being tested in humans against malaria, influenza, herpes, and HIV.

Experimental recombinant vector vaccines: Experimental vaccines similar to DNA vaccines, but they use an attenuated virus or bacterium to introduce microbial DNA to cells of the body. Vector refers to the virus or bacterium used as the carrier. They use the harmless shell of one microbe to deliver genetic material of a disease-causing microbe. The genetic material contains the code for making vaccine antigen inside some of the body's cells, using those cells as factories. Recombinant vector vaccines closely mimic a natural infection and do a good job of stimulating the immune system. Researchers are working on both bacterial- and viral-based recombinant vector vaccines for HIV, rabies, and measles.

Combination vaccines: Some vaccines come in combinations. Most of us are familiar with the DTP (diphtheria, tetanus, pertussis) and the MMR (measles, mumps, rubella) vaccines that children in the United States receive. Combination vaccines reduce visits to the doctor, save time and money, and spare children extra needle sticks.

Table 4.1. Vaccine Types and Diseases They Protect Against

Vaccine Type: Live, attenuated vaccines

Disease: Measles, mumps, rubella, polio (Sabin vaccine), yellow fever

Advantages: Produce a strong immune response

Often give lifelong immunity with one or two doses

Disadvantages: Remote possibility that the live microbe could mutate back to a virulent form

Must be refrigerated to stay potent

Vaccine Type: Inactivated or killed vaccines

Disease: Cholera, flu, hepatitis A, Japanese encephalitis, plague, polio (Salk vaccine), rabies

Advantages: Safer and more stable than live vaccines

Don't require refrigeration: more easily stored and transported

Disadvantages: Produce a weaker immune response than live vaccines

Usually require additional doses, or booster shots

Vaccine Type: Toxoid vaccine

Disease: Diphtheria, tetanus

Advantages: Teaches the immune system to fight off bacterial toxins

Vaccine Type: Subunit vaccines

Disease: Hepatitis B, pertussis, pneumonia caused by *Streptococcus pneumoniae*

Advantages: Targeted to very specific parts of the microbe

Fewer antigens, so lower chance of adverse reactions

Disadvantages: When developing a new vaccine, identifying the best antigens can be difficult and time consuming

Vaccine Type: Conjugate vaccines

Disease: *Haemophilus influenzae* type B, pneumonia caused by *Streptococcus pneumoniae*

Advantages: Allow infant immune systems to recognize certain bacteria

Vaccine Type: DNA vaccines

Disease: In clinical testing

Advantages: Produce a strong antibody and cellular immune response

Relatively easy and inexpensive to produce

Disadvantages: Still in experimental stages

Vaccine Type: Recombinant vector vaccines

Disease: In clinical testing

Advantages: Closely mimic a natural infection, stimulating a strong immune response

Disadvantages: Still in experimental stages

Infant Immunizations Not Shown to Be Harmful to Children's Immune Systems

The current immunization schedule calling for infants to get up to 20 vaccinations by the age of two does not increase the risk of contracting type 1 diabetes or various infections, such as pneumonia and meningitis, says a report from the National Academies' Institute of Medicine. The evidence is inconclusive as to whether the immunization schedule increases the risk of asthma. The committee that wrote the report said there is no need for a federal review of the schedule for infant immunizations at this time.

The increase in vaccine number and doses given to infants in recent years has led to concerns among some parents about possible adverse effects from immunizing infants so heavily. One concern is related to the higher incidence of diseases associated with immune system dysfunction, such as asthma and type 1 diabetes—an insulin-dependent form of the disease previously referred to as juvenile diabetes. Although genetic factors are known to affect the risk of developing these diseases, the increase in their incidence seems more likely to be the result of environmental factors. Immunization has been proposed as one possible adverse environmental modifier of immune function.

"Like any drug, no vaccine is 100 percent safe, but this report should at least assure parents that getting so many immunizations during infancy is not causing diabetes or increasing the risk of certain serious infections," said committee chair Marie McCormick, Professor and Chair, Department of Maternal and Child Health, Harvard School of Public Health, Boston.

The immunization schedule in this country has grown complex over the last 20 years. In 1980, infants were vaccinated against four diseases—diphtheria, tetanus, pertussis, and polio. Today, most healthy infants get up to 15 shots of five vaccines by the time they are six months old, and up to 5 additional shots of seven more vaccines by age two. These immunizations protect against 11 diseases in total—diphtheria, tetanus, pertussis, polio, measles, mumps, rubella, hepatitis B, *Haemophilus influenzae* type b (commonly referred to as Hib disease), varicella, and pneumococcus.

Despite the rise in the number of both vaccines and vaccine doses, exposure to vaccine antigens—those portions of a foreign substance that trigger an immune response—is lower than it used to be. This reduced antigen load is explained, in part, by the removal of two vaccines from the immunization schedule. Smallpox vaccine, which was discontinued in 1971, contained approximately 200 potentially antigenic substances. In addition, a new, streamlined form of pertussis vaccine approved for use in 1991 reduced the number of potential antigens from approximately 3,000 to between two and five. Furthermore, vaccines added to the immunization schedule during the past two decades have relatively few antigens. The new hepatitis B vaccine, for example, contains only one antigen.

The committee reviewed eight studies of the relationship between multiple vaccinations and type 1 diabetes—the autoimmune form of the disease in which the body produces antibodies against its own insulin-secreting pancreatic islet cells. All eight studies consistently demonstrated that multiple immunizations had no effect on the incidence of type 1 diabetes, leading the committee to reject the notion that multiple vaccinations cause an increased risk of the disease.

Likewise, the committee said multiple immunizations do not increase the risk of young children developing various infections, ranging from colds and ear infections to pneumonia and meningitis. The committee based its decision on the results of seven studies, which despite some variations and limitations, consistently showed that multiple vaccinations either had no effect on the risk of infection or provided some degree of protection against infection.

The committee looked at five studies examining multiple vaccinations and their potential to cause allergic diseases—a hypersensitivity of the immune system to relatively harmless agents in the environment, like pollens, dust mites, insect venom, and specific foods. Some, but not all, of these studies suggested that certain vaccines increase the risk of developing allergic disorders. Methodological weaknesses and inconsistent findings among the studies, however, led the committee to conclude that there is inadequate evidence to either accept or reject a causal relationship between multiple immunizations and increased risk of allergic diseases, particularly asthma.

Although the committee's review of clinical and epidemiological studies found no link between childhood immunizations and immune system dysfunction, its evaluation of basic science research yielded weak evidence of biological mechanisms by which vaccinations might increase the risk of diabetes or allergies. However, there is strong evidence of mechanisms by which vaccinations could increase the risk for infections. While such biological evidence can never prove causality, it can guide further investigation.

Given that about 25 percent of parents in a recent survey agreed with the statement that getting too many vaccines is not good for a baby and can weaken the immune system, the committee recommended that the U.S. Department of Health and Human Services convene an expert panel to examine parents' perceptions of vaccine risks and benefits in order to develop better communication tools for them and their doctors.

Additional Information

National Immunization Program
NIP Public Inquiries
1600 Clifton Rd. N.E., MSE-05
Atlanta, GA 30333
Toll-Free English: 800-232-2522
Toll-Free Spanish: 800-232-0233
Website: http://www.cdc.gov/nip
E-mail: NIPINFO@cdc.gov

Every Child by Two
Phone: 202-783-7034
Website: http://www.ecbt.org/index.htm
E-mail: info@ecbt.org

National Academy of Sciences
500 Fifth St. N.W.
Washington, DC 20001
Toll-Free: 800-624-6242
Phone: 202-334-2000
Website: http://national-academies.org

Chapter 5

Disorders of the Immune System

Allergic Diseases

The most common types of allergic diseases occur when the immune system responds to a false alarm. In an allergic person, a normally harmless material, such as grass pollen or house dust, is mistaken for a threat and attacked.

Allergies such as pollen allergy are related to the antibody known as immunoglobulin E (IgE). Like other antibodies, each IgE antibody is specific; one acts against oak pollen, another against ragweed.

Autoimmune Diseases

Sometimes the immune system's recognition apparatus breaks down, and the body begins to manufacture T cells and antibodies directed against its own cells and organs. Misguided T cells and autoantibodies, as they are known, contribute to many diseases. For instance, T cells that attack pancreas cells contribute to diabetes, while an autoantibody known as rheumatoid factor is common in people with rheumatoid arthritis. People with systemic lupus erythematosus (SLE) have antibodies to many types of their own cells and cell components.

No one knows exactly what causes an autoimmune disease, but multiple factors are likely to be involved. These include elements in

Excerpted from "Understanding the Immune System: How It Works," National Institute of Allergy and Infectious Diseases (NIAID), NIH Publication No. 03–5423, September 2003.

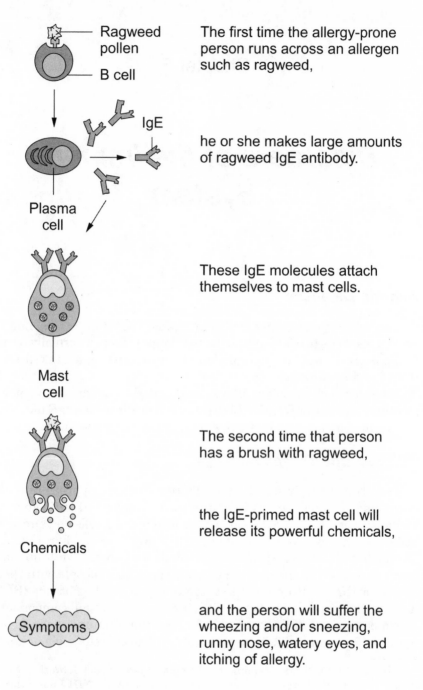

The first time the allergy-prone person runs across an allergen such as ragweed,

he or she makes large amounts of ragweed IgE antibody.

These IgE molecules attach themselves to mast cells.

The second time that person has a brush with ragweed,

the IgE-primed mast cell will release its powerful chemicals,

and the person will suffer the wheezing and/or sneezing, runny nose, watery eyes, and itching of allergy.

Figure 5.1. Allergic Disease and IgE Antibody

the environment, such as viruses, certain drugs, and sunlight, all of which may damage or alter normal body cells. Hormones are suspected of playing a role, since most autoimmune diseases are far more common in women than in men. Heredity, too, seems to be important. Many people with autoimmune diseases have characteristic types of self marker molecules.

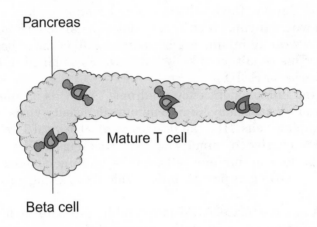

Figure 5.2. *Misguided T cells can attack insulin-producing cells of the pancreas, contributing to diabetes.*

Immune Complex Diseases

Immune complexes are clusters of interlocking antigens and antibodies. Normally, immune complexes are rapidly removed from the bloodstream. Sometimes, however, they continue to circulate, and eventually become trapped in the tissues of the kidneys, lungs, skin, joints, or blood vessels. There they set off reactions with complement—a group of at least 20 distinct serum proteins—that lead to inflammation and tissue damage. Immune complexes work their mischief in many diseases. These include malaria and viral hepatitis, as well as many autoimmune diseases.

Immunodeficiency Disorders

When the immune system is missing one or more of its components, the result is an immunodeficiency disorder. Immunodeficiency disorders can be inherited, acquired through infection, or produced unintentionally by drugs such as those used to treat people with cancer or those who have received transplants.

Temporary immune deficiencies can develop in the wake of common virus infections, including influenza, infectious mononucleosis, and measles. Immune responses can also be depressed by blood transfusions, surgery, malnutrition, smoking, and stress.

Some children are born with poorly functioning immune systems. Some have flaws in the B cell system and cannot produce antibodies. Children whose thymus is either missing or small and abnormal, lack T cells. Very rarely, infants are born lacking all of the major immune defenses. This condition is known as severe combined immunodeficiency disease or SCID.

Acquired immunodeficiency syndrome (AIDS) is an immunodeficiency disorder caused by human immunodeficiency virus (HIV) that infects immune cells. HIV can destroy or disable vital T cells, paving the way for a variety of immunologic shortcomings. HIV also can hide for long periods in immune cells. As the immune defenses falter, a person with AIDS falls prey to unusual, life-threatening infections and rare cancers.

A contagious disease, AIDS is spread by intimate sexual contact, transfer of the virus from mother to infant during pregnancy, or direct blood contamination. There is no cure for AIDS, but newly developed antiviral drugs can slow the advance of the disease, at least for a time. Researchers also are testing HIV vaccines in clinical studies.

Cancers of the Immune System

The cells of the immune system, like other cells, can grow uncontrollably, resulting in cancer. Leukemias are caused by the proliferation of white blood cells, or leukocytes. The uncontrolled growth of antibody-producing plasma cells can lead to multiple myeloma. Cancers of the lymphoid organs, known as lymphomas, include Hodgkin's disease.

Chapter 6

Influence of Alcohol and Gender on Immune Response

Decades of research have shown that women's and men's immune systems function differently. During the reproductive years, women have a stronger immune response than men. This gender difference is believed to be controlled by differences in the blood levels of gonadal steroid hormones—including the female hormone estrogen which stimulates immune responses, and the male hormone testosterone which is immunosuppressive. In both males and females, alcohol exposure suppresses immune responses; however, it is unclear whether there are significant gender differences in this suppression. Chronic exposure to alcohol alters the production of this same set of hormones (i.e., estrogen and testosterone), and hence alcohol's effects on immunity could involve an indirect mechanism in which alcohol alters hormone levels, and in turn, the hormones regulate immune responses.

Alcohol and Immune Responses

An overwhelming amount of evidence reveals that both acute and chronic alcohol exposure suppresses all branches of the immune system, including early responses to infection and the tumor surveillance system.[14, 21, 52, 54] For example, there is a decrease in the ability to recruit and activate germ-killing, white blood cells [19, 66] and an increase in the incidence of breast cancer in people who consume alcohol.[72, 75]

Excerpted from "Influence of Alcohol and Gender on Immune Response," by Elizabeth J. Kovacs, Ph.D., and Kelly A.N. Messingham, Ph.D., National Institute on Alcohol Abuse and Alcoholism (NIAAA), June 2003.

Some experts suspect that alcohol exerts an all or nothing effect on immune response—that is, the presence or absence of alcohol, rather than its amount, dictates the immune response.[48, 51] Other researchers believe that low doses of alcohol—the amount equivalent to a glass of wine—can confer health benefits, including protection against damage to the cardiovascular[40] and immune systems.[49] Such benefits, if they are present, may be attributable to antioxidants in alcoholic beverages such as red wine. In any case, health experts agree that the beneficial effects of antioxidants in some alcoholic beverages are lost if the level of alcohol consumption is elevated.[39]

There are several mechanisms by which alcohol impedes immune function. First, alcohol impairs the ability of white blood cells known as neutrophils to migrate to sites of injury and infection, a process called chemotaxis.[4] In addition, removing germ fighting, white blood cells (macrophages) and proteins that act as messengers between immune cells (cytokines) from an animal that has not been given alcohol and culturing them in the presence of alcohol, or isolating these cells from humans or animals after administering alcohol, has been shown to alter production of these macrophages and cytokines.[19, 64, 65]

Gender Differences in Immune Response Following Alcohol Exposure

To date, only a handful of studies have directly examined gender differences in the effects of alcohol on inflammatory and immune responses.[34, 43, 44, 61-63] These studies were conducted in rodents and employed different methods, including varying the quantity and duration of alcohol exposure. These reports show that in the absence of alcohol exposure, inflammatory and immune responses are stronger in females than in males.[34, 60, 63] However, the increased immunity in females is nullified by alcohol exposure. For example, in one study, proliferation of white blood cells was suppressed in alcohol exposed female rats;[34] however, investigation also showed that alcohol induced an increase in antibody production. In two other studies, female rats were less able to fight infection when intoxicated.[44, 63] The mechanisms driving these effects remain uncertain. One possibility is that gender differences in inflammatory and immune responses following alcohol exposure stem from alcohol induced changes in the production of gonadal steroid hormones, such as estrogen and testosterone.

In general, estrogen stimulates immune responses and testosterone is immunosuppressive.[7, 9, 33, 52, 71] During their reproductive years, females have more vigorous cellular and humoral immune responses than do males. This heightened immunity in females is evidenced by a more developed thymus, higher antibody concentrations, and a greater ability to reject tumors and transplanted tissues. (The thymus is a gland located in the upper chest that is involved in the maturation of immune cells.) Ironically, the enhanced immune function in women of reproductive age is associated with a higher prevalence of autoimmune disorders than is found in postmenopausal women or in men. (Although estrogen is present in males, its concentration is too low to affect immune response.)

The effects of alcohol on production of the gonadal steroid hormones are well documented.[23, 28, 29, 30, 70] In women, chronic alcohol exposure causes an initial increase in estrogen levels, followed by a marked decrease.[28, 29] In men, chronic alcohol consumption causes a decrease in testosterone.[23] The alcohol induced decrease in testosterone levels is significant enough to cause shrinkage (atrophy) of the testes, impotence, and loss of secondary sex characteristics.[70]

Estrogen and Cytokines

From the limited information available, it is thought that fluctuations in estrogen may alter immune cell function, in part, by increasing or decreasing the production of cytokines.[7, 9, 56, 71] There are several pieces of evidence for this idea. First, researchers found that removing the ovaries of adult rodents (eliminating the primary source of estrogen) lowered the level of cytokine production by certain types of white blood cells.[12, 15, 20, 26] This lower level of cytokine production was comparable to that of males and could be restored by administering estrogen.[31]

In other studies, drugs known as estrogen receptor antagonists inhibited the effect of estrogen on immune cells in animals.[32, 74] While receptor antagonists are bound to the same receptors that normally interact with estrogen, they block the binding of the hormone. Thus, it is possible to alter immune responses by blocking estrogen at one of its sites of action in white blood cells.

Further evidence that estrogen affects immune cell function, in part, by altering production of cytokines comes from cell culture studies in which estrogen was added to a culture of white blood cells.[7] The effects of estrogen on cytokine production by immune target cells may involve direct interaction (binding) of the hormone and hormone receptors within those cells.[37] The idea of direct effects of estrogen on target cells is supported by the existence of estrogen receptors not only in reproductive tissues including the uterus, ovaries, and testes, where one would expect the hormone's actions to occur, but also in white blood cells.[5, 35, 73]

Alcohol, Stress Responses, and Immunity

Like other stressors, alcohol stimulates a neuroendocrine network known as the hypothalamic-pituitary-adrenal (HPA) axis, resulting in a dampening of the immune response.[24] This process begins with activation of the hypothalamus (near the base of the brain), which produces a molecule called corticotropin-releasing hormone (CRH). This triggers the pituitary gland (below the hypothalamus) to secrete adrenal corticotropic hormone (ACTH). Finally, ACTH stimulates the adrenal glands (above the kidneys) to release glucocorticoids (cortisol in humans and corticosterone in rodents). These steroid hormones, which direct the activity of many cell types, are transmitted throughout the body in the blood. At high levels, they suppress inflammatory and immune responses.[16, 36] Several studies have documented that under resting (baseline) conditions and in response to stress, females have higher levels of glucocorticoids than do men.[13, 41] Furthermore, estrogen stimulates glucocorticoid production in females,[8, 38] whereas testosterone suppresses its production in both male and female subjects.[11, 13, 38] Alcohol exposure stimulates glucocorticoid production in both males and females.[24, 55] Thus, there are two possible pathways by which alcohol-induced changes in steroid hormones could suppress immune responses in females, whereas there is only one such potential pathway in males. Further study will be required to determine if and how the two pathways interact to mediate alcohol induced effects on immune function in females.

Gender, Alcohol, and Liver Damage

Epidemiologic evidence clearly indicates that the adverse consequences of alcohol consumption, including severe liver disease such as alcoholic cirrhosis, develop more quickly and require lower levels of alcohol exposure for females than for males.[2, 22, 46, 58, 69] At any given level of alcohol intake, women are at higher risk than men of developing liver disease.[2, 17, 46, 58] It has been shown that a daily alcohol ingestion of as low as two drinks per day increases the risk of developing cirrhosis in women, although at least four drinks per day are required to increase this risk in men.[2, 27, 46, 67, 68] These observations were made taking into account differences in body weight, fat distribution, body water, and other potentially confounding variables.

42

It is possible that gender differences in alcohol-related liver disease could be explained by gender differences in:

- The breakdown and elimination of alcohol and its byproducts, including the resulting differences in acetaldehyde levels within the liver.[45, 68]

- The level of activation of inflammatory and immune cells within the liver in response to alcohol ingestion, including Kupffer cells. [1, 42, 47, 53] (Kupffer cells are star shaped immune cells that reside in the microscopic blood vessels of the liver. They are phagocytic, meaning that they are capable of ingesting other cells and foreign particles. Alcohol exposure can cause the digestive tract to leak, which can result in the release of endotoxins—bacterial cell wall products—from the gut into the blood. These endotoxins travel through the blood to the liver, where they can activate Kupffer cells.) Upon stimulation, these cells produce free oxygen radicals and cytokines, which damage and destroy liver cells.[1]

- The amount of alcohol that is metabolized in the stomach (first-pass metabolism). Some research has indicated that women breakdown less alcohol in the stomach than men do, leading to higher blood alcohol levels—and hence greater risk to the liver—for a given dose of alcohol.[3, 57]

Summary

Taken together, these studies show clearly that there are dramatic suppressive effects of both acute and chronic alcohol exposure on inflammation and immunity, regardless of gender. This results in decreased ability of the immune system to fight infections and tumors. The decrease in immunity after consumption of larger quantities of alcohol is in marked contrast to the effects of very low levels of some alcoholic beverages (such as a single glass of red wine), which contain immune protective antioxidants. By depressing estrogen levels, chronic or acute alcohol exposure may cause females to lose the important boost to the immune system that estrogen normally provides. This could act additively or synergistically with an elevation in immunosuppressive glucocorticoids (through activation of the HPA axis) to attenuate immune response, thus leading to a weakened ability to fight infections and tumors. Finally, although chronic alcohol exposure causes liver damage in both males and females, it takes less alcohol and shorter periods of consumption to raise the risk of liver damage for females than for males. Like the observed gender differences in alcohol induced immune suppression, this effect may involve the combined effect of stimulating glucocorticoid production and inhibiting estrogen production.

Further studies will be required to determine whether the alcohol induced changes in gonadal steroid hormone production are sufficient to explain the observed gender differences in immune function. These will require using a similar model system in which both males and females are given alcohol at doses designed to raise blood alcohol levels to the same extent, after which immune responses can be examined. Because of the complexity of studying these parameters in humans, it may be necessary to conduct these studies in animal models of alcohol exposure.

References

1. Adachi, Y.; Bradford, B.U.; Guo, W.; et al. Inactivation of Kupffer cells prevents early alcohol-induced liver injury. *Hepatology* 20:453–460, 1994.

2. Ashley, M.J.; Olin, J.S.; Le Riche, W.H.; et al. Morbidity in alcoholics: Evidence for accelerated development of disease in women. *Archives of Internal Medicine* 137:883–887, 1977.

3. Baraona, E.; Abittan, C.S.; Dohmen, K.; et al. Gender differences in pharmacokinetics of alcohol. *Alcoholism: Clinical and Experimental Research* 25:502–507, 2001.

4. Bautista, A.P. Free radicals, chemokines, and cell injury in HIV-1 and SIV infections and alcoholic hepatitis. *Free Radical Biology Medicine* 31:1527–1532, 2001.

5. Benten, W.P.; Stephan, C.; Lieberherr, M.; et al. Estradiol signaling via sequestrable surface receptors. *Endocrinology* 142:1669–1677, 2001.

6. Brezel, B.S.; Kassenbrock, J.M.; and Stein, J.M. Burns in substance abusers and in neurologically and mentally impaired patients. *Journal of Burn Care & Rehabilitation* 9:169–171, 1988.

7. Burger, D., and Dayer, J.M. Cytokines, acute phase proteins, and hormones: IL-1 and TNF-alpha production in contact-mediated activation of monocytes by T lymphocytes. *Annals of the New York Academy of Sciences* 966:464–473, 2002.

8.   Burgess, L., and Handa, R.J. Chronic estrogen induced alterations in adrenocorticotropin and corticosterone secretion, and glucocorticoid receptor-mediated functions in female rats. *Endocrinology* 131:1261–1269, 1992.

9.   Cannon, J.G., and St. Pierre, B.A. Gender differences in host defense mechanisms. *Journal of Psychiatric Research* 31:99–113, 1997.

10. Carey, M.P.; Deterd, C.H.; De Koenig, J.; et al. The influence of ovarian steroids on hypothalamic-pituitary-adrenal regulation in the female rat. *Journal of Endocrinology* 144:311–321, 1995.

11. Carlstrom, K., and Stege, R. Adrenocortical function in prostatic cancer patients: Effects of orchidectomy or different modes of estrogen treatment on basal steroid levels and on the response to exogenous adrenocorticotropic hormone. *Urology International* 45:160–163, 1990.

12. Chao, T.C.; Van Alten, P.J.; Greager, J.A.; et al. Steroid sex hormones regulate the release of tumor necrosis factor by macrophages. *Cellular Immunology* 160:43–49, 1995.

13. Chasari, A.; Carino, M.; Perone, M.; et al. Sex and strain variability in the rat hypothalamic-pituitary-adrenal axis function. *Journal of Endocrinological Investigation* 18:25–33, 1995.

14. Cooke, R.T. Alcohol abuse, alcoholism, and damage to the immune system–A review. *Alcoholism: Clinical and Experimental Research* 22:1927–1942, 1998.

15. D'Agostino, P.; Milano, S.; Barbera, C; et al. Sex hormones modulate inflammatory mediators produced by macrophages. *Annals of the New York Academy of Sciences* 876:426–429, 1999.

16. Da Silva, J.A.P. Sex hormones and glucocorticoids: Interactions with the immune system. *Annals of the New York Academy of Sciences* 699:158–165, 2002.

17. Dawson, D.A. Consumption indicators of alcohol dependence. *Addiction* 89:345–350, 1994.

18. De Weerdt, O., and Gooren, L.J. Patterns of serum cortisol in ovariectomized females with and without androgen administration. *Hormone Metabolism Research* 28:82–84, 1992.

19. Deaciuc, I.V. Alcohol and cytokine networks. *Alcohol* 14:421–430, 1997.

20. Deshpande, R.; Khalili, H.; Pergolizzi, R.G.; et al. Estradiol down–regulates LPS-induced cytokine production and NF-kB activation in murine macrophages. *American Journal of Reproductive Immunology* 38:46–54, 1997.

21. Diaz, L.E.; Montero, A.; Gonzalez-Gross, M.; et al. Influence of alcohol consumption on immunological status: A review. *European Journal of Clinical Nutrition* 56 (Suppl. 3):S50–S52, 2002.

22. Diehl, A.M. Liver disease in alcohol abusers: Clinical perspective. *Alcohol* 27:7–11, 2002.

23. Emanuele, M.A., and Emanuele, N. Alcohol and the male reproductive system. *Alcohol Research & Health* 25:282–287, 2001.

24. Eskandari, F., and Sternberg, E.M. Neural-immune interactions in health and disease. *Annals of the New York Academy of Sciences* 966:20–27, 2002.

25. Faunce, D.E.; Gregory, M.S.; and Kovacs, E.J. Effects of acute ethanol exposure on cellular immune responses in a murine model of thermal injury. *Journal of Leukocyte Biology* 62:733–740, 1997.

26. Frazier-Jessen, M.R., and Kovacs, E.J. Estrogen modulation of JE/monocyte chemoattractant protein-1 mRNA expression in murine macrophages. *Journal of Immunology* 154:1838–1845, 1995.

27. Frezza, M.; Di Padova, D.; Pozzato, G.; et al. High blood alcohol levels in women. The role of decreased gastric alcohol dehydrogenase activity and first-pass metabolism. *New England Journal of Medicine* 322:95–99, 1990.

28. Gavaler, J.S., and Van Thiel, D.H. The association between moderate alcoholic beverage consumption and serum estradiol and testosterone levels in normal postmenopausal women: Relationship to the literature. *Alcoholism: Clinical and Experimental Research* 16:87–92, 1992.

29. Gavaler, J.S.; Deal, S.R.; Van Thiel, D.H.; et al. Alcohol and estrogen levels in postmenopausal women: The spectrum of effect. *Alcoholism: Clinical and Experimental Research* 17:786–90, 1993.

30. Gill, J. The effects of moderate alcohol consumption on female hormone levels and reproductive function. *Alcohol and Alcoholism* 35:417–423, 2000.

31. Gregory, M.S.; Faunce, D.E.; Duffner, L.A.; et al. Estrogen mediates the gender difference in post-burn immunosuppression. *Journal of Endocrinology* 146:129–138, 2000a.

32. Gregory, M.S.; Faunce, D.E.; and Kovacs, E.J. The gender difference in cell-mediated immunity following thermal injury is mediated in part by elevated levels of interleukin-6. *Journal of Leukocyte Biology* 67:319–326, 2000b.

33. Grossman, C.J. Possible underlying mechanisms of sexual dimorphism in the immune response, fact and hypothesis. *Journal of Steroid Biochemistry* 34:241–251, 1989.

34. Grossman, C.J.; Neinabar, M.; Mendenhall, C.L.; et al. Sex differences in the effects of alcohol on immune response in male and female rats. *Alcoholism: Clinical and Experimental Research* 17:832–840, 1993.

35. Gulshan, S.; McCruden, A.B.; and Stimson, W.H. Oestrogen receptors in macrophages. *Scandinavian Journal of Immunology* 31:691–697, 1990.

36. Guyre, P.M., and Goulding, N. Glucocorticoids, lipocortin and the immune response. *Current Opinion in Immunology* 5:108–113, 1993.

37. Hall, J.M.; Couse, J.F.; and Korach, K.S. The multifaceted mechanisms of estradiol and estrogen receptor signaling. *Journal of Biological Chemistry* 276:36869–36872, 2001.

38. Handa, R.J.; Nutley, K.M.; Lorens, S.A.; et al. Androgen regulation of adrenocorticotrophins and corticosterone secretion in the male following novelty and foot shock stress. *Physiology and Behavior* 55:117–124, 1994.

39. Hanna, E.; Dufour, M.C.; Elliott, S.; et al. Dying to be equal: Women, alcohol and cardiovascular disease. *British Journal of Addiction* 87:1593–1597, 1992.

40. Holman, C.D.J.; English, D.R.; Milne, E.; et al. Meta-analysis of alcohol and all cause mortality: A validation of NHMRC recommendations. *Medical Journal of Australia* 164:141–145, 1996.

41. Kant, G.J.; Lenox, R.H.; Bunnell, B.N.; et al. Comparison of stress responses in male and female rats: Pituitary cyclic AMP and plasma prolactin, growth hormone and corticosterone. *Psychoneuroendocrinology* 8:421–428, 1983.

42. Kono, H.; Wheeler, M.D.; Rusyn, I.; et al. Gender differences in early alcohol-induced liver injury: Role of CD14, NF-kB, and TNF-a. *American Journal of Physiology: Gastrointestinal and Liver Physiology* 278:G652–G661, 2000.

43. Lee, S., and Rivier, C. Gender differences in the effect of prenatal alcohol exposure on the hypothalamic-pituitary-adrenal axis response to immune signals. *Psychoneuroendocrinology* 21:145–155, 1996.

44. Li, X.; Grossman, C.J.; Mendenhall, C.L.; et al. Host response to mycobacterial infection in the alcoholic rat: Male and female dimorphism. *Alcohol* 16:207–212, 1998.

45. Li, T.K.; Beard, J.D.; Orr, W.E.; et al. Variation in ethanol pharmacokinetics and perceived gender and ethnic differences in alcohol elimination. *Alcoholism: Clinical and Experimental Research* 24:415–416, 2000.

46. Loft, S.; Olesen, K.; and Dossing, M. Increased susceptibility to liver disease in relation to alcohol consumption in women. *Scandinavian Journal of Gastroenterology* 22:1251–1256, 1987.

47. McClain, C.J.; Hill, D.B.; Song, A.; et al. Monocyte activation in alcoholic liver disease. *Alcohol* 27:53–61, 2002.

48. McGill, V.; Kowal-Vern, A.; Fisher, S.G.; et al. The impact of substance use on mortality and morbidity from thermal injury. *Journal of Trauma* 38:931–934, 1995.

49. Mendenhall, C.L.; Theus, S.A.; Roselle, G.A.; et al. Biphasic in vivo immune function after low- versus high-dose alcohol consumption. *Alcohol* 14:255–260, 1997.

50. Messingham, K.A.N.; Heinrich, S.A.; and Kovacs, E.J. Estrogen restores cellular immunity in injured male mice via suppression of interleukin-6 production. *Journal of Leukocyte Biology* 70: 887–895, 2001.

51. Messingham, K.A.N.; Fauce, D.E.; and Kovacs, E.J. Alcohol, injury, and cellular immunity. *Alcohol* 28:137–149, 2002.

52. Morell, V. Zeroing in on how hormones affect the immune system. *Science* 269:773–775, 1995.

53. Nanji, A.A.; Jokelainen, K.; Fotouhinia, M.; et al. Increased severity of alcoholic liver injury in female rats: Role of oxidative stress,

endotoxin, and chemokines. *American Journal of Physiology: Gastrointestinal and Liver Physiology* 281:G1348–G1356, 2001.

54.   Nelson, S., and Kolls, J.K. Alcohol, host defense and society. *Nature Reviews Immunology* 2:205–209, 2002.

55.   Ogilvie, K.; Lee, S.; Weiss, B.; et al. Mechanisms mediating the influence of alcohol on the hypothalamic-pituitary-adrenal axis responses to immune and nonimmune signals. *Alcoholism: Clinical and Experimental Research* 22 (Suppl. 5):243S–247S, 1998.

56.   Olsen, N.J., and Kovacs, W.J. Gonadal steroids and immunity. *Endocrinology Reviews* 17:369–384, 1996.

57.   Pozzato, G.; Moretti, M.; Frazin, F.; et al. Ethanol metabolism and aging: The role of "first pass metabolism" and gastric alcohol dehydrogenase activity. *Journal of Gerontology* 50:B135–B141, 1995.

58.   Schenker, S. Medical consequences of alcohol abuse: Is gender a factor? *Alcoholism: Clinical and Experimental Research* 21:179–181, 1997.

59.   Smith, G.S., and Kraus, J.F. Alcohol and residential, recreational, and occupational injuries: A review of the epidemiologic evidence. *Annual Review of Public Health* 9:99–121, 1988.

60.   Spitzer, J.A. Gender differences in some host defense mechanisms. *Lupus* 8:380–383, 1999.

61.   Spitzer, J.A., and Spitzer, J.J. Lipopolysaccharide tolerance and ethanol modulate hepatic nitric oxide production in a gender-dependent manner. *Alcohol* 21:27–35, 2000.

62.   Spitzer, J.A., and Zhang, P. Gender differences in neutrophil function and cytokine-induced neutrophil chemoattractant generation in endotoxic rats. *Inflammation* 20:485–498, 1996a.

63.   Spitzer, J.A., and Zhang, P. Gender differences in phagocytic responses in the blood and liver, and the generation of cytokine-induced neutrophil chemoattractant in the liver of acutely ethanol-intoxicated rats. *Alcoholism: Clinical and Experimental Research* 20:914–920, 1996b.

64.   Szabo, G. Monocytes, alcohol use, and altered immunity. *Alcoholism: Clinical and Experimental Research* 22(Suppl. 5):216S–219S, 1998.

65. Szabo, G. Consequences of alcohol consumption on host defense. *Alcohol and Alcoholism* 34:830–841, 1999.

66. Szabo, G.; Chavan, S.; Mandrekar, P.; et al. Acute alcohol consumption attenuates interleukin-8 (IL-8) and monocyte chemoattractant peptide-1 (MCP-1) induction in response to ex vivo stimulation. *Journal of Clinical Immunology* 19:67–76, 1999.

67. Taylor, J.L.; Dolhert, N.; Friedman, L.; et al. Alcohol elimination and simulator performance of male and female aviators: A preliminary report. *Aviation Space and Environmental Medicine* 67:407–413, 1996.

68. Thomasson, H.R. Gender differences in alcohol metabolism. In: Galanter, M., ed. *Recent Developments in Alcoholism: Women and Alcoholism.* New York: Plenum Press, 1995. pp. 163–179.

69. Thurman, R.G. Sex-related liver injury due to alcohol involves activation of Kupffer cells by endotoxin. *Canadian Journal of Gastroenterology* 14(Suppl. D):129D–135D, 2000.

70. Van Thiel, D.H.; Gavaler, J.S.; Rosenblum, E.R.; et al. Effects of ethanol on endocrine cells: Testicular effects. *Annals of the New York Academy of Sciences* 492:287–302, 1987.

71. Verthelyi, D. Sex hormone as immunomodulators in health and disease. *International Immunopharmacology* 1:983–993, 2001.

72. Warner-Smith, S.A.; Speigelman, D.; Yaun, S.S.; et al. Alcohol and breast cancer in women: A pooled analysis of cohort studies. *JAMA: Journal of the American Medical Association* 279:535–540, 1998.

73. Weusten, J.J.; Blankenstein, M.A.: Gmelig-Meyling, F.H.; et al. Presence of oestrogen receptors in human blood mononuclear cells and thymocytes. *Acta Endocrinologica* 112:409–414, 1986.

74. Wu, A.H.; Pike, M.C.; and Stram, D.O. Meta-analysis: Dietary fat intake, serum estrogen levels, and the risk of breast cancer. *Journal of the National Cancer Institute* 91:529–534, 1999.

75. Zhang, Y.; Kreger, B.E.; Dogran, J.F.; et al. Alcohol consumption and risk of breast cancer: The Framingham study revisited. *American Journal of Epidemiology* 149:93–101, 1999.

Chapter 7

Immunology Research

Scientists are now able to mass-produce immune cell secretions, both antibodies and lymphokine, as well as specialized immune cells. The ready supply of these materials not only has revolutionized the study of the immune system itself, but also has had an enormous impact on medicine, agriculture, and industry.

Monoclonal antibodies are identical antibodies made by the many descendants (clones) of a single B cell. Because of their unique specificity for different molecules, monoclonal antibodies are promising treatments for a range of diseases. Researchers make monoclonal antibodies by injecting a mouse with a target antigen and then fusing B cells from the mouse with another long-lived cell. The resulting hybrid cell becomes a type of antibody factory, turning out identical copies of antibody molecules specific for the target antigen.

Mouse antibodies are foreign to people, and might trigger their own immune response when injected into a human. Therefore, researchers have begun to study humanized monoclonal antibodies. To construct these molecules, scientists take the antigen-binding portion of a mouse antibody and attach it to a human antibody scaffolding, greatly reducing the foreign portion of the molecule.

Because they recognize very specific molecules, monoclonal antibodies are used in diagnostic tests to identify invading pathogens or

Excerpted from "Understanding the Immune System: How It Works," National Institute of Allergy and Infectious Disease (NIAID), NIH Publication No. 03–5423, September 2003.

changes in the body's proteins. In medicine, monoclonal antibodies can attach to cancer cells, blocking the chemical growth signals that cause the cells to divide out of control. In other cases, monoclonal antibodies can carry potent toxins into select cells, killing the cell while leaving its neighbors untouched.

Genetic Engineering

Genetic engineering allows scientists to pluck genes—segments of the hereditary material called deoxyribonucleic acid (DNA)—from one type of organism and combine them with genes of a second organism. In this way relatively simple organisms such as bacteria or yeast can be induced to make quantities of human proteins, including hormones such as insulin as well as lymphokine and monokine. They can also manufacture proteins from infectious agents, such as the hepatitis virus or human immunodeficiency virus (HIV), for use in vaccines.

Gene Therapy

Genetic engineering also holds promise for gene therapy—replacing altered or missing genes or adding helpful genes. Severe combined immunodeficiency disease (SCID) is a prime candidate for gene therapy. SCID is caused by the lack of an enzyme due to a single missing gene. A genetically engineered version of the missing gene can be introduced into cells taken from the patient's bone marrow. After treated marrow cells begin to produce the enzyme, they can be injected back into the patient.

Cancer is another target for gene therapy. In pioneering experiments, scientists are removing cancer-fighting lymphocytes from the cancer patient's tumor, inserting a gene that boosts the lymphocytes' ability to make quantities of a natural anticancer product, then growing the restructured cells in quantity in the laboratory. These cells are injected back into the patient, where they can seek out the tumor and deliver large doses of the anticancer chemical.

Immune Regulation

Research into the delicate checks and balances that control the immune response is increasing knowledge of normal and abnormal immune functions. Someday it may be possible to treat diseases such as systemic lupus erythematosus by suppressing parts of the immune system that are overactive.

By transplanting immature human immune tissues or immune cells into SCID mice, scientists have created a living model of the human immune system. This animal model promises to be immensely valuable in helping scientists understand the immune system and manipulate it to benefit human health.

Summary

Although scientists have learned much about the immune system, they continue to study how the body launches attacks that destroy invading microbes, infected cells, and tumors while ignoring healthy tissues. New technologies for identifying individual immune cells are now letting scientists quickly determine which targets are triggering an immune response. Improvements in microscopy are permitting the first observations of B cells, T cells, and other cells as they interact within lymph nodes and other body tissues.

In addition, scientists are rapidly unraveling the genetic blueprints that direct the human immune response as well as those that dictate the biology of bacteria, viruses, and parasites. The combination of new technology and expanded genetic information will no doubt teach us even more about how the body protects itself from disease.

Part Two

Diagnosis of Immune System Disorders

Chapter 8

Getting a Proper Diagnosis of Autoimmune Disease

For people with autoimmune diseases, getting a proper diagnosis can be one of the most difficult challenges they face. The American Autoimmune Related Diseases Association (AARDA) conducted a survey of autoimmune disease patients and found that the majority of those eventually diagnosed with serious autoimmune diseases had significant problems in getting a correct diagnosis. Many were incorrectly diagnosed with a variety of conditions that have no specific blood test to confirm the diagnosis. Many were told that their symptoms were in their heads or that they were under too much stress. Further, the survey revealed that 45 percent of autoimmune disease patients had been labeled hypochondriacs in the earliest stages of their illnesses.

To help people having confusing, undiagnosed symptoms to obtain a correct diagnosis, AARDA urges them to take these steps:

1. **Do your own family medical history.** Take an inventory of your family's health problems, expanding your research beyond your immediate family to cousins, aunts, uncles, and other relatives. Since current research points to a genetic component in most autoimmune diseases, you should know the health histories of your first degree relatives, including grandparents and cousins, if possible. Once you know your family history,

you can communicate it effectively to your doctor who can then assess the possibilities with a degree of accuracy and order appropriate tests.

2. **Keep a symptoms list.** People with autoimmune diseases often suffer from a number of symptoms that on the surface seem unrelated. In addition, they may have suffered from other seemingly unrelated symptoms throughout their lives. Therefore, it is important to make a list of every major symptom you have experienced so that you can present it clearly to your doctor. List the symptoms in the order of concern to you. When the nurse calls you into the exam room, review your list—or, better yet (in most cases), give the list to the nurse to record in your chart. When you see your doctor, be sure to mention at the very start of your visit the symptom that bothers you the most. This is often the problem to which your doctor will pay the most attention. Unless your problem list is lengthy, or the doctor notes a serious problem which takes higher priority, she/he usually will be able to answer all your questions. Know in advance what questions are truly important to you. In this way, you will not spend a lot of time discussing things that confuse the issue of your current needs.

3. **Seek referrals to good physicians.** Talk to your family and friends. If you are having trouble getting a proper diagnosis, see whether someone you know and trust can recommend an internist in your community who is also a good diagnostician. It is always good to ask around. Check your community resources—attend health agency meetings and community health meetings sponsored by local hospitals, and talk with the health care professionals at those meetings and elsewhere. Because there is no medical specialty of "autoimmunologist," it can be difficult to determine the type of doctor you may need to see. One thought is to identify the medical specialist that deals with your major symptom and then check with a major medical center for a referral to that specialty department. A number of agencies dealing specifically with autoimmune diseases maintain referral lists.

4. **Inquire about the physician's and hospital's experience with autoimmune disease.** All patients want to receive the highest quality treatment, but it is difficult to evaluate physicians and hospitals to who they entrust their care. It is a good

idea to ask the physician whether he or she takes care of patients with the specific disease that has been diagnosed. Generally speaking, the larger number of patients with a particular autoimmune disease treated by the physician, the better. Also, a specialist should be adept at managing the therapies used to treat a particular autoimmune disease.

5. **Obtain a thorough clinical examination.** Tests vary for different autoimmune diseases, and no single test can ascertain whether a patient has an autoimmune disease. When facing test situations, a patient might ask: What is the purpose of this test? Are there any alternatives? Is this an outpatient or inpatient procedure? Can I anticipate any pain, discomfort, or claustrophobia; and if so, can I take medication to make me more comfortable? How much does the procedure cost, and is it covered by my health insurance? Who will get the test results, and what will they tell me about my condition? The patient needs to understand that, although diagnostic criteria define a disease, they are sometimes uncertain. Making an autoimmune diagnosis is an exercise in the art of medicine as well as the science of medicine.

6. **Get a second, third, fourth opinion if necessary.** Sort out your options for treatment at the beginning before symptoms worsen, but check first to see whether your insurance will pay for a consultation. Since autoimmunity has just begun to be recognized as the underlying cause of some 100 known autoimmune diseases and because symptoms can be vague and not visibly apparent, many doctors do not think to test for autoimmune diseases initially. If a doctor does not take your symptoms seriously, dismisses them as stress related (when you do not feel as though you are under any excess stress), or refers you to a psychologist, find another doctor. You know you are not feeling well, so do not be intimidated. When trying to get a correct diagnosis, it is important to be assertive.

7. **Partner with your physicians to manage your disease.** Once your have settled on your treatment plan, keep in mind that your health is best managed through a partnership—you and your medical team. Do not be afraid to ask questions: What are the treatment options? What are the advantages and disadvantages of each? How long will the treatment last? Establish a dialogue based on mutual respect.

8. **Learn to deal with the long-term effect of autoimmune disease.** The complicated process of obtaining a diagnosis and developing an appropriate plan of treatment may mean that you will be subjected to a great deal of uncertainty. Accept that patients with autoimmune disease and their families very likely will need to adapt to a somewhat different life style. Some people are using the Internet as a way to communicate their symptoms with others. Doing so can help advance your own personal research, may provide clues to what disease you are experiencing, and can be a means of uncovering good resources for finding a good diagnostician. Sharing your situation with others can have enormous benefit, including eliciting the kind of emotional support that is so necessary for people with undiagnosed autoimmune diseases. If you do not have your own computer, many libraries provide access to the Internet through their computers. Ask your librarian whether this is available to you, and do not hesitate to ask for help if getting online is not clear to you. Also, contact your hospital community education department, a nurse at the health department, or a nonprofit disease-specific organization to find out about support groups.

Additional Information

American Autoimmune-Related Diseases Association, Inc. (AARDA)
22100 Gratiot Ave.
East Detroit, MI 48021
Toll-Free: 800-598-4668 (for literature requests)
Phone: 586-776-3900
Fax: 586-776-3903
Website: http://www.aarda.org
E-mail: aarda@aarda.org

Chapter 9

Immune Function Blood Tests

One of the many functions of the body is to protect itself from the invasion of foreign substances. This protective role is acted out by the immune system which is a complex network of specialized cells and organs. The success of this system in defending the body relies on an incredibly elaborate interplay of T-cells, B-cells, natural killer cells, and accessory cells. It is one of the most difficult systems to understand because of its complexity. By combining a series of tests utilizing both in vivo (in the body) and in vitro (in the lab) measurements of immune function, along with determination of cell numbers, one is better able to understand the function of the immune system of a given individual. The easiest way to evaluate the function of various cells of the immune system is by drawing blood from the arm.

Along with looking at the immune function, other tests may be done. These tests, referred to as safety bloods (labs), include a complete blood count (CBC)/differential, full chemistries, and a urinalysis. The CBC consists of the white blood cell count, differential, hemoglobin, hematocrit, and platelet count. The differential is the percent of the various types of white cells; lymphocytes, granulocytes, and several others. The full chemistries look at the functioning of the liver, kidneys, heart, and many other important workings of the body. The urinalysis also helps determine the function of the kidneys. There is

---

Excerpted from "Laboratory Test Information: NIAID and Clinical Center HIV Program," National Institute of Allergy and Infectious Diseases (NIAID), 10/9/2003.

some overlap of safety bloods and immune function studies. The normal levels (values) presented are what are used at the National Institutes of Health (NIH). They may vary slightly when compared to those done at another laboratory.

Immune Function Studies

White Blood Cells (WBC, Leukocytes)

White blood cells (WBC) are produced in the bone marrow and stored in various lymphoid tissues such as the thymus, lymph nodes, spleen, tonsils, etc. White blood cells play a major role in defending the body against infections and foreign invaders such as bacteria, fungi, viruses, and parasites. There are five types of white blood cells: neutrophils, lymphs, monocytes, eosinophils, and basophils. Normal Value: 3300–9600/cubic millimeter (cu mm).

Polymorphonuclear Granulocytes (Polys, Neutrophils)

Polys are mature white blood cells with bands being the less mature polys. Neutrophils (polys and bands) are considered scavenger cells and are the first to arrive at a site of infection or injury. The main function of neutrophils is phagocytosis, meaning that they ingest, and then kill bacteria and foreign matter. When the total neutrophil count (polys + bands) drops to less than 1000/cu mm, there is an increased risk for bacterial and certain fungal infections and severe risk when less than 500/cu mm. Neutropenia is the term used for a low neutrophil count. If the neutrophil count drops too low, dosage of the medication may be reduced or stopped until the count returns to normal. The drug, Neupogen®, may be prescribed in certain conditions to boost the neutrophil count. Normal Value: 40–78% of WBC or 1200–7800/cu mm.

Lymphocytes (Lymphs)

Lymphocytes are small white blood cells that bear the major responsibility for carrying out the activities of the immune system. They are able to specifically identify foreign substances as being mutant (defective) cells and cause their destruction and elimination. There are two major classes of lymphocytes, B-lymphocytes and T-lymphocytes. There is also the natural killer cell that falls under the classification of lymphocytes. Normal Value: 14–49% of WBC or 420–4900/cu mm.

B Lymphocytes

B cells are programmed to produce substances called immunoglobulins also known as antibodies. Each B cell produces a specific antibody for a specific antigen (foreign substance) much like a specific key is made for a specific lock. When an antibody locks with an antigen it usually renders the antigen harmless and marks it for destruction. There are five classes of immunoglobulins (Ig): IgG, IgM, IgA, IgD, and IgE. Each has a different role in the immune defense scheme.

- IgG is the most abundant immunoglobulin in blood. It coats microorganisms making them more desirable for ingestion and destruction by other white blood cells.

- IgM is the largest of the immunoglobulins and is also found in the bloodstream. It is very effective in killing bacteria.

- IgA is found mainly in body fluids such as tears, saliva, respiratory, and gastrointestinal secretions. Its function is seen as guarding the entrances into the body. These are the three immunoglobulins that are measurable in the peripheral blood.

- IgE and IgD are found in small amounts in the blood stream and are not easily measurable.

Normal values of immunoglobulins:

- IgG: 650–1600 milligrams per deciliter (mg/dl)
- IgM: 50–320 mg/dl
- IgA: 65–415 mg/dl

T Lymphocytes

T cells do not produce antibodies, but have a very major role in the immune response. They have two functions:

1. Acting as regulators of the immune system.

2. Directly attacking cells that are malignant or defective.

There are two main types of T cells that vary in respect to their function.

- T4 cells or CD4+ cells, also called the helper/inducer cells. These cells are essential for the activation of B cells, other T cells,

63

natural killer cells, and monocytes/macrophages when they detect that the body has been invaded by viruses, parasites, or fungi.

* T8 cells or CD8+ are the other subset of T lymphocytes and are known as the suppressor/cytotoxic T cells. Their main function is to down regulate (turn off) antibody production by the B cell and to suppress or turn off the cells once the infection is under control. The cytotoxic T cells kill cells that are infected by virus and also kill tumor cells.

Normal values:

* T4 Cells: 600–1200/cu mm, 40–60%
* T8 Cells: 150–600/cu mm, 15–20%

Natural Killer Cells (NK Cells)

Natural killer cells are a type of lymphocyte that does not carry the markers to become B cells or T cells. Like cytotoxic T cells they attack and kill tumor cells and protect against a wide variety of infectious microbes. They are natural killers because they do not need additional stimulation or need to recognize a specific antigen in order to attack and kill.

Branched Chain Deoxyribonucleic Acid (bDNA)

Branched chain DNA (bDNA) is a sensitive, rapid, quantitative, and reproducible means of measuring viral particles of the HIV genetic material ribonucleic acid (RNA) that are circulating in the blood plasma. This assay is done by spinning down and removing the viral particles that are present in the plasma. The genetic material is extracted and undergoes a number of steps which involve attaching probes to the RNA, binding an amplifier (bDNA) to the probes, and labeling the amplifier so that a chemiluminescence agent can bind allowing the amplified probes to be measured. The chemiluminescent agent gives off light that is then measured. The measurement of the light intensity is directly proportional to the viral particles present in the plasma indicating the amount of viral burden. This test rapidly detects changes in virus levels, and along with other immune-based tests, permits researchers and clinicians to respond with changes in therapy.[2]

Reverse Transcriptase Polymerase Chain Reaction (RT PCR)

RT PCR also measures the quantity of the genetic material, RNA of the HIV virus, in the blood plasma. This test is different from bDNA in that the genetic material is being measured and not the amplifier probe. The technique involves spinning out all particles from the plasma and removing all DNA. DNA copies are then made from the HIV RNA. The DNA copies that are made from the HIV RNA are proportional to the amount of genomic RNA present in the original plasma sample.[2] The DNA copies then undergo an amplification process. This process is repeated 20–30 times, eventually amplifying even tiny amounts of material into detectable quantities in order to determine the amount of HIV RNA present in the plasma sample. Sensitivity for detecting viral RNA in the plasma is close to 100%, and reliability makes the technique excellent for quantification of viral burden over time.[1] Limitations of RT PCR are contamination of the sample and false positive results. For this reason, controls are always run with samples.

Measurement: 50 HIV RNA copies/ml is the smallest number of viral particles that can be measured with this test. If the test is 50 copies, viral activity may be present but not measurable.

References

1. Barrick B, and Vogel S. Applications of Laboratory Diagnostics in HIV Nursing. In Grady C, Boenning-Betchel C, Boland M (eds): *Nursing Clinics of North America*, Philadelphia; W.B. Saunders, 1996, p 41.

2. Davey, R.T. Jr. and Lane, H.C. Laboratory methods in the diagnosis and prognostic staging of infection with human immunodeficiency virus type 1. *Reviews of Infectious Diseases*. 12: 912, 1990.

Chapter 10

Antibody Blood Tests

Chapter Contents

Section 10.1

What Is an Antibody Test and Why Is It Done?

"Antibody Tests: What Are They? Why Are They Done?" © 2005 American Association for Clinical Chemistry. Reprinted with permission. For additional information about clinical lab testing, visit the Lab Tests Online website at http://www.labtestsonline.org.

What is an antibody test?

Antibodies are part of the body's immune system. They are immunoglobulin proteins that help protect us against microscopic invaders such as viruses, bacteria, chemicals, or toxins.

There are five different classes of immunoglobulins (IgM, IgG, IgE, IgA, and IgD). The three most frequently measured are IgM antibodies which are produced early in an infection; IgG antibodies which are created later and can remain in the bloodstream for decades; and IgE antibodies which are primarily associated with allergies.

Each antibody produced is unique. It is created to recognize a specific chemical structure on the invader cell or particle. This target structure is called an antigen. Once the antibody attaches to the invader, it serves as a flag for the rest of the immune system, making it a target for destruction.

The first time someone is exposed to a particular antigen it may take the immune system up to two weeks to make an antibody blueprint and to produce enough of that specific antibody (primarily IgM at this point) to fight the initial infection. After the immediate threat has passed, the body saves the blueprint along with a small supply of the antibody (a mixture of IgM and IgG). This supply, which helps the immune system remember, can be measured in the blood (or sometimes in the CSF—cerebral spinal fluid) as an IgG antibody titer. The next time the body is exposed to the same antigen it will respond much more strongly and quickly to provide primarily IgG antibody protection.

Vaccines are useful because they eliminate the normal time delay in initial antibody production. Using either a weakened microorganism, or a protein that the body recognizes as the same antigen, vaccines provide a safe initial exposure to the microorganisms that cause common diseases in humans. Vaccines provoke an immune response to create antibodies against these diseases and to stockpile enough of them to provide long-term protection (immunity). Additional booster vaccinations are sometimes used to raise the concentration of antibodies in the blood to a level where they are considered to be sufficiently protective. Since antibody concentrations tend to fall over time, boosters may be given several years to decades later to maintain protection. In some infections, such as human immunodeficiency virus (HIV) or hepatitis C, antibodies do not destroy the infection.

Appropriate antibody creation and targeting depends on the body's ability to distinguish between itself and others and to correctly identify threats. Sometimes a person's immune system may build IgE antibodies against foreign substances that do not usually cause a response in most people, leading to food, respiratory, or animal allergies. In addition, their system may react to antigens in donated blood that is given during a blood transfusion, or to antigens on transplanted body organs, resulting in rejection.

Normally, a person's immune system learns to identify and ignore the antigens on their own organs, tissues, and cells, but sometimes it may mistakenly identify a part of its own body as foreign and create autoantibodies. This autoimmune response can affect a single organ (like the thyroid) or be systemic, and it can lead to an autoimmune disorder.

Why are antibody tests done?

Antibody concentrations are measured to:

- Document exposure to an infectious or foreign agent.
- Evaluate protection level (immune status) against a particular microorganism.
- Diagnose an autoimmune condition.
- Diagnose the reason for a transfusion reaction or a rejection of a transplanted organ.
- Diagnose an allergy.
- Monitor the course of an infection or autoimmune process.

One test will not determine all of a person's various antibody levels; antibodies are as individual as the diseases they target. Antibody tests are ordered singly or in combinations, depending on symptoms, and on what information the doctor is trying to gather. If he suspects a current infection, two samples (called acute and convalescent samples) may be taken a few weeks apart to look for rising antibody levels.

Testing may involve the measurement of individual antibody IgM and/or IgG concentrations. In the case of allergies, individual IgE antibody levels are measured (such as an IgE test for a peanut allergy or a ragweed allergy) to determine whether or not a person is allergic to that substance.

There really is not a normal antibody concentration. People produce antibodies at different rates, and may store them at variable levels for decades. The result reported and its interpretation by the doctor depends on the particular antibody being tested and the specific circumstances. Results may be reported as detected or not-detected in the case of antibodies causing chronic infections (such as HIV), where any amount of antibody is considered meaningful. They may be reported as greater than a particular cutoff level if immunity is being checked (above that level—which varies depending on the microorganism involved—a person is usually considered to be protected), or as immune or non-immune. Or results may be reported as a number, a concentration that may indicate a current or previous infection. High amounts of IgM and low amounts of IgG indicate recent exposure to infection whereas low IgM and high IgG indicate exposure some time ago.

Antibody titers are sometimes used to determine how significant a positive antibody level is. These titers involve increasing (serial) dilutions of the sample being tested. The highest dilution that is still positive is reported as a "1 to dilution rate" ratio (for instance 1:40 or 1:320, etc.). This is still used to report some antibody levels, especially in the case of autoimmune conditions. Antibody titer is a term that is also sometimes used generically to refer to antibody concentrations.

High levels of individual IgE antibodies may help diagnose an allergy, but they do not necessarily correlate to the severity of the symptoms the patient may be experiencing.

Section 10.2

Antinuclear Antibody (ANA) Test

The antinuclear antibody (ANA) test is used to help diagnose systemic lupus erythematosus (SLE) and drug-induced lupus, but may also be positive in cases of scleroderma, Sjögren syndrome, Raynaud disease, juvenile chronic arthritis, rheumatoid arthritis, antiphospholipid antibody syndrome, autoimmune hepatitis, and many other autoimmune and non-autoimmune diseases. For this reason, SLE, which is commonly known as lupus, can be tricky to diagnose correctly. Because the ANA test result may be positive in a number of these other diseases, additional testing can help to establish a diagnosis of SLE. The doctor may run other tests that are considered subsets of the general ANA test and that are used in conjunction with patient symptoms and clinical history to rule out a diagnosis of other autoimmune diseases.

When is it ordered?

Because autoimmune diseases can be difficult to diagnose, this test offers a reliable first step for identifying SLE and some other autoimmune disorders with a wide variety of symptoms. These symptoms, including painful or swollen joints, unexplained fever, extreme fatigue, and a red rash, may come and go over time and may be mild or severe. It may take months or years for these symptoms to show a pattern that might suggest SLE or any of the other autoimmune diseases.

What does the test result mean?

A positive test result may suggest an autoimmune disease, but further specific testing is required to assist in making a final diagnosis. ANA test results can be positive in people without any known autoimmune disease. While this is not common, the frequency of a false positive ANA result increases as people get older.

About 95% of SLE patients have a positive ANA test result. If a patient has symptoms of SLE, such as arthritis, a rash, and autoimmune thrombocytopenia (a low number of blood platelets), then she/he probably has SLE. In these cases, a positive ANA result can be useful to support SLE diagnosis. If needed, two subset tests, anti-dsDNA and anti-Sm, can help to show that the condition is SLE. If anti-dsDNA autoantibodies are found, this supports the diagnosis of SLE. Higher amounts of anti-Sm are more specific for SLE.

A positive ANA can also mean that the patient has drug-induced lupus. This condition is associated with the development of autoantibodies to histones. An anti-histone test can be given to support the diagnosis of drug-induced lupus.

Other conditions in which a positive ANA test result may be seen include:

- **Sjögren syndrome:** Between 40% and 70% of patients with this condition have a positive ANA test result. While this finding supports the diagnosis, it is not required for diagnosis. Again, your doctor may want to test for two subsets of ANA, the ribonucleoproteins SSA and SSB. The frequency of autoantibodies to SSA in patients with Sjögren syndrome can be 90% or greater if the test is done by enzyme immunoassay.

- **Scleroderma:** About 60% to 90% of patients with scleroderma have a positive ANA finding. In patients who may have this condition, the subset tests can help distinguished two forms of the disease, limited versus diffuse. The diffuse form is more severe. Limited disease is most closely associated with the anticentromere pattern of ANA staining (anti-centromere test), while the diffuse form is associated with autoantibodies to the anti–Scl-70.

- **Others:** A positive result on the ANA also may show up in patients with Raynaud disease, juvenile chronic arthritis, or antiphospholipid antibody syndrome, but a doctor needs to rely on clinical symptoms and history for diagnosis.

A negative ANA result makes SLE an unlikely diagnosis. Unless an error in the testing is suspected, it is not necessary to immediately repeat a negative ANA test. However, because autoimmune diseases change over time, it may be worthwhile to repeat the ANA test in the future.

Aside from rare cases, further autoantibody (subset) testing is not necessary if a patient has a negative ANA result.

Please note: Numerically reported test results are interpreted according to the test's reference range, which may vary by the patient's age, sex, as well as the instrumentation or kit used to perform the test. A specific result within the reference (normal) range—for any test—does not ensure health just as a result outside the reference range may not indicate disease. To learn the reference range for your test, consult your doctor or laboratorian. Lab Tests Online recommends you consult your physician to discuss your test results as a part of a complete medical examination.

Is there anything else I should know?

More specific subsets of the general ANA test are used to help pinpoint the specific autoimmune disease; these autoantibody tests include anti-dsDNA, anti-Sm, Sjögren syndrome antigen (SSA, SSB), Scl-70 antibodies, anti-centromere, anti-histone, and anti-RN.

Some drugs and infections as well as other conditions mentioned can give a false positive result for the ANA test. These drugs may bring on a condition that includes SLE symptoms, called drug-induced lupus. When the drugs are stopped, the symptoms usually go away. Although many medications have been reported to cause drug-induced lupus, those most closely associated with this syndrome include hydralazine, isoniazid, procainamide, and several anticonvulsants.

Section 10.3

C-Reactive Protein

"C-Reactive Protein: The Test," © 2005 American Association for Clinical Chemistry. Reprinted with permission. For additional information about clinical lab testing, visit the Lab Tests Online website at http://www .labtestsonline.org.

The C-reactive protein (CRP) test is sometimes used in patients with inflammatory bowel disease and some forms of arthritis and autoimmune diseases to assess how active the inflammation is and to monitor the treatment. The CRP test is also used to monitor patients after surgery or other invasive procedures to detect the presence of an infection during the recovery period. CRP tests are not specific enough to diagnose a particular disease. Rather, CRP is a general marker of infection and inflammation that alerts medical professionals that further testing and treatment may be necessary.

When is it ordered?

Because CRP increases in cases of inflammation, the test is ordered when acute inflammation is a risk (such as from an infection after surgery) or suspected based on patient symptoms. It is also ordered to help evaluate conditions, such as rheumatoid arthritis and lupus. The test may be repeated to determine whether treatment of an inflammatory disease is effective since CRP levels drop as inflammation subsides.

CRP also is used to monitor wound healing and to monitor patients who have surgical cuts (incisions), organ transplants, or burns as an early detection system for possible infections.

What does the test result mean?

A high or increasing amount of CRP in the blood suggests an acute infection or inflammation. In a healthy person, CRP is usually less than 10 milligrams/liter (mg/L). Most infections and inflammations result in CRP levels above 100 mg/L.

If the CRP level in the blood drops, it means that the person is getting better and inflammation is being reduced. When the results fall below 10 mg/L, the inflammation is no longer clinically active.

Please Note: Numerically reported test results are interpreted according to the test's reference range, which may vary by the patient's age, sex, as well as the instrumentation or kit used to perform the test. A specific result within the reference (normal) range—for any test—does not ensure health just as a result outside the reference range may not indicate disease. To learn the reference range for your test, consult your doctor or laboratorian. Lab Tests Online recommends you consult your physician to discuss your test results as a part of a complete medical examination.

Is there anything else I should know?

Another test to monitor inflammation is called the erythrocyte sedimentation rate (ESR). Both tests give similar information about the presence of inflammation. However, CRP appears and then disappears sooner than changes in the ESR. Thus, the CRP level may fall to normal if a person has been treated successfully, such as for a flare-up of arthritis, but the ESR may still be abnormal for a while longer.

Section 10.4

Erythrocyte Sedimentation Rate (ESR)

"ESR: The Test," © 2005 American Association for Clinical Chemistry. Reprinted with permission. For additional information about clinical lab testing, visit the Lab Tests Online website at http://www.labtestsonline.org.

The erythrocyte sedimentation rate (ESR), or sedimentation rate, is an easy, inexpensive, nonspecific test that has been used for many years to help diagnose conditions associated with acute and chronic inflammation, including infections, cancers, and autoimmune diseases. ESR is said to be nonspecific because increases do not tell the doctor exactly where the inflammation is in the body or what is causing it, and also because it can be affected by other conditions besides inflammation. For this reason, ESR is typically used in conjunction with other tests.

ESR is helpful in diagnosing two specific inflammatory diseases, temporal arteritis and polymyalgia rheumatica. A high ESR is one of the main test results used to confirm the diagnosis. It is also used to monitor disease activity and response to therapy in both of these diseases.

When is it ordered?

A physician usually orders an ESR test (along with others) to evaluate a patient who has symptoms that suggest polymyalgia rheumatica or temporal arteritis, such as headaches, neck or shoulder pain, pelvic pain, anemia, unexplained weight loss, and joint stiffness. There are many other conditions that can result in a temporary or sustained elevation in the ESR, and some that will cause a decrease.

Since ESR is a nonspecific marker of inflammation and is affected by other factors, the results must be used along with the doctor's other clinical findings, the patient's health history, and results from other appropriate laboratory tests. If the ESR and clinical findings match, the doctor may be able to confirm or rule out a suspected diagnosis. A single elevated ESR, without any symptoms of a specific disease, will usually not give the physician enough information to make a medical decision.

Before doing an extensive workup looking for disease, a doctor may want to repeat the ESR test after a period of several weeks or months. If a doctor already knows the patient has a disease like temporal arteritis (where changes in the ESR mirror those in the disease process), she/he may order the ESR at regular intervals to assist in monitoring the course of the disease. In the case of Hodgkin disease, for example, a sustained elevation in ESR may be a predictor of an early relapse following chemotherapy.

What does the test result mean?

Doctors do not base their decisions solely on ESR results. You can have a normal result and still have a problem.

- A very high ESR usually has an obvious cause, such as an acute infection. The doctor will use other follow-up tests, such as cultures, depending on the patient's symptoms.

- Moderately elevated ESR occurs with inflammation, but also with anemia, infection, pregnancy, and old age.

- A rising ESR can mean an increase in inflammation or a poor response to a therapy; a decreasing ESR can mean a good response.

A common cause of high ESR is anemia, especially if it is associated with changes in the shape of the red cells; however, some changes in red cell shape (such as sickle cells in sickle cell anemia) lower ESR. Kidney failure will also increase ESR. Persons with multiple myeloma or Waldenström macroglobulinemia (tumors that make large amounts of immunoglobulins) typically have very high ESR even if they do not have inflammation.

Although a low ESR is not usually important, it can be seen with polycythemia (a condition where a patient makes too many red blood cells), with extreme leukocytosis (patient has too many white blood cells), and with some protein abnormalities.

Please Note: Numerically reported test results are interpreted according to the test's reference range, which may vary by the patient's age, sex, as well as the instrumentation or kit used to perform the test. A specific result within the reference (normal) range—for any test—does not ensure health just as a result outside the reference range may not indicate disease. To learn the reference range for your test, consult your doctor or laboratorian. Lab Tests Online recommends you consult your physician to discuss your test results as a part of a complete medical examination.

Is there anything else I should know?

ESR and C-reactive protein (CRP) are both markers of inflammation. Generally, ESR does not change as rapidly as does CRP, either at the start of inflammation or as it goes away. CRP is not affected by as many other factors as is ESR, making it a better marker of inflammation. However, because ESR is an easily performed test, many doctors still use ESR as an initial test when they think a patient has inflammation.

Females tend to have higher ESR, and menstruation and pregnancy can cause temporary elevations.

Drugs such as dextran, methyldopa (Aldomet), oral contraceptives, penicillamine procainamide, theophylline, and vitamin A can increase ESR, while aspirin, cortisone, and quinine may decrease ESR.

Section 10.5

Rheumatoid Factor

"Rheumatoid Factor: The Test," © 2005 American Association for Clinical Chemistry. Reprinted with permission. For additional information about clinical lab testing, visit the Lab Tests Online website at http://www .labtestsonline.org.

The test for rheumatoid factor (RF) is used to help diagnose rheumatoid arthritis (RA). The test may also be used to help diagnose an arthritis-related condition called Sjögren syndrome. About 80% to 90% of patients with this syndrome have high amounts of RF in their blood.

When is it ordered?

The test for RF is ordered when a person has signs of RA. Symptoms may include stiffness in the joints for a long time in the morning, swelling, nodules under the skin, and evidence on x-rays of swollen joint capsules and loss of cartilage and bone if the disease has progressed.

If a person still has symptoms of RA and the first RF test is negative, the test may need to be repeated. The levels vary with the degree of symptoms and inflammation and may be negative in periods of remission or inactive disease.

The RF test also may be ordered to help diagnose Sjögren syndrome. Symptoms include extremely dry mouth and eyes, dry skin, and joint and muscle pain. Many connective tissue disorders are autoimmune diseases, and RA and other diseases, such as Raynaud syndrome, scleroderma, autoimmune thyroid disorders, and systemic lupus erythematosus, are common among people with Sjögren syndrome.

What does the test result mean?

The presence of RF indicates that the person may have rheumatoid arthritis (RA). Positive RF test results are found in the majority of cases of rheumatoid arthritis. In addition, more than 50% of patients with high levels of RF in their blood have Sjögren syndrome. Many patients with RA also have Sjögren syndrome. (Women more often have both of these diseases. About two to three times as many women as men have RA, and women have 90% of the cases of Sjögren syndrome.)

If a person has a positive RF test result but does not have RA or Sjögren syndrome, there may be another reason, such as endocarditis; systemic lupus erythematosus (lupus); tuberculosis; syphilis; sarcoidosis; cancer; viral infection; or disease of the liver, lung, or kidney. Also, the test may be positive if skin or kidney grafts have been received from a person who does not have an identical genetic profile with the patient.

A negative RF test result means: that the person does not have RA; it is too early in the disease progression to detect RF; or possibly, the person is in a remission phase. If the symptoms appear to be those of RA or Sjögren syndrome, the doctor may order the RF test again as the condition progresses.

Please Note: Numerically reported test results are interpreted according to the test's reference range, which may vary by the patient's age, sex, as well as the instrumentation or kit used to perform the test. A specific result within the reference (normal) range—for any test—does not ensure health just as a result outside the reference range may not indicate disease. To learn the reference range for your test, consult your doctor or laboratorian. Lab Tests Online recommends you consult your physician to discuss your test results as a part of a complete medical examination.

Is there anything else I should know?

The RF test has a high false positive rate, and the result must be used along with the patient's symptoms and history to make a diagnosis of RA, Sjögren syndrome, or another condition.

Interfering factors for the RF test generally include having many vaccinations, lipemia (a large amount of fats in the blood), or specimen handling. Methyldopa, a blood pressure drug, can increase the amount of RF detected by the test.

Section 10.6

Serum Angiotensin Converting Enzyme (SACE)

"ACE: The Test," © 2005 American Association for Clinical Chemistry. Reprinted with permission. For additional information about clinical lab testing, visit the Lab Tests Online website at http://www.labtestsonline .org.

Serum angiotensin converting enzyme (SACE, or angiotensin-converting enzyme—ACE) is primarily ordered to help diagnose and monitor sarcoidosis. It is often ordered as part of an investigation into the cause of a group of troubling, chronic symptoms that may or may not be due to sarcoidosis. SACE will be elevated in 50–80% of patients with active sarcoidosis. If it is initially elevated in someone with sarcoidosis, SACE can be ordered at regular intervals to monitor the course of the disease and the effectiveness of corticosteroid treatment.

When is it ordered?

SACE is ordered when a person has signs or symptoms such as granulomas, a chronic cough or shortness of breath, red watery eyes, and/or joint pain that may be due to sarcoidosis or to another disorder.

This is especially true for individuals between 20 and 40 years of age, when sarcoidosis is most frequently seen. The doctor may order SACE, along with other tests such as an acid-fast bacillus (AFB) culture or sputum culture (tests that can detect mycobacterial and fungal infections), when she/he wants to differentiate between sarcoidosis and another granulomatous condition.

If a person has been diagnosed with sarcoidosis, and the initial SACE levels were elevated, the doctor may order SACE testing at regular intervals to monitor changes over time.

What does the test result mean?

If someone is under 20 years of age, then high ACE levels are usually normal, not significant. For those over 20 years of age, ACE blood levels are a nonspecific indicator. They do not tell why the levels are elevated, what organs and/or body systems are involved, or to what degree. SACE does not cause granulomas, but it often reflects their presence.

If SACE levels are high, other diseases have been ruled out, and there are clinical findings consistent with sarcoidosis, then it is likely that the person has an active case of sarcoidosis. About 20–50% of the time, however, sarcoidosis can be present without elevated ACE levels. This may be due to the disease being in an inactive state, due to an early detection of sarcoidosis—the levels have not risen yet, or due to the fact that the cells are just not excreting increased amounts of SACE. SACE levels are also less likely to be elevated in those with chronic sarcoidosis.

What is often important with sarcoidosis is initially high levels of SACE, then decreasing levels, indicating spontaneous or therapy induced remission. Falling levels usually indicate a favorable prognosis. Rising levels of SACE on the other hand, may indicate either an early disease process, or disease activity that is not responding to therapy.

Please Note: Numerically reported test results are interpreted according to the test's reference range, which may vary by the patient's age, sex, as well as the instrumentation or kit used to perform the test. A specific result within the reference (normal) range—for any test—does not ensure health just as a result outside the reference range may not indicate disease. To learn the reference range for your test, consult your doctor or laboratorian. Lab Tests Online recommends you consult your physician to discuss your test results as a part of a complete medical examination.

Is there anything else I should know?

ACE conversion of angiotensin I to angiotensin II is a normal regulatory process in the body. This process has been targeted by the development of drugs called ACE inhibitors that are commonly used in treating hypertension and diabetes. These drugs inhibit the conversion process, keeping the blood vessels more dilated and the blood pressure lower. ACE inhibitors are useful in managing hypertension, but they are not monitored with ACE blood tests. They may however interfere with ACE measurements ordered for other reasons.

Hemolysis (broken red blood cells) and hyperlipidemia (excess fats) in the blood sample may falsely decrease ACE levels. Decreased ACE levels may also be seen in patients with:

- Chronic obstructive pulmonary disease (COPD)
- Cystic fibrosis
- Emphysema
- Lung cancer
- Starvation
- Steroid drug therapy
- Hyperthyroidism.

ACE has been found in moderately increased levels in a variety of diseases and disorders such as:

- HIV
- Certain fungal diseases
- Diabetes mellitus
- Hyperthyroidism
- Lymphoma
- Alcoholic cirrhosis
- Gaucher disease (a rare inherited lipid metabolism disorder).

The SACE test, however, is not routinely used to diagnose or monitor these conditions (it has not been shown to be clinically useful).

Section 10.7

Protein Electrophoresis and Immunofixation Electrophoresis

Electrophoresis is used to identify the presence or absence of aberrant proteins and to identify when different groups of proteins are increased or decreased in serum or urine. It is frequently ordered to detect and identify monoclonal proteins (an excessive production of one specific immunoglobulin). Protein electrophoresis and immunofixation electrophoresis are ordered to help detect, diagnose, and monitor the course and treatment of conditions associated with these abnormal proteins, including multiple myeloma and a few related diseases.

Protein is usually excreted in the urine in minute amounts. When it is present in moderate to large amounts, it often indicates a problem with the kidneys. The primary reason protein electrophoresis and immunofixation electrophoresis are ordered on urine is to look for monoclonal protein production. This protein may show up in both the serum and urine, or it may only be seen in the urine. An example of this is Bence Jones protein, which is the free light chain component of antibodies. (Normally, antibodies are composed of four parts, two identical heavy chains and two identical light chains. Sometimes, in multiple myeloma, only one or the other is produced, or it may be produced in excess.) The small size of Bence Jones protein allows it to pass through the kidneys and enter the urine.

Urine protein electrophoresis may also be ordered to help diagnose the cause and estimate the severity of protein excretion due to kidney damage or disease. This damage or disease may be due to diabetes, chronic inflammation, an autoimmune condition, or a malignancy. Electrophoresis is not usually necessary to assess the loss of small to moderate amounts of protein due to temporary conditions, such as a urinary tract infection or an acute inflammation.

When is it ordered?

Protein electrophoresis may be ordered when a doctor is investigating symptoms that suggest multiple myeloma, such as bone pain, anemia, fatigue, unexplained fractures, and recurrent infections. It may also be ordered as a follow-up to other laboratory tests, such as an abnormal total protein and/or albumin level, elevated urine protein levels, elevated calcium levels, and low white or red blood cell counts. Immunofixation electrophoresis is usually ordered when the protein electrophoresis test shows the presence of an abnormal protein band that may be an immunoglobulin.

Electrophoresis tests are most frequently ordered when a doctor suspects a disease or condition that causes a monoclonal protein to be produced. Once a disease or condition has been diagnosed, electrophoresis may be ordered at regular intervals to monitor the course of the disease and the effectiveness of treatment. As a disease progresses, the amount of protein increases; with treatment, it decreases. Monoclonal protein production may be due to a malignant disease, such as multiple myeloma, but it may also be due to a monoclonal gammopathy of undetermined significance (MGUS). Most patients with MGUS have a benign course, but they must continue to be monitored regularly as some may develop multiple myeloma after a number of years.

Serum protein electrophoresis may also be ordered when symptoms suggest an inflammatory condition, an autoimmune disease, an acute or chronic infection, a kidney or liver disorder, or a protein-losing condition, even if the total protein and/or albumin concentrations are apparently normal. Urine protein electrophoresis may be ordered when there is protein detected in the urine or when the doctor suspects a monoclonal protein may be present.

What does the test result mean?

Protein electrophoresis and immunofixation electrophoresis tests give the doctor a rough estimate of how much of each protein is present. The value of protein electrophoresis lies in the proportions of proteins and in the patterns they create on the electrophoresis graph. The value of immunofixation electrophoresis is in the identification of the presence of a particular type of immunoglobulin.

For example, certain conditions or diseases may be associated with decreases or increases in various serum proteins:

- **Albumin decreased**—with malnutrition and malabsorption, pregnancy, kidney disease (especially nephrotic syndrome), liver disease, inflammatory conditions, and protein-losing syndromes

- **Albumin increased**—with dehydration

- **Alpha 1 globulin decreased**—in congenital emphysema (a_1-antitrypsin deficiency, a rare genetic disease) or severe liver disease

- **Alpha 1 globulin increased**—in acute or chronic inflammatory diseases

- **Alpha 2 globulin decreased**—with hyperthyroidism or severe liver disease, hemolysis (red blood cell breakage)

- **Alpha 2 globulin increased**—with kidney disease (nephrotic syndrome), acute or chronic inflammatory disease

- **Beta globulin decreased**—with malnutrition, cirrhosis

- **Beta globulin increased**—with hypercholesterolemia, iron deficiency anemia, some cases of multiple myeloma or MGUS

- **Gamma globulin decreased**—variety of genetic immune disorders, and in secondary immune deficiency

- **Gamma globulin increased**—

  - **Polyclonal:** chronic inflammatory disease, rheumatoid arthritis, systemic lupus erythematosus, cirrhosis, chronic liver disease, acute and chronic infection, recent immunization

  - **Monoclonal:** Waldenström macroglobulinemia, multiple myeloma, monoclonal gammopathies of undetermined significance (MGUS)

Please Note: Numerically reported test results are interpreted according to the test's reference range, which may vary by the patient's age, sex, as well as the instrumentation or kit used to perform the test. A specific result within the reference (normal) range—for any test—does not ensure health just as a result outside the reference range may not indicate disease. To learn the reference range for your test, consult your doctor or laboratorian. Lab Tests Online recommends you consult your physician to discuss your test results as a part of a complete medical examination.

Is there anything else I should know?

Immunizations within the previous six months can increase immunoglobulins as can drugs such as phenytoin (Dilantin), procainamide, oral contraceptives, methadone, and therapeutic gamma globulin. Aspirin, bicarbonates, chlorpromazine (Thorazine), corticosteroids, and neomycin can affect protein electrophoresis results.

Section 10.8

Nephelometry: Measuring Immunoglobulins

"Quantitative Immunoglobulins–Nephelometry," © 2005 A.D.A.M., Inc.
Reprinted with permission.

Definition: Nephelometry is a laboratory technique used to obtain a measurement of the amount of IgM, IgG, and IgA immunoglobulins accurately and rapidly. The test uses a specialized instrument to measure the movement of particles in a solution (turbidity) caused by the interaction of immunoglobulins in the serum and anti-immunoglobulin that has been added to the serum.

How the Test Is Performed

Blood is drawn from a vein (venipuncture), usually from the inside of the elbow or the back of the hand. The puncture site is cleaned with antiseptic, and a tourniquet (an elastic band) or blood pressure cuff is placed around the upper arm to apply pressure and restrict blood flow through the vein. This causes veins below the tourniquet to distend (fill with blood). A needle is inserted into the vein, and the blood is collected in an airtight vial or a syringe. During the procedure, the tourniquet is removed to restore circulation. Once the blood has been collected, the needle is removed, and the puncture site is covered to stop any bleeding.

Infant or Young Child

The area is cleansed with antiseptic and punctured with a sharp needle or a lancet. The blood may be collected in a pipette (small glass tube), on a slide, onto a test strip, or into a small container. Cotton or a bandage may be applied to the puncture site if there is any continued bleeding.

How to Prepare for the Test

You may be asked to fast for 4 hours before the test.

How the Test Will Feel

When the needle is inserted to draw blood, some people feel moderate pain, while others feel only a prick or stinging sensation. Afterward, there may be some throbbing.

Why the Test Is Performed

The test provides a rapid and accurate measurement of the amounts of immunoglobulins (Ig) M, G, and A. (Immunoglobulin D has no known clinical significance, and IgE must be measured by more sensitive techniques such as radioimmunoassay or enzyme-linked immunoassay.)

Normal Values

- IgG: 560 to 1800 milligrams/deciliter (mg/dL)
- IgM: 45 to 250 mg/dL
- IgA: 100 to 400 mg/dL

What Abnormal Results Mean

Increased levels of IgG may indicate:

- Chronic infection
- Hyperimmunization
- IgG multiple myeloma
- Liver disease
- Rheumatoid arthritis
- Rheumatic fever.

Decreased levels of IgG may indicate:

- Agammaglobulinemia (very rare)
- Amyloidosis
- Leukemia
- Preeclampsia.

Increased levels of IgM may indicate:

- Infectious mononucleosis

- Lymphosarcoma
- Macroglobulinemia
- Rheumatoid arthritis.

Decreased levels of IgM may indicate:

- Agammaglobulinemia (very rare)
- Amyloidosis
- Leukemia.

Increased levels of IgA may indicate:

- Chronic infections, especially involving the gastrointestinal tract
- Inflammatory bowel disease
- Rheumatic fever.

Decreased levels of IgA may indicate:

- Agammaglobulinemia (very rare)
- Protein-losing gastroenteropathy
- Hereditary IgA deficiency.

What the Risks Are

- Excessive bleeding
- Fainting or feeling light-headed
- Hematoma (blood accumulating under the skin)
- Infection (a slight risk any time the skin is broken)
- Multiple punctures to locate veins

Special Considerations

Nephelometry determines the total amount of each immunoglobulin but cannot distinguish monoclonal antibodies. Other tests such as immunoelectrophoresis or immunofixation can be used to make these distinctions.

Veins and arteries vary in size from one patient to another and from one side of the body to the other. Obtaining a blood sample from some people may be more difficult than from others.

Chapter 11

Genetic Testing

What Is Genetic Testing?

A genetic test is the analysis of human deoxyribonucleic acid (DNA), ribonucleic acid (RNA), chromosomes, proteins, or certain metabolites in order to detect alterations related to a heritable disorder. This can be accomplished by directly examining the DNA or RNA that makes up a gene (direct testing), looking at markers co-inherited with a disease-causing gene (linkage testing), assaying certain metabolites (biochemical testing), or examining the chromosomes (cytogenetic testing).

Although genetic testing shares some features in common with other kinds of laboratory testing, in many ways it is unique and requires special considerations.

Points to Consider

- Genetic testing may be used for medical management and for personal decision-making.

- Genetic test results usually apply not only to the patient, but also to other family members.

Reprinted with permission from GeneTests: Medical Genetics Information Resource (database online). Educational Materials: What Is Genetic Testing?; Uses of Genetic Testing; and Who Should Have a Genetics Consultation? Copyright 2004 University of Washington, Seattle. Available at http://www.genetests .org.

- Genetic testing may be performed in the context of a genetics consultation and should include informed consent, test interpretation, and follow-up medical and psychosocial services as indicated.

- Because most genetic disorders are rare, genetic testing is often done only by specialized laboratories.

- Intense research efforts in molecular genetics result in the rapid development and availability of new genetic tests; therefore, healthcare providers need to continuously update their knowledge.

- Additional costs may be incurred for services necessary for genetic testing to yield meaningful results. These may include:

  - multiple test methodologies
  - testing other family members
  - a genetics consultation.

Clinical Tests

Clinical tests are those in which specimens are examined and results reported to the provider or patient for the purpose of diagnosis, prevention, or treatment in the care of individual patients.

Points to Consider

- United States laboratories performing clinical tests must be Clinical Laboratory Improvement Amendments (CLIA) approved.

- There is a charge for clinical tests; cost varies by complexity.

- Test results are reported in writing.

- The time between specimen submission and reporting of results varies between laboratories and may be based in part on the complexity of the testing.

Research Tests

Research tests are those in which specimens are examined for the purpose of understanding a condition better, or developing a clinical test.

Points to Consider

- Laboratories performing research testing are not subject to CLIA regulation.

- The cost of research testing is generally covered by the researcher.

- Test results are generally not given to patients or their providers.

- Rarely, a research laboratory will share, at the patient's request, potentially useful findings with a clinical laboratory so the patient's test results can be confirmed and a formal report issued.

- Requests for participation in research may be denied at the laboratory's discretion if the laboratory has sufficient samples or the family does not fit the research project goals.

Investigational Tests

Investigational tests are deemed to be of value, but not yet scientifically valid or generally accepted by the medical community as accurate and useful.

Points to Consider

- Test results may or may not be shared, and it may be a long time before results are available.

- If test results are shared with the provider or patient, the laboratory must be CLIA approved.

- There may or may not be a cost for testing.

Uses of Genetic Testing

Diagnostic Testing

Diagnostic testing is used to confirm or rule out a known or suspected genetic disorder in a symptomatic individual.

Points to Consider

- DNA testing may yield diagnostic information at a lower cost and with less risk than other procedures.

- Diagnostic testing is appropriate in symptomatic individuals of any age.

- Confirming a diagnosis may alter medical management for the individual.

- Diagnostic testing of an individual may have reproductive or psychosocial implications for other family members as well.

- Establishing a diagnosis may require more than one type of genetic test.

- DNA testing may not always be the best way to establish a clinical diagnosis.

Predictive Testing

Predictive testing is offered to asymptomatic individuals with a family history of a genetic disorder. Predictive testing is of two types: presymptomatic (eventual development of symptoms is certain when the gene mutation is present, e.g., Huntington disease) and predispositional (eventual development of symptoms is likely but not certain when the gene mutation is present, e.g., breast cancer).

Points to Consider

- Predictive testing is medically indicated if early diagnosis allows interventions which reduce morbidity or mortality.

- Even in the absence of medical indications, predictive testing can influence life planning decisions.

- Because predictive testing can have psychological ramifications, careful patient assessment, counseling, and follow-up are important.

- Many laboratories will not proceed with predictive testing without proof of informed consent and genetic counseling.

- Identification of the specific gene mutation in an affected relative or establishment of linkage within the family should precede predictive testing.

- Predictive testing of asymptomatic children at risk for adult onset disorders is strongly discouraged when no medical intervention is available.

Carrier Testing

Carrier testing is performed to identify individuals who have a gene mutation for a disorder inherited in an autosomal recessive or X-linked recessive manner. Carriers usually do not themselves have symptoms related to the gene mutation. Carrier testing is offered to individuals who have family members with a genetic condition, family members of an identified carrier, and individuals in ethnic or racial groups known to have a higher carrier rate for a particular condition.

Points to Consider

- Identifying carriers allows reproductive choices.

- Genetic counseling and education should accompany carrier testing because of the potential for personal and social concerns.

- Molecular genetic testing of an affected family member may be required to determine the disease-causing mutation(s) present in the family.

- In some situations, DNA testing may not be the primary way of determining carrier status.

- Carrier testing can improve risk assessment for members of racial and ethnic groups more likely to be carriers for certain genetic conditions.

Prenatal Testing

Prenatal testing is performed during a pregnancy to assess the health status of a fetus. Prenatal diagnostic tests are offered when there is an increased risk of having a child with a genetic condition due to maternal age, family history, ethnicity, a suggestive multiple marker screen, or fetal ultrasound examination. Routine prenatal diagnostic test procedures are amniocentesis and chorionic villus sampling (CVS). More specialized procedures include placental biopsy, periumbilical blood sampling (PUBS), and fetoscopy with fetal skin biopsy.

Points to Consider

- A laboratory that performs the disease-specific test of interest must be identified before any prenatal diagnostic test procedure is offered.

- All prenatal diagnostic test procedures have an associated risk to the fetus and the pregnancy; therefore, informed consent is required, most often in conjunction with genetic counseling.

- In most cases, before prenatal diagnosis using molecular genetic testing can be offered, specific gene mutation(s) must be identified in an affected relative or carrier parent(s).

- Prenatal testing for adult-onset conditions is controversial. Individuals seeking prenatal diagnosis for these conditions should be referred to a professional trained in genetic counseling for a complete discussion of the issues.

Preimplantation Testing (Preimplantation Genetic Diagnosis)

Preimplantation testing is performed on early embryos resulting from in vitro fertilization in order to decrease the chance of a particular genetic condition occurring in the fetus. It is generally offered to couples with a high chance of having a child with a serious disorder. Preimplantation testing provides an alternative to prenatal diagnosis and termination of affected pregnancies.

Points to Consider

- Preimplantation testing is only performed at a few centers and is only available for a limited number of disorders.

- Preimplantation testing is not possible in some cases due to difficulty in obtaining eggs or early embryos and problems with DNA analysis procedures.

- Due to possible errors in preimplantation diagnosis, traditional prenatal diagnostic methods are recommended to monitor these pregnancies.

- The cost of preimplantation testing is very high and is usually not covered by insurance.

Newborn Screening

Newborn screening identifies individuals who have an increased chance of having a specific genetic disorder so that treatment can be started as soon as possible.

Points to Consider

- Newborn screening programs are usually legally mandated and vary from state to state.

- Newborn screening is performed routinely at birth, unless specifically refused by the parents in writing.

- Screening tests are not designed to be diagnostic, but to identify individuals who may be candidates for further diagnostic tests.

- Many parents do not realize that newborn screening has been done (or which tests were included), even if they signed a consent form when their child was born.

- Education is necessary with positive screening results in order to avoid misunderstandings, anxiety, and discrimination.

Who Should Have a Genetics Consultation?

Individuals and families who are concerned about a genetic disease may benefit from a genetic consultation whether or not testing is available for that condition. Many people are seeking information and coping strategies as much as test results.

Reasons for referral for a genetics consultation are often grouped by age: preconception/prenatal, pediatric, and adult. Common reasons for referral follow, but these lists are not exhaustive. Consult your local genetics clinic to determine whether a genetics referral is appropriate.

Common Reasons for a Preconception/Prenatal Genetics Consultation

- Mother will be 35 years or older at delivery
- Abnormal results from a triple marker screen or fetal ultrasound
- Personal or family history of a known or suspected genetic disorder, birth defect, or chromosomal abnormality
- Exposure to a known or suspected teratogen
- Mother has a medical condition known or suspected to affect fetal development
- Two or more pregnancy losses
- Close biological relationship of parents
- Ethnic predisposition to certain genetic disorders

Common Reasons for a Pediatric Genetics Consultation

- Abnormal newborn screening results
- One or more major malformations in any organ system
- Abnormalities in growth
- Mental retardation or developmental delay
- Blindness or deafness
- Presence of a known or suspected genetic disorder or chromosomal abnormality

- Family history of a known or suspected genetic disorder, birth defect, or chromosomal abnormality

Common Reasons for an Adolescent/Adult Genetics Consultation

- Mental retardation
- Personal or family history of hereditary cancers
- Personal or family history of a known or suspected genetic condition or chromosomal abnormality
- Blindness or deafness
- Development of a degenerative disease
- Risk assessment for pregnancy planning

Additional Information

National Human Genome Research Institute
31 Center Drive, MSC 2152
9000 Rockville Pike
Bethesda, MD 20892-2152
Phone: 301-402-0911
Fax: 301-402-2218
Website: http://www.genome.gov

Chapter 12

Allergy Tests

Also known as: Radioallergosorbent (RAST) test, allergy screen

The Test

How is it used?

The allergen-specific immunoglobulin E (IgE) antigen test is done to screen for an allergy (a type 1 hypersensitivity) to a specific substance or substances in response to acute or chronic allergy-like symptoms in the patient.

The allergen-specific IgE antibody test may be done (instead of other medically supervised allergy testing) when the patient has significant dermatitis or eczema, is taking necessary histamines or antidepressants that would make other testing more difficult, or if a dangerous allergic reaction could be expected to follow another test.

The allergen-specific IgE antibody test may also be done to monitor immunotherapy or to see if a child has outgrown an allergy, although it can only be used in a general way; the level of IgE present does not correlate to the severity of an allergic reaction, and someone who has outgrown an allergy may have a positive IgE for many years afterward.

"Allergy Test: The Test, Common Questions," © 2005 American Association for Clinical Chemistry. Reprinted with permission. For additional information about clinical lab testing, visit the Lab Tests Online website at http://www.labtestsonline.org.

When is it ordered?

The allergen-specific IgE antibody test is usually ordered when you have signs or symptoms that suggest that you have an allergy to one or more substances or foods.

What does the test result mean?

Normal negative results indicate that you probably do not have a true allergy, an IgE-mediated response to that specific allergen, but the results of allergen-specific IgE antibody tests must always be interpreted and used with caution and the advice of your doctor. Even if your IgE test is negative, there is still a small chance that you do have an allergy.

Elevated results usually indicate an allergy, but even if your specific IgE test was positive, you may or may not ever have an actual physical allergic reaction when exposed to that substance. And the amount of specific IgE present does not necessarily predict the potential severity of a reaction. Your clinical history and other allergy tests, done under close medical supervision, may be necessary to confirm an allergy diagnosis.

Please note: Numerically reported test results are interpreted according to the test's reference range, which may vary by the patient's age, sex, as well as the instrumentation or kit used to perform the test. A specific result within the reference (normal) range—for any test—does not ensure health just as a result outside the reference range may not indicate disease. To learn the reference range for your test, consult your doctor or laboratorian. Lab Tests Online recommends you consult your physician to discuss your test results as a part of a complete medical examination.

Is there anything else I should know?

Sometimes your doctor will look at other blood tests for an indirect indication of an ongoing allergic process, including your total IgE level, or your complete blood count (CBC) and white blood cell differential (specifically at your eosinophils and basophils). Elevations in these tests may suggest an allergy, but they may also be elevated for other reasons.

Common Questions

What other tests are available for allergy testing?

Skin prick or scratch tests, patch tests, and oral food challenges are usually done by an allergist or dermatologist. Your doctor may also try eliminating foods from your diet and then reintroducing them to find out what you are allergic to. It is important that these tests be done under close medical supervision, as a life-threatening anaphylactic reaction is possible.

My allergy test was negative, but I am having symptoms. What else could it be?

You could have a genetic hypersensitivity problem, like Celiac disease's sensitivity to gluten, or an enzyme deficiency, such as lactase deficiency causing lactose intolerance. It could also be an allergy-like condition that is not mediated by IgE for which there are no specific laboratory tests. Or it could be another disease that is causing allergy-like symptoms. It is important to investigate your individual situation with your doctor's assistance.

My allergy symptoms are generally mild. How serious is this really?

Allergic reactions are very individual. They can be mild or severe, vary from exposure to exposure, worsen or stabilize over time, involve the whole body, and can sometimes be fatal.

Will my allergies ever go away?

Although children do outgrow some allergies, adults usually do not. Allergies that cause the worst reactions, such as anaphylaxis caused by peanuts, do not usually go away. Avoidance of the allergen, and advance preparation for accidental exposure in the form of medications such as antihistamines and portable epinephrine injections, is the safest course. Immunotherapy can help decrease symptoms for some unavoidable allergies, but they will not work for food, and the treatment which usually consists of years of regular injections, may need to be continued indefinitely.

Why am I told to avoid melons and bananas when my allergy is to ragweed?

There are cross-reactions between some airborne and fruit pollens. Your body thinks it is detecting ragweed and creates an allergic reaction to the melon.

Chapter 13

Laboratory Tests Used to Diagnose and Evaluate Lupus

Lupus is characterized by abnormalities in many laboratory test results. These abnormalities are different for every patient and vary significantly during the course of a patient's disease. The serial evaluation of an individual's tests along with the physician's observations and the patient's history determine the diagnosis of systemic lupus erythematosus (SLE), its course, and the treatment regimen. All laboratory values must be interpreted in light of the patient's present status, other correlating laboratory test results, and coexisting illnesses. This chapter briefly describes the major tests used to diagnose and evaluate SLE. Rheumatologists, manuals of laboratory and diagnostic tests, or hospital clinical laboratory departments may have further information on possible interpretations of results from these tests and their implications for SLE.

Tests for Blood Cell Abnormalities

Blood cell abnormalities often accompany SLE. People suspected of having lupus are usually tested for anemia, leukopenia, and thrombocytopenia.

Anemia

Tests for anemia include those for hemoglobin, hematocrit, and red blood cell (RBC) count. In addition, the levels of iron, total iron-binding

"Lupus: A Patient Care Guide for Nurses and Other Health Professionals— Laboratory Tests Used to Diagnose and Evaluate SLE," National Institute of Arthritis and Musculoskeletal and Skin Diseases (NIAMS), May 2001.

capacity, and ferritin may be tested. At any time during the course of the disease, about 40% of patients with SLE will be anemic. The anemia may be caused by iron deficiency, gastrointestinal (GI) bleeding, medications, or autoantibody formation to RBCs. When first diagnosed, about 50% of patients have a form of anemia in which the concentration of hemoglobin and the size of the RBCs are normal. This is called normochromic anemia, normocytic anemia, or anemia of chronic disease. Autoimmune hemolytic anemia, with a positive Coombs test, is much less common.

Leukopenia and Thrombocytopenia

Abnormalities in the white blood cell (WBC) and platelet counts are an important indicator of SLE. Leukopenia, a decrease in the number of WBCs, is very common in active SLE and is found in 15–20% of patients. Thrombocytopenia, or a low platelet count, occurs in 25–35% of patients with SLE.

Measurements of Autoimmunity

The presence of certain autoantibodies have diagnostic value for SLE. The most specific tests are those that detect high levels of these autoantibodies. The most common and specific tests for autoantibodies and other elements of the immune system are listed first.

Antinuclear Antibody (ANA)

A screening test for ANA is standard in assessing SLE because it is positive in close to 100% of patients with active SLE. However, it is also positive in 95% of patients with mixed connective tissue disease, in more than 90% of patients with systemic sclerosis, in 70% of patients with primary Sjögren syndrome, in 40–50% of patients with rheumatoid arthritis, and in 5–10% of patients with no systemic rheumatic disease. Patients with SLE tend to have high titers of ANA. False-positive results are found during chronic infectious diseases, such as subacute bacterial endocarditis, tuberculosis, hepatitis, and malaria. The sensitivity and specificity of ANA determinations depend on the technique used.

Anti-Sm (Samarium)

Anti-Sm is an immunoglobulin specific against samarium (Sm), a ribonucleoprotein found in the cell nucleus. This test is highly specific for SLE; it is rarely found in patients with other rheumatic diseases. However, only 30% of patients with SLE have a positive anti-Sm test.

Anti-nDNA (Native Deoxyribonucleic Acid)

Anti-nDNA is an immunoglobulin specific against native (double-stranded) DNA. This test is highly specific for SLE; it is not found in patients with other rheumatic diseases. Sixty to eighty percent of patients with active SLE have a positive anti-nDNA test. For many patients with anti-nDNA, the titer is a useful measure of disease activity. The presence of anti-nDNA is associated with a greater risk of lupus nephritis.

Anticytoplasmic Antibodies (Ro [SSA] La [SSB])

These immunoglobulins, commonly found together, are specific against RNA proteins. Anti-Ro is found in 30% of SLE patients and 70% of patients with primary Sjögren syndrome. Anti-La is found in 15% of lupus patients and 60% of patients with primary Sjögren syndrome. Anti-Ro is highly associated with photosensitivity; both are associated with neonatal lupus.

Complement

Complement proteins constitute a serum enzyme system that helps mediate inflammation. Complement components are triggered into an activated form by such immunologic events as interaction with immune complexes. Complement components are identified by numbers (C1, C2, etc.). Genetic deficiencies of C1q, C2, and C4, although rare, are commonly associated with SLE. A test to evaluate the entire complement system is called CH50. The most commonly measured complement components are the serum level of C3 and C4. These tests are particularly useful in evaluating kidney involvement and in monitoring the disease over time.

Erythrocyte Sedimentation Rate (ESR) and C-Reactive Protein (CRP)

Tests for ESR and CRP are nonspecific tests to detect generalized inflammation. Levels are generally increased in patients with active lupus and decline when corticosteroids or nonsteroidal anti-inflammatory drugs (NSAIDs) are used to reduce inflammation.

Antiphospholipid Antibodies (APLs)

APLs are autoantibodies that react with phospholipids. Recent data indicate that APLs recognize a number of phospholipid-binding plasma proteins (e.g., prothrombin, ß2-glycoprotein I) or protein-phospholipid complexes rather than phospholipids alone. APLs are present in 30–40% of lupus patients. A positive APL test plus the presence of arterial and venous thrombosis and thromboembolism, or recurrent fetal deaths, or thrombocytopenia, is called APL syndrome. APL syndrome affects about a third of lupus patients with APLs (10–15% of all lupus patients). APLs and APL syndrome may also occur in patients without lupus (primary APL syndrome). APLs are detected in the following three types of laboratory assays.

- **Syphilis Serology:** Certain blood tests for syphilis may be falsely positive in lupus patients. Chronically false-positive VDRL or rapid plasma reagin (RPR) tests may occur in patients with lupus.

- **Anticardiolipin Antibody (ACA):** Sensitive enzyme-linked immunoabsorbent assays (ELISA) using cardiolipin as the putative antigen are commonly used to detect APLs. In patients with APL syndrome, most antibodies detected in anticardiolipin ELISAs are directed against cardiolipin-bound ß2-glycoprotein I.

- **Lupus Anticoagulant:** Lupus anticoagulants are APLs that inhibit certain coagulation tests, such as the activated partial thromboplastin time (aPTT), dilute Russell viper venom time (dRVVT), and kaolin clotting time (KCT). Although the antibodies act as anticoagulants in these laboratory assays, they are not clinically associated with hemorrhage, but with thrombosis and other manifestations of the APL syndrome. Most lupus anticoagulant antibodies are directed against prothrombin or ß2-glycoprotein I.

Tests for Kidney Disease

Measurement of Glomerular Filtration Rate

The glomerular filtration rate is a measure of the efficiency of kidneys in filtering blood to excrete metabolic products. Typically this is done by collecting a 24-hour urine sample for measurement of creatinine clearance. Impairment of renal function by lupus nephritis results in reduced levels of creatinine clearances.

Urinalysis

Urinalysis can indicate the presence or extent of renal disease. For example, proteinuria can be a reliable indicator of renal disease. The presence of RBCs, WBCs, and cellular casts, particularly red cell casts, in the urine also indicates renal disease.

Measurement of Serum Creatinine Concentration

Creatinine is a waste product of muscle metabolism that is excreted by the kidney. Loss of renal function as a consequence of lupus nephritis causes increases in serum levels of creatinine. The concentration of creatinine in the serum can be used to assess the degree of renal impairment.

Kidney Biopsy

Kidney biopsy can be used to determine the presence of immune complexes and the presence, extent, and type of inflammation in the glomeruli. Diagnosis of the extent and type of inflammation may help to determine a treatment program for lupus.

Part Three

Inherited Immune Deficiency Diseases

Chapter 14

Primary Immune Deficiency (PID)

The 10 Warning Signs of Primary Immunodeficiency

1. Eight or more new ear infections within a year.

2. Two or more serious sinus infections within a year.

3. Two or more months on antibiotics with little effect.

4. Two or more pneumonias within a year.

5. Failure of an infant to gain weight or grow normally.

6. Recurrent deep abscesses in the skin or organs.

7. Persistent thrush in mouth or on skin, after age one.

8. Need for intravenous antibiotics to clear infections.

9. Two or more deep-seated infections such as meningitis, osteo-myelitis, cellulitis, or sepsis.

10. A family history of primary immunodeficiency.

Source: These warning signs were developed by the Jeffrey Modell Foundation Medical Advisory Board and are reprinted with permission.

This chapter includes excerpts from "Primary Immunodeficiency," National Institute of Child Health and Human Development (NICHD), June 1999. Reviewed in February 2005 by Dr. David A. Cooke, M.D., Diplomate, American Board of Internal Medicine. Also, excerpts from *Patient and Family Handbook For The Primary Immune Deficiency Diseases, Third Edition.* Copyright © 2001 The Immune Deficiency Foundation. Reprinted with permission.

Introduction to Primary Immunodeficiency

Most of us are no strangers to infections. Just about everyone has had a cold, cough, infected cut, the flu, or chicken pox. Some people have had first-hand experience with infections that are even more serious—pneumonia and meningitis. Usually, we expect to recover quickly from an infection. We count on our body's immune defenses (sometimes with the help of antibiotics) to get rid of any germs that cause infection, and to protect us against new germs in the future.

However, some people are born with an immune defense system that is faulty. They are missing some, or in the worst cases, almost all of the body's immune defense weapons. Such people are said to have a primary immunodeficiency (PI). Over 80 types of PI have been identified. Each type has somewhat different symptoms, depending on which parts of the immune defense system are deficient. Some deficiencies are deadly, while some are mild. But they all have one thing in common: they may open the door to multiple infections.

Individuals with PI—many of them infants and children—get one infection after another. Ear, sinus, and other infections may not improve with treatment as expected, but keep coming back or occurring with less common but severe infections, such as recurrent pneumonia. Besides being painful, frightening, and frustrating, these constant infections can cause permanent damage to the ears or to the lungs. In the more severe forms of PI, germs which cause only mild infections in people with healthy immune systems may cause severe or life-threatening infections.

Although infections are the hallmark of PIs, they are not always the only health problem, or even the main one. Some PIs are associated with other immune system disorders such as anemia, arthritis, or autoimmune diseases. Other PIs involve more than the immune system; some, for instance, are associated with symptoms involving the heart, digestive tract, or the nervous system. Some PIs retard growth and increase the risk of cancer.

PI diseases were once thought to be rare, mostly because only the more severe forms were recognized. Today physicians realize that PIs are not uncommon. They are sometimes relatively mild, and they can occur in teenagers and adults as often as in infants and children. Very serious inherited immunodeficiencies become apparent almost as soon as a baby is born. Many more are discovered during the baby's first year of life. Others—usually the milder forms—may not show up until people reach their twenties and thirties. There are even some inherited immune deficiencies that never produce symptoms.

The exact number of persons with a PI is not known. It is estimated that each year about 400 children are born in the United States with a serious PI. The number of Americans now living with a primary immunodeficiency is estimated to be between 25,000 and 50,000.

As new laboratory tests become more widely available, more cases of PI are being recognized. At the same time, new types of PI are being discovered and described. Currently, the World Health Organization lists over 80 PIs and the numbers are increasing. Among the rarest forms of immune deficiency is severe combined immune deficiency (SCID). SCID has been reported in small numbers, while some deficiencies, like DiGeorge syndrome, are diagnosed more commonly. At the other extreme, an immune disorder called selective immunoglobulin A (IgA) deficiency may occur in as many as one in every 300 persons. This figure is an estimate, based on studies of blood from blood donors, since most people with IgA deficiency are healthy and never realize they have this disorder.

Today, thanks to rapid advances in medicine, many PI diseases can be successfully treated or even cured. With proper treatment, most people with PIs are not only surviving once-deadly diseases, they are usually able to lead normal lives. Children usually can go to school, mix with playmates, and take part in sports. Most adults with PI are leading productive lives in their communities.

Successfully combatting PI depends on prompt detection. Physicians, parents, and adult patients alike need to recognize when infections are more than ordinary, so that treatment can be started in time to prevent permanent damage or life-threatening complications.

Inheritance of Primary Immunodeficiency Diseases

PI diseases are usually inherited. Like anything that is inherited, these diseases are the result of altered or mutated genes that can be passed on from parent to child or can arise as genes are being copied.

One or both parents, usually healthy themselves, may carry a gene (or genes) that is somehow defective or mutated, so that it no longer produces the right protein product. If their child inherits a defective gene and does not have a normal gene to compensate, the child may show signs of immunodeficiency. The loss of just one small molecule, if it is an important one, can impair the body's immune system.

Sometimes close relatives—brothers, sisters, cousins—also inherit the defective gene. If they do not inherit a normal gene copy, they may also have immunodeficiency. In some PIs, some relatives may have only mild symptoms while others may have no symptoms at all.

It is also possible to develop, or acquire, an immunodeficiency disorder during one's lifetime. This can be the result of immune system damage due to an infection, as is the case with AIDS—the acquired immune deficiency syndrome. AIDS is caused by infection with HIV, the human immunodeficiency virus which infects immune cells and destroys the immune system. When HIV is transmitted from a mother to her baby, congenital AIDS may occur; but the disease is viral and not inherited. An immunodeficiency can also develop as the unintended side effect of certain drug or radiation treatments, such as those given to cancer or transplant patients.

The focus of this chapter is primary immunodeficiency disease that is heritable. It is carried through the genes; you cannot catch it like a cold.

Genes and Primary Immunodeficiency (PI)

In recent years, scientists have succeeded in identifying the genes that are responsible for many PI diseases. These include X-linked agammaglobulinemia, X-linked hyper-IgM syndrome, Wiskott-Aldrich syndrome, ataxia telangiectasia, four forms of chronic granulomatous disease, and several forms of SCID. The search for other genes that cause PI is underway and more are being discovered.

Sometimes the same, or similar symptoms can be the product of different defective genes on different chromosomes. For example, SCID can be caused by mutations in different genes. One genetic defect blocks activation of B cells and T cells. Another genetic defect prevents immune cells from getting rid of toxic chemicals. In every case, however, the end result is the same: major immune defenses are non-functional.

Once researchers have identified the defective gene, they try to find out what it normally does, what protein it makes, and how that protein contributes to the immune response. Some proteins, for example, relay signals that tell immune cells to multiply and mature. Other proteins help the immune system to eliminate excess or unwanted cells. The next step is to ascertain what happens when the protein is missing or distorted, and how the faulty protein causes disease. Learning about a disease-causing gene and its protein product raises the exciting prospect of finding a cure for the disease. One possibility might be to replace a mutated gene through gene therapy. Another way might be to supply the missing protein as a medicine.

Signs and Symptoms

The most common problem in PI disease is an increased susceptibility to infection. For people with PI, infections may be common, severe, lasting, or hard to cure.

Even healthy youngsters may get frequent colds, coughs, and ear-
aches. For example, many infants and young children with normal
immunity have one to three ear infections per year. However, children
with PI can get one infection after another. Or, they get two or three
infections at a time. Weakened by infection, the child may fail to gain
weight or fall behind in growth and development.

Despite the usual antibiotics, the infections of PI often drag on and
on, or they keep coming back. One common problem is chronic sinusitis (infection and inflammation of the sinuses, air passages in bones
of the cheeks, forehead, and jaw). Another common problem is chronic
bronchitis (infection and inflammation of the airways leading to the
lungs).

Serious infections, especially bacterial infections, may cause a
youngster to be hospitalized repeatedly. Pneumonia is an infection of
the smallest airways and air sacs in the lungs, which prevents oxygen from reaching the blood and makes breathing hard. Meningitis,
an infection of the membranes that surround the brain and spinal
cord, causes fever and severe headache and can lead to seizures, coma,
and even death. Osteomyelitis is an infection that invades and destroys bones. Cellulitis is a serious infection of connective tissues just
beneath the skin.

Some people with PI develop blood poisoning, an infection that
flourishes in the bloodstream and spreads rapidly through the body.
Some people may develop deep abscesses—pockets of pus that form
around infections in the skin or in body organs.

Some children with PI are infected with germs that a healthy immune system would hold in check. These are known as opportunistic
infections because the germs take advantage of the opportunity af-
forded by a weakened immune system. Such an unusual infection may
be the tip-off to an immunodeficiency. For example, *Pneumocystis
carinii* is a microscopic parasite that infects many healthy people
without making them sick. But when the immune system is compromised, *Pneumocystis* can produce a severe form of pneumonia.

Toxoplasma is a widespread parasite that usually produces no disease. In persons with a weakened immune system, it causes toxoplasmosis, which can be a life-threatening infection of the brain that can
cause confusion, headaches, fever, paralysis, seizures, and coma.

Patterns of Inheritance

Although many PI diseases can be traced to a single gene, others cannot. No family pattern is evident, and they are said to occur sporadically.

A sporadic disorder might be the result of several disabled genes interacting, interactions between particular forms of genes, and environmental influences. It might develop from gene changes that occur during a person's lifetime. It might be due to new mutations in germ cells or an inheritance pattern that has not been recognized yet.

Some PIs are X-linked, others autosomal recessive. At least one is autosomal dominant. Some PIs have more than one pattern of inheritance. For example, a group of diseases known as common variable immunodeficiency (CVID) can be inherited as autosomal recessive, autosomal dominant, or X-linked. However, most cases of CVID are sporadic.

Besides all the infections, some immunodeficiency diseases produce other immune system problems, including autoimmune disorders. Autoimmune disorders develop when the immune system gets out of control and mistakenly attacks the body's own organs and tissues.

Finally, an immunodeficiency can be just one part of a complex syndrome with a telltale combination of signs and symptoms. For example, children with DiGeorge syndrome not only have an underdeveloped thymus gland (and a corresponding lack of T cells), they typically have congenital heart disease, malfunctioning or underdeveloped parathyroid glands, and characteristic facial features. Young boys with Wiskott-Aldrich syndrome, in addition to being prone to infections, develop bleeding problems and a skin rash.

Diagnosing PI

Sometimes the signs and symptoms of a PI are so severe, or so characteristic, that the diagnosis is obvious. In most cases, it is not clear if a long string of illnesses are just ordinary infections, or if they are the result of an immunodeficiency.

Many conditions can produce an immunodeficiency, at least temporarily, and most children who seem to have too many infections are not, in fact, suffering from an immunodeficiency. Experts estimate that half of the children who see a doctor for frequent infections are normal. Another 30 percent may have allergies, and 10 percent have some other type of serious disorder. Just 10 percent turn out to have a primary or secondary immunodeficiency.

When a pattern of frequent infections suggests an immunodeficiency, the doctor begins by exploring the patient's history and the family's history, and then conducts a physical examination.

- **The patient's history:** What infections has the patient had in the past or has now? Have they been unusually frequent, or severe, or long-lasting? Have they failed to respond to standard treatments? When a child who is immunologically normal develops a string of infections, they are usually mild and short-lived, and between infections the child recovers completely.

- **Physical examination:** Is the child well-nourished and growing well? A severely immunodeficient child is likely to look sickly and pale. Very often the child is underweight and lags behind in growth and development. The doctor will listen for changes in the lungs and look for rashes, sores, thrush in the mouth, an enlarged spleen or liver, and swollen joints. Some immunodeficient children may lack palpable tonsils or lymph nodes in the neck.

- **Family history:** Have any family members or relatives ever been diagnosed with PI or shown an unusual susceptibility to infections? Have there been any infant deaths from infections? Were only boys affected?

Evaluating Immune Responses

To find out if illness can be traced to an immunodeficiency, laboratory tests are necessary. These tests, most of which can be performed on a sample of blood, probe the soundness of the various parts of the immune system. Are all the right immune cells present, in adequate numbers, and are they working properly? Are there normal amounts and types of antibodies?

Screening starts out with a few relatively simple and inexpensive routine tests. In fact, just two routine tests—complete blood count and quantitative immunoglobulins—will detect most, but not all, immunodeficiencies.

If antibodies are normal—or if the patient's infections seem to be caused by viruses or fungi—the T cells should be checked. If the T cells are present in normal numbers and function normally, phagocyte function should be evaluated.

The most common screening tests include:

- **Blood count:** A complete blood count (CBC) shows levels of red blood cells and white blood cells as well as platelets. A differential count itemizes the different types of white blood cells, including lymphocytes and neutrophils.

- **Quantitative immunoglobulins:** This standard laboratory test measures various immunoglobulin levels in the blood. In addition to total immunoglobulins, it shows levels of the different immunoglobulin types (IgG, IgM, and IgA).

- **Antibody responses:** Are immunoglobulins working properly? A blood test can show if the blood contains antibodies to the usual childhood immunizations, i.e., tetanus, measles, pertussis, or diphtheria. Sometimes a person may be given a booster shot, or a specific immunization such as a tetanus shot, to see if she or he responds by producing antibodies.

- **Complement:** A laboratory test using a sample of blood indicates how effectively the complement system is working.

- **Skin tests:** These tests, which are similar to TB skin tests, show how well T cells are functioning. Tiny amounts of several standard, reaction-provoking antigens (including mumps and *Candida*) are injected into the skin. A person with a healthy immune system usually develops local swelling within 24 to 48 hours. However, these tests are not as accurate in very young infants.

When screening tests indicate an immunodeficiency—or when they fail to explain a stubborn infection—additional tests will likely be needed. There are dozens of sophisticated tests that allow doctors to identify and count subsets of B cells and T cells, and to assess subtle abnormalities in antibodies, immune cells, and immune tissues. Tests can also probe the characteristics of infectious germs.

Evaluating Infections

If an infection proves resistant to standard treatments, the doctor will want to find out exactly what germs are involved. Samples of mucus, sputum, stool, or a small surgically removed sample of the infected tissue can be cultured in the laboratory. This allows germs to grow until they are plentiful enough to study in detail. Once the germ is identified, it becomes possible to select the most effective treatment.

The infection itself often provides a good clue to the nature of an immune defect. Common bacteria typically elicit antibodies, while viruses and fungi stimulate T cells. Thus, sinus infections and respiratory infections, which are most often due to bacteria, suggest an antibody deficiency. Infections caused by a variety of viruses and fungi, or by *Pneumocystis*, point to a T cell defect. Recurrent infections involving the skin or soft tissues can often be traced to problems with phagocytes. Blood-borne infections caused by encapsulated bacteria, including meningitis, may be linked to complement deficiencies.

An experienced physician will also find clues in particular combinations of details, such as age and sex, along with the physical findings. For example, a young infant suffering from diarrhea, pneumonia, thrush, and exhibiting failure to thrive may well have SCID. A 4-year-old with swollen lymph glands, skin problems, pneumonia, and bone infections may have chronic granulomatous disease (CGD). A 10-year old with sinus and respiratory infections, an enlarged spleen, and signs of autoimmune problems is apt to have common variable immunodeficiency.

Prenatal Diagnosis

Some PIs can be detected even before birth. Prenatal testing may be sought by families that have already had a child with a PI.

Cells for prenatal diagnosis can be obtained in several ways. In amniocentesis at about 14 weeks of pregnancy or later, a small amount of amniotic fluid containing cells shed by the fetus is removed from the uterus. In chorionic villus sampling, cells are taken from the chorion—the tissue that becomes the placenta—as early as 9–10 weeks of pregnancy. After about the 18th week of pregnancy, it is possible to obtain a sample of blood from the fetus.

Prenatal tests make it possible to identify abnormalities in cells, or in the case of some deficiencies, of enzymes. In disorders where a gene mutation has been identified, DNA from fetal cells can be checked for the gene defect.

In some cases, test results make it possible to be ready to treat the baby with a bone marrow transplant soon after birth. Intrauterine bone marrow transplantation of the fetus is also being studied.

Primary Immune Deficiency Diseases in America: The First National Survey of Patients and Specialists

Background: Immune Deficiency Diseases

Primary immune deficiency diseases represent a class of disorders in which there is an intrinsic defect in the human immune systems (rather than immune disorders that are secondary to infection, chemotherapy, or some other external agent). In some cases, the body fails to produce any, or enough, antibodies to fight infection. In other cases, the cellular defenses against infection fail to work properly. There are more than 80 different primary immune deficiency diseases recognized by the World Health Organization.

Medical recognition of primary immune deficiency disease is only fifty years old. Although these disorders may have existed in antiquity, it was not until the development of antibiotics that infections could be controlled long enough to recognize there was an underlying defect in the immune system. Also, the parallel development of gamma globulin in World War II provided a replacement therapy for the antibody deficiency forms of immune deficiency.

Although primary immune deficiency diseases are often described as rare disorders, the true population prevalence of these diseases, either individually or in the aggregate, is not well established. The major health surveys conducted by the government in the United States, the *National Health Interview Survey* and the *National Health and Nutrition Examination Survey*, do not collect information on primary immune deficiency diseases. No comprehensive population survey has even been undertaken by the federal government to estimate the prevalence or the population characteristics of these diseases in the United States. Hence, although these diseases are clinically described in the medical literature, there is no comprehensive portrait available of the patient with primary immune deficiency disease.

Survey of Patients with Primary Immune Deficiency Diseases

The Immune Deficiency Foundation undertook the first national survey of the state of primary immune deficiency diseases in the United States. The survey has a number of objectives. First, the survey sought to provide an estimate of the general magnitude of primary immune deficiency in the American population, if not a precise estimate of population prevalence. Second, the survey sought to describe the general population characteristics of persons with these disorders. Third, the survey sought to describe the health of persons with primary immune deficiency diseases, both with and without treatment. Fourth, the survey sought to identify problems in access to treatment in this population. All of these goals are related to the primary objective of the Immune Deficiency Foundation (IDF)—improving the diagnosis and treatment of persons with primary immune deficiency diseases. The survey was designed for IDF by Schulman, Ronca and Bucuvalas, Inc. (SRBI), a national public opinion research organization. SRBI analyzed the survey data prepared their report for the Foundation.

Characteristics of the PID Patient Population

An estimate of the relative distribution of the primary immune deficiency diseases by diagnosis is provided by the specialist survey. The specialists were asked how many patients they were seeing by major diagnosis. Since the survey of physicians is limited to a sample of specialists who see primary immune deficiency diseases, these counts provide an estimate of the relative prevalence of the individual disorders, not a population count of these diseases. Moreover, since the sample is restricted to specialists, the more serious and complex disorders may be disproportionately represented in the sample.

Despite the non-probability sampling procedures for the patient survey, the geographic distribution of the patient sample closely mirrors the total population of the United States. Among the nearly 3,000 patients in the sample, the place of birth is reported in all 50 states and the District of Columbia. There is a somewhat higher proportion of patients born in the Mid-Atlantic region (21%) than the total population

Table 14.1. Commonly Reported Primary Immune Deficiency Diseases

Condition	Number of Patients
Common Variable Immune Deficiency	5,291
Selective IGA Deficiency	5,237
IgG Subclass Deficiency	4,943
X-linked Agammaglobulinemia	811
Severe Combined Immune Deficiency	798
Complement Disorders	725
Ataxia Telangiectasia	502
Hyper IgM	391
Wiskott-Aldrich Syndrome	369

Source: IDF Survey of Specialists

(15%); while a somewhat lower proportion of patients from the East North Central region (13%) than the total population (17%). In the other seven census divisions, the patient and population distributions are virtually identical. There are almost no cases in the sample of patients born outside of the United States

Like the geographic distribution, the gender distribution of persons with primary immune deficiency diseases mirrors the general population. Among patients with primary immune deficiency diseases, 48% are male and 52% are female. Primary immune deficiency diseases are no longer child disorders. About 10% of patients are under six years of age. Twenty percent are aged six to twelve. And, another 10% are adolescents, aged thirteen to seventeen. Sixty percent of patients with primary immune deficiency diseases are adults, aged 18 or older. Indeed, a quarter of patients are aged 45 or older. Five percent are aged 65 or older

Diagnosis

Only 12% of patients were initially diagnosed with a primary immune deficiency disease before one year of age.

One reason for late diagnosis is the absence of a family history of these disorders. Only 2% of patients had a father with a primary immune deficiency disease and 4% had a mother with one of these diseases. It is somewhat more common for patients to have a brother (8%) or sister (5%) with this disorder. About one in ten patients (11%) report other family members with a history of these diseases. But, three-quarters

Table 14.2. Age at Diagnosis with PID

Age at Diagnosis	Percent of Patients with a PID
Less than one	12%
1–5	26%
6–11	12%
12–17	8%
18–39	23%
40–64	18%
65+	2%

Source: IDF Patient Survey N=2,651

(76%) of patients with primary immune deficiency diseases have no family history of PID.

The importance of early diagnosis of these diseases is demonstrated by medical history prior to diagnosis. Although most patients are diagnosed before age twelve, 70% of patients report being hospitalized prior to diagnosis.

Table 14.3. Times Hospitalized before Diagnosis

Times in Hospital before Diagnosis	Percent of Patients Diagnosed with PID
None	30%
One	17%
2–5	32%
6–10	10%
11–20	6%
21+	5%

Source: IDF Patient Survey N=2,708

Table 14.4. Conditions before Diagnosis

Condition	Percent of Patients Reporting
Arthritis	17%
Bronchitis	55%
Cancer	2%
Diarrhea	30%
Ear Infections	51%
Hepatitis	3%
Malabsorption	9%
Meningitis	4%
Pneumonia	51%
Sepsis	5%
Sinusitis	68%

Source: IDF Patient Survey N=2,807

Treatment with Intravenous Gammaglobulin (IVIG)

Seven out of ten (70%) patients with primary immune deficiency disease report that they have been treated with intravenous gammaglobulin (IVIG) for their disorder.

A small proportion of persons with primary immune deficiency diseases began IVIG use in the late 1970s and early 1980s in clinical trials. In the three years prior to the survey, the proportion of immune deficient patients beginning IVIG use was 8%, 10%, and 12% respectively. This represents an increase in the total population of immune deficient patients on IVIG at 15% per annum. This is probably identical to the annual increase in the immune deficient population in the United States.

The impact of treatment, including IVIG therapy, on primary immune deficiency diseases is reflected in the prevalence of serious and chronic conditions before and after diagnosis.

* Arthritis (from 17% to 20%), which is age-related, and hepatitis (from 2.9% to 3.7%) are the only conditions that are more common after diagnosis than before.

* There is a small, but statistically significant decline in the rate of sinusitis (from 68% to 65%), malabsorption (from 9% to 8%), and sepsis (from 5% to 4%) after diagnosis.

Table 14.5. IVIG Use (Ever) by Diagnosis

PID Diagnosis	Percent of PID Patients
Common Variable	92%
IgG Subclass	74%
IgA Subclass	41%
X-Linked Agammaglobulinemia	94%
Severe Combined	80%
CGD	12%
Hyper IgM	89%
DiGeorge	24%
Wiskott-Aldrich	75%
Ataxia	47%
Other	70%

Source: IDF Patient Survey

• There is a much more dramatic decline after diagnosis in pneumonia (from 51% to 27%), ear infections (from 51% to 27%), bronchitis (from 55% to 40%), and chronic diarrhea (from 30% to 24%).

Although seventy percent of patients had been hospitalized prior to diagnosis, nearly half (48%) reported no hospitalization since diagnosis. Another 14% reported only one hospitalization since diagnosis. By contrast, about one in ten patients reported 11–20 (4%) or more than 20 hospitalizations (5%) since diagnosis.

Current Health

More than two-thirds of patients with primary immune deficiency diseases describe their current health status as good to excellent.

Table 14.6. Patient Described Current Health Status

Status	Percent of PID Patients
Excellent	10%
Very Good	24%
Good	34%
Only Fair	22%
Poor/Very Poor	8%
Deceased	2%

Source: IDF Patient Survey N=2,683

Most patients with primary immune deficiency diseases report only slight (28%) or no physical limitations (42%) as a result of health.

Table 14.7. Current Physical Limitation

Limitations	Percent
None	42%
Slight	28%
Moderate	21%
Severe	9%

Source: IDF Patient Survey N=2,647

Three-quarters of patients with immune deficiency diseases (76%) report no hospital nights in the past year (2001).

Table 14.8. Hospital Nights in Past Year

Number of nights	Percent
15+	6%
8–14	4%
3–7	8%
1–2	6%
None	76%

Source: IDF Patient Survey N=2,426

Conclusions

Primary immune deficiency diseases are a set of comparatively rare genetic disorders. Nonetheless, the survey suggests that approximately 50,000 persons in the United States have been diagnosed with one of these diseases. Hence, primary immune deficiency diseases are more common in the United States than some better known genetic disorders, including hemophilia (less than 15,000), cystic fibrosis (30,000), and Huntington disease (30,000), among others.

Half of all persons with primary immune deficiency diseases are not diagnosed until they are adolescents or older. In some cases, this may represent adult or delayed onset of symptomatic disease. In other cases, however, this represents late diagnosis of the condition despite unusual, serious, or repeated infections. One problem for early diagnosis is that the vast majority of patients have no family history of immune deficiency disease.

The cost of late diagnosis is a heavy burden of disease for the patient. The majority of patients suffered two or more hospitalizations before diagnosis. The majority experienced repeated ear infections, bronchitis, and pneumonias before diagnosis, which may cause permanent limitations. In addition, some suffered serious infections and potentially life-threatening infections before diagnosis including sepsis, meningitis, and hepatitis.

Treatment significantly reduces the burden of disease among persons with primary immune deficiency diseases. The prevalence of pneumonia, bronchitis, diarrhea, and repeated ear infections drops significantly after diagnosis. Nearly half of persons with primary immune deficiency diseases have had no hospitalizations since diagnosis.

Two-thirds of persons with primary immune deficiency diseases describe their current health as good, very good, or excellent. Most say their health causes no limitations or only slight limitations on work, play, and other activities. Three-quarters have had no hospitalizations in the past year.

The most common form of treatment for primary immune deficiency diseases is intravenous gammaglobulin (IVIG). Seven out of ten patients report being treated with IVIG for their condition. The proportion of PID patients being treated with IVIG has been increasing at a rate of about fifteen percent per annum in recent years.

Most patients are covered by some form of health insurance or health plan, most commonly through employer group insurance. Nonetheless, a quarter of persons with primary immune deficiency disease report experiencing insurance problems as a result of their condition. In addition, over half report using savings, selling property, or borrowing to pay for treatment. As a result of cost or lack of coverage, nearly two out of five patients with primary immune deficiency disease has missed needed doctor or hospital visits, failed to fill prescriptions, or reduced the amount or frequency of their treatment.

Despite a generally positive outlook after diagnosis for most patients with primary immune deficiency diseases, the survey finds that a significant portion of the patient population faces barriers to timely and effective treatment of their condition. In addition, a significant number of patients with primary immune deficiency disease are only diagnosed after multiple hospitalizations. The long-term outlook for most patients with primary immune deficiency diseases is good, but could be greatly improved by earlier diagnosis and better access to appropriate care and treatment.

Immune Deficiency Foundation
40 W. Chesapeake Ave., Suite 308
Towson, MD 21204
Toll-Free: 800-296-4433
Website: http://www.primaryimmune.org
E-mail: idf@primaryimmune.org

Chapter 15

Ataxia-Telangiectasia

What Is Ataxia-Telangiectasia (A-T)?

A Multi-System Disease

Ataxia-telangiectasia (A-T) is a progressive, degenerative disease that affects a startling variety of body systems. Children with A-T appear normal at birth, and the first signs of the disease usually appear during the second year of life. These first signs are usually a wobbly lack of balance and slurred speech caused by ataxia, which means a lack of muscle control.

Ataxia

The onset of this ataxia marks the beginning of progressive degeneration of a part of the brain known as the cerebellum, which gradually leads to a general lack of muscle control, and eventually confines the patient to a wheelchair. Because of the worsening ataxia, children with A-T lose their ability to write and speech also becomes slowed and slurred. Even reading eventually becomes impossible as eye movements become difficult to control.

This chapter includes text from the following Ataxia-Telangiectasia Children's Project, Inc. documents: "What Is A-T?" © 2005 Ataxia-Telangiectasia Children's Project, Inc. Reprinted with permission; and "How Is A-T Inherited?" and "Diagnosing A-T," © 2000 Ataxia-Telangiectasia Children's Project, Inc. Reprinted with permission.

Telangiectasia

Soon after the onset of the ataxia, the A-T patient usually shows another clinical hallmark of A-T: telangiectasia—tiny, red, spider veins which appear in the corners of the eyes or on the surface of the ears and cheeks exposed to sunlight. Although surface telangiectasia are harmless, their unique appearance with ataxia is what led to naming this disease ataxia-telangiectasia.

Immune System Problems

For most (about 70 percent) of children with A-T there is another clinical hallmark: immunodeficiency that usually brings recurrent respiratory infections. In many patients, these infections can become life-threatening. Because of deficient levels of IgA and IgE immunoglobulins, the natural infection fighting agents in the blood, children with A-T are highly susceptible to lung infections that do not respond to typical antibiotic treatments. For these A-T patients, the combination of a weakened immune system and the progressive ataxia can ultimately lead to pneumonia as a common cause of death.

Predisposition to Cancer

Children with A-T tend to develop malignancies of the blood system almost 1,000 times more frequently than the general population. Lymphoma and leukemia are particularly common types of cancer, although the frequencies of most cancers are elevated. Ironically, another facet of the disease is an extreme sensitivity to radiation, which means that A-T patients cannot tolerate the therapeutic radiation usually given to cancer patients.

Other Features of A-T

Other features of ataxia-telangiectasia that may affect some children are: mild diabetes mellitus, premature graying of the hair, difficulty swallowing causing choking and/or drooling, and slowed growth. Even though A-T is a multi-system disorder, the children afflicted have and maintain normal or even above-normal intelligence. Their dispositions seem to remain equable and help them to maintain a healthy outlook on life despite the progression of their disabilities.

How Frequent Is A-T?

Ataxia-telangiectasia respects no racial, economic, geographic, or educational barriers. Both males and females are equally affected.

Epidemiologists estimate the frequency of A-T as 1 in 40,000 births. But it is believed that many children with A-T, particularly those who die at a young age, are never properly diagnosed. Therefore, this disease may actually be much more common.

The Prognosis

A-T is presently incurable and unrelenting. If they are lucky enough not to develop cancer, most A-T children are dependent on wheelchairs by the age of ten, not because their muscles are too weak, but because they cannot control them. Later, A-T patients usually die from respiratory failure or cancer by their teens or early twenties. A few A-T patients live into their forties, but they are extremely rare.

What Treatments Are Available?

There is no cure for A-T, and there is currently no way to slow the progression of the disease. At this time, treatments are directed only toward partially alleviating some symptoms as they appear. Because A-T is a rare, orphan disease, very little research data is available on pharmaceutical therapies that may aid these children. Physical, occupational, and speech therapy are used to help maintain flexibility, gamma-globulin injections help supplement the immune systems of A-T patients, and high-dose vitamin regimes are being undertaken with some moderate results.

How Is A-T Inherited?

Every person's body is made up of millions of tiny structures called cells. Each cell comes with a full set of instructions that tell the cell what to do and how to make the body work. The instructions are called genes, and they are made from a chemical called deoxyribonucleic acid (DNA). Genes usually come in pairs, and determine everything about the body. For example, certain genes determine eye color, while other genes determine blood type.

Genes are often called the units of heredity because the information they contain is passed from one generation to the next. We all get one gene in each pair from our mother and the other gene in the pair from our father. In this way our bodies work with a combination of instructions inherited from both our parents. Parents have no control over which genes get passed to their children.

Ataxia-telangiectasia is called a recessive genetic disease, because parents do not exhibit symptoms, but they each carry a recessive gene which may cause A-T in their offspring. Therefore, the genetic path of A-T is impossible to predict, and an A-T child is almost always a shock to parents. The recessive gene may lie dormant for many generations until suddenly two people with the defective gene have children.

Each time two such A-T carriers have a child together, there is a 1-in-4 chance (25% risk) of having a child affected with A-T. And every healthy sibling of an A-T patient has a 2-in-3 chance (66% risk) of being a carrier, like his parents.

Diagnosing A-T

The Clinical Presentation of A-T

A-T almost always includes the onset of cerebellar ataxia between the ages of two and five years. Other, less consistent features may include: dysarthria and drooling, oculocutaneous telangiectasia, progressive apraxia of eye movements, characteristic hypotonic facies, absence or dysplasia of the thymus gland, recurrent pulmonary infections, susceptibility to neoplasia, slowed growth, endocrine abnormalities, and progeric changes in the hair and skin.

Common Errors in the Diagnosis of A-T

To a physician at the A-T Clinical Center who has seen hundreds of cases of A-T, the diagnosis can usually be made on purely clinical grounds and often on inspection. But, because most physicians have never seen a case of A-T, mistakes are likely to occur.

For example, perhaps because of the disorder's name, physicians examining ataxic children frequently rule out A-T if telangiectasia are not seen. However, telangiectasia often do not appear until the age of six, and sometimes much older. Similarly, a history of recurrent sinopulmonary infections would heighten suspicion, but about 30 percent of A-T cases do not have immune problems.

The most common early misdiagnosis is that of static encephalopathy (so-called ataxic cerebral palsy). Even though truncal and gait ataxia, almost always the presenting symptom in A-T, is slowly and steadily progressive, it may be compensated for by the normal development of motor skills between the ages of 2 and 5 years, which may mask the progression of ataxia so that an impression of improvement is often reported. As a result, until the progression of the disease becomes apparent, clinical diagnosis will often be incorrect and uncertain unless the patient has an affected sibling.

Once the progression of the disease becomes apparent, Friedreich ataxia becomes the most common misdiagnosis. However, Friedreich ataxia usually has a later onset and the typical pes cavus and kyphoscoliosis are highly characteristic. The spinal signs involving posterior and lateral columns along with the positive Romberg sign distinguish this type of spinal ataxia from the primary cerebellar ataxia of A-T.

Laboratory Markers of A-T

Fortunately, any differential diagnostic difficulty should be easily resolved by reference to the laboratory. The most consistent laboratory marker of A-T is an elevated serum alpha-fetoprotein after the age of two years. Diagnostic support may also be offered by a finding of low serum IgA, IgG, and/or IgE. However, these findings vary from patient to patient and are not abnormal in all cases.

The presence of spontaneous chromosome breaks and rearrangements in lymphocytes in vitro and in cultured skin fibroblasts, although not always present, is also an important laboratory marker of A-T. And finally, reduced survival of lymphocyte and fibroblast cultures after exposure to ionizing radiation will confirm a diagnosis of A-T, although this technique is usually a research procedure and is not routinely available to the physician.

Possible Markers of A-T

- elevated serum alpha-fetoprotein after two years of age
- elevated plasma carcinoembryonic antigen
- low serum levels of IgA, IgG2, and/or IgE (in 70 percent of cases)
- presence of spontaneous chromosome breaks and rearrangements in lymphocytes in vitro and in cultured fibroblasts
- reduced survival of lymphocyte and fibroblast cultures after exposure to ionizing radiation

Possible Symptoms of A-T

Note that tremendous clinical variability is seen among A-T patients, and therefore, many of the following symptoms will not be seen in any one patient.

- progressive cerebellar ataxia (although ataxia may appear static between the ages of two and five years

- progressive oculocutaneous telangiectases appearing by the age of six years
- susceptibility to neoplasia
- characteristic hypotonic facies
- progressive apraxia of eye movements (slow initiation)
- absence or dysplasia of thymus gland
- recurrent sinopulmonary infection
- choreoathetosis (abnormal body movements)
- slowed growth
- cerebellar dysarthria and drooling
- equable disposition
- endocrine abnormality
- proneness to insulin-resistant diabetes in adolescence
- progeric changes in hair, skin, and vascular system
- cortical cerebellar degeneration, involving mainly the Purkinje and granule cells

Additional Information

A-T Children's Project
668 S. Military Trail
Deerfield Beach, FL 33442-3023
Toll-Free: 800-5-HELP-A-T (800-543-5728)
Phone: 954-481-6611
Fax: 954-725-1153
Website: http://www.atcp.org
E-mail: info@atcp.org

Chapter 16

Chediak-Higashi Syndrome

Definition: Chediak-Higashi syndrome is an inherited disorder of the immune system that results in chronic infection, decreased pigmentation in skin and eyes, neurological disease, and early death.

Causes, Incidence, and Risk Factors

Chediak-Higashi is inherited as an autosomal recessive disease. Mutations have been found in the *CHS1* gene. The primary defect in this disease is in intracellular granules. For example, a granule that contains melanin is not made properly in skin giving the pigmentary differences in patients. A neutrophil granule defect (an abnormality in the granules found in certain types of white blood cells that are essential for killing some bacteria, fungi, and viruses) causes the immune problems.

This is one of a group of disorders called oculocutaneous albinism which means decreased pigment in the eye and skin. Children who have inherited the disorder have partial albinism when compared to family members. There may be a silvery sheen to their hair, light-colored eyes, jerky eye movements (nystagmus), and increased infections in their lungs, skin, and mucus membranes.

More serious than the pigmentation problems are the effects of this disease on the immune and nervous systems of the body. Surviving adults develop unsteady gaits (ataxia) and nerve abnormalities in the limbs (peripheral neuropathy) causing motor and sensory changes and weakness. Infection with certain viruses such as Epstein-Barr virus (EBV) can cause a fatal illness resembling a blood cancer, lymphoma.

Symptoms

- Jerky eye movements (nystagmus)
- Decreased vision
- Sensitivity to bright light (photophobia)
- Albinism (a lighter complexion than unaffected family members)
- Silvery sheen to hair which may be fair in color
- Frequent infections (skin, oral, respiratory)
- Mental retardation
- Tremor, abnormal walking gait, seizures, numbness
- Muscle weakness

Signs and Tests

- Blood smear that shows giant granules in the white blood cells that are positive with stains for peroxidases
- Giant granules are also found in cells from biopsy of skin, muscle, nervous system
- Blood platelet or white blood cell levels are abnormally low
- Physical examination may show enlarged spleen, liver, or jaundice
- Genetic testing may show mutations in the *CHS1* gene
- Electroencephalogram (EEG) may show seizures
- Brain magnetic resonance imaging (MRI) or computed tomography (CT) scan may show small brain due to atrophy
- Electromyogram (EMG) or nerve conduction velocity testing may show delayed nerve conduction
- Presence of red light reflex of the eye (frequently seen in albinism)
- Tests show abnormal immune function

Treatment

There is no specific treatment for Chediak-Higashi syndrome. Bone marrow transplants appear to have been successful in several patients. Infections are treated with antibiotics and abscesses are surgically drained when appropriate. Antiviral drugs such as acyclovir have been tried during the terminal phase of the disease. Cyclophosphamide and prednisone have been tried.

Expectations (Prognosis)

The frequent infections of Chediak-Higashi syndrome cannot be prevented. The terminal phase of the illness is not treatable.

Complications

- Frequent infections especially with Epstein-Barr virus
- Lymphoma-like cancer
- Early death

Calling Your Health Care Provider

Call your health care provider if you have a family history of this disorder and you are planning to have children.

Call for an appointment with your health care provider if your child shows symptoms of Chediak-Higashi syndrome.

Prevention

Genetic counseling is recommended for prospective parents with a family history of Chediak-Higashi. Prenatal diagnosis may be available for this disease.

Support Group

Chediak-Higashi Syndrome Association
One South Road
Oyster Bay, NY 11771
Toll-Free: 800-789-9477
Phone: 516-922-4022
Website: http://www.chediak-higashi.org
E-mail: dappell@hpsnetwork.org

135

Chapter 17

Chronic Granulomatous Disease

Chronic granulomatous disease (CGD) is a genetically determined (inherited) disease characterized by an inability of the body's phagocytic cells to kill certain microorganisms. As a result of this defect in phagocytic cell killing, patients with CGD have an increased susceptibility to infections caused by certain bacteria and fungi.

The term phagocytic cell is a general term used to describe any white blood cell in the body that can phagocytose, or ingest, microorganisms. In general, there are two main categories of phagocytic cells, or phagocytes:

1. Polymorphonuclear leukocytes (also called neutrophils or granulocytes)

2. Mononuclear phagocytes (also called monocytes when in the blood and macrophages when in tissues)

Very complex interactions are necessary for normal function of phagocytic cells. First, the phagocyte must be able to migrate to the site of microbial invasion, whether that is under the skin, under a mucous membrane, or in an internal organ such as the lung or liver. Then the phagocyte must be able to ingest the microorganism, whether bacteria or fungus, and bring it into the interior of the phagocyte. After ingestion,

---

a series of complex interactions, including metabolic and mechanical changes, must occur within the phagocyte in order for it to kill the bacteria or fungus.

Although phagocytic cells from patients with CGD can move normally and ingest microorganisms normally, they are unable to kill certain bacteria and fungi because of abnormal metabolism within the cell. Hydrogen peroxide and other oxygen-containing compounds are produced during phagocytosis in normal phagocytes. These oxygen-containing compounds are needed to kill certain bacteria and fungi once these microorganisms are inside the phagocytic cells. The phagocytic cells of patients with CGD are unable to process oxygen properly and create the oxygen-containing compounds needed for killing. As a result, these patients lack an important mechanism to kill certain bacteria.

Some bacterial species, such as the *pneumococcus* and *streptococcus*, produce oxygen-containing compounds such as hydrogen peroxide. When these bacteria are ingested by the phagocytic cells of patients with CGD, the bacterium contributes its own hydrogen peroxide to the defective phagocytic cell. As a result, the defect is overcome, and the phagocytic cell can kill these organisms using the hydrogen peroxide contributed by the bacteria itself. Thus, patients with CGD do not have an increased susceptibility to infection with these organisms. They are only susceptible to organisms, such as staphylococci and fungi, which cannot produce hydrogen peroxide and other oxygen-containing compounds. These microbes cannot supply the missing chemical needed by the phagocytic cell for normal killing.

Patients with CGD have normal antibody production, normal T-cell function, and a normal complement system; in short, the rest of their immune system is normal.

Clinical Presentation

Children with chronic granulomatous disease (CGD) are usually healthy at birth. However, sometime in their first few months or years of life, they develop recurrent infections, infections that are difficult to treat, or infections that are caused by unusual organisms such as fungi. The infections may involve any organ system or tissue of the body, but the skin, lungs, lymph nodes, liver, or bones are the usual sites of infection. Infected lesions may have prolonged drainage, delayed healing, and residual scarring.

Pneumonia is a recurrent and common problem in patients with CGD. Many of the lung infections are chronic. In some instances, patients develop lung abscesses. Abscesses of other organs, such as the liver and spleen, can also occur. Infections of the lymph nodes are also relatively common and may affect the lymph nodes of the neck, axilla, or groin. Osteomyelitis (bone infections) frequently involves the small bones of the hands and feet. Although osteomyelitis requires prolonged therapy, complete healing and return of function usually occurs.

Some infections may result in the formation of localized, swollen collections of infected tissue. In some instances, these swellings may cause obstruction of the intestine or urinary tract. They often contain microscopic collections of cells called granulomas. In fact, it is the granuloma formation that was the basis for the name of the disease.

Diagnosis

The diagnosis of chronic granulomatous disease (CGD) is usually first suspected because of serious infections. Abscesses of the lung, the liver, the region around the anus, and the small bones of hand and feet are often the first clues to the diagnosis. In addition, infections caused by an unusual microbial species such as *Serratia, Nocardia, Burkholderia*, and *Aspergillus* may provide a valuable clue to the diagnosis.

The diagnosis of CGD is made by analyzing the metabolic function and killing capacity of the patient's phagocytic cells. Blood from CGD patients is obtained and the phagocytes are isolated. A number of tests are performed to test the metabolic machinery of the cell and determine if the patient's cells can metabolize oxygen correctly and produce hydrogen peroxide and other oxygen-containing compounds. Confirmation of a diagnosis of CGD may be done by measuring the ability of the phagocytes to kill *staphylococci* or other bacteria. These tests are usually done in specialized laboratories.

Inheritance Pattern

Chronic granulomatous disease (CGD) is a genetically determined disease, and therefore, can be inherited or passed on in families. There are two patterns for transmission. One form of the disease is inherited in a sex-linked (or X-linked) recessive manner; i.e., it is carried on one of the sex chromosomes or X chromosome. Other forms of the disease are inherited in an autosomal recessive fashion; they are carried on chromosomes other than the X chromosome. It is important to understand the type of inheritance so families can understand why a child has been affected, the risk that subsequent children may be affected, and the implications for other members of the family.

139

Treatment

A mainstay of therapy is the early diagnosis of infection and prompt, aggressive use of appropriate antibiotics. Initial therapy with antibiotics aimed at the most likely offending organisms may be necessary while waiting for results of cultures.

A careful search for the cause of infection is important so that sensitivity of the microorganism to antibiotics can be determined. Intravenous antibiotics are usually necessary for treating serious infections in CGD patients and clinical improvement may not be obvious for a number of days in spite of treatment with the appropriate antibiotics. Granulocyte transfusions may also be helpful for some CGD patients when aggressive antibiotic therapy fails and the infection is life-threatening.

Patients with CGD have such frequent infections, especially as young children, that continuous oral antibiotics (prophylaxis) are often recommended. CGD patients who receive prophylactic antibiotics may have infection-free periods and prolonged intervals between serious infections. The most frequently recommended agent for prophylaxis is a combination of trimethoprim and sulfamethoxazole.

A natural product of the immune system, gamma interferon, is also used to treat patients with CGD in order to boost their immune system. Patients with CGD who are treated with gamma interferon may have fewer infections and when infections do occur they may be less serious.

Many physicians suggest that swimming should be confined to well chlorinated pools since fresh water lakes and salt water swimming may expose patients to organisms which are not virulent (or infectious) for normal swimmers but may be infectious for CGD patients. *Aspergillus* is present in many samples of marijuana, so CGD patients should be discouraged from smoking pot. Patients should also avoid dusty conditions, especially spoiled or moldy grass, hay, and compost. Since early treatment of infections is very important, patients are urged to consult their physicians about even minor infections.

Expectations

The quality of life for many patients with chronic granulomatous disease (CGD) has improved remarkably with knowledge of the phagocytic cell abnormality and appreciation of the need for early, aggressive antibiotic therapy when infections occur.

Recurrent hospitalization may be required in CGD patients since multiple tests are often necessary to locate the exact site and cause of infections, and intravenous antibiotics are usually needed for treatment of serious infections. Disease-free intervals are increased by prophylactic antibiotics and treatment with gamma interferon. Serious infections tend to occur less frequently when patients reach their teenage years. In fact, many patients with CGD complete high school, attend college, and are living relatively normal lives.

Additional Information

Immune Deficiency Foundation
40 W. Chesapeake Ave., Suite 308
Towson, MD 21204
Toll-Free: 800-296-4433
Website: http://www.primaryimmune.org
E-mail: idf@primaryimmune.org

Chapter 18

Digeorge Syndrome

The DiGeorge syndrome is a primary immune deficiency disease which is caused by abnormal development of certain cells and tissues of the neck during growth and differentiation of the fetus. As part of the developmental defect, the thymus gland may be affected and T-lymphocyte function may be impaired. Tissues which are dependent upon a single group of embryonic cells for their normal fetal development are called fields. Although the tissues and organs that ultimately develop from a field may appear to be unrelated in the fully formed child, they are related in that they have developed from the same embryonic or fetal tissues. Most patients with the DiGeorge syndrome have a small deletion in a specific part of chromosome number 22 at position 22q11.2. Thus, another name for the syndrome is the 22q11.2 deletion syndrome.

The field, or region, of the developing embryo that is affected in the DiGeorge syndrome controls the development of the face, parts of the brain, the thymus, the parathyroid glands, the heart, and the aorta. The original control of the development of this field is found in a group of cells that originate in the back of the neck of the developing embryo. In order for the components of the field to develop properly, cells must migrate out from the neck during fetal development to areas of the developing face, thymus, parathyroid glands, and heart.

If this does not occur, normal facial, thymus, parathyroid, and heart development may not occur. The anomalies seen in the DiGeorge syndrome are the consequence of abnormal development of this field.

Patients with the DiGeorge syndrome do not all show the same organ involvement. A given organ may be uninvolved, or so mildly involved, that the organ appears to be normal. Patients with the DiGeorge syndrome may have any or all of the following:

- **Facial appearance**—affected children may have an upward bowing of their mouth, an underdeveloped chin, eyes that slant somewhat downward, low set ears, and defective upper portions of their ear lobes. These facial characteristics vary greatly from child to child and may not be very prominent in many affected children.

- **Parathyroid gland abnormalities**—affected children may have underdeveloped parathyroid glands (hypoparathyroidism). The parathyroids are small glands found in the neck near the thyroid gland (hence the name parathyroid). They function to control the normal metabolism and blood levels of calcium. Children with the DiGeorge syndrome may have trouble maintaining normal levels of calcium, and this may cause them to have seizures (convulsions). In some cases, the parathyroid abnormality is relatively mild or not present at all. The parathyroid defect may become less severe with time.

- **Heart defects**—affected children may have a variety of heart (or cardiac) defects. For the most part, these anomalies involve the aorta and the part of the heart from which the aorta develops. As with other organs affected in the DiGeorge syndrome, heart defects vary from child to child. In some children, heart defects may be very mild or absent.

- **Thymus gland abnormalities**—affected infants and children may have abnormalities of their thymus. The thymus gland is normally located in the upper area of the front of the chest. However, the thymus begins its development high in the neck during the first three months of development in the uterus. As the thymus matures and gets bigger, it drops down into the chest to its ultimate location under the breastbone and over the heart. The thymus controls the development and maturation of one kind of lymphocyte, the T-lymphocyte (T for thymus). T-lymphocytes are essential for resistance to certain viral and fungal infections. T-lymphocytes also help B-lymphocytes to develop into plasma cells and produce immunoglobulins or antibodies. Patients with the DiGeorge syndrome may have defects in their T-lymphocyte function, and as a result, they have an increased susceptibility to viral, fungal, and bacterial infections. As with the other defects in the DiGeorge syndrome, the T-lymphocyte defect varies from patient to patient. In addition, small or mild deficiencies may disappear with time.

- **Miscellaneous clinical features**—in addition to other features, patients with the DiGeorge syndrome may occasionally have a variety of other developmental abnormalities including cleft palate, poor function of the palate, delayed acquisition of speech, and difficulty in feeding and swallowing. In addition, some patients have learning disabilities and hyperactivity.

Diagnosis

The diagnosis of the DiGeorge syndrome is usually made on the basis of signs and symptoms which are present at birth or develop soon after birth. Some children may have the facial features that are characteristic of the DiGeorge syndrome. Affected children may also show signs of low blood calcium levels as a result of their hypoparathyroidism. This may show up as low blood calcium on a routine blood test, or the infant may be jittery or have seizures (convulsions). Affected children may also show signs and symptoms of a heart defect. They may have a heart murmur that shows up on a routine physical exam, they may show signs of heart failure, or they may have low oxygen content of their arterial blood and appear blue or cyanotic. Finally, affected children may show signs of infection because of the underdevelopment of their thymus gland and low T-lymphocyte function. Some children have signs or symptoms at birth or while they are in the hospital nursery; others may not show signs or symptoms until they are a few weeks or months older.

There is a great amount of variation in the DiGeorge syndrome from child to child. In some children, all of the different organs and tissues are affected. These children have the characteristic facial characteristics, low blood calcium from hypoparathyroidism, heart defects, and a deficiency in their T-lymphocyte number and function. In other children, all of the different organs and tissues may not be affected and the organs and tissues that are affected may be affected to different degrees. Not only do children differ in the organs and tissues that are affected, but they also differ from each other in terms of how severely a given organ or tissue is affected.

In the past, the diagnosis of DiGeorge syndrome was usually made when at least three of the characteristic findings described were present. However, many mild cases were missed. In recent years, the genetic basis for the syndrome has been discovered. Over 90% of patients with the clinical diagnosis of the DiGeorge syndrome have a small deletion of a specific portion of chromosome number 22 at position 22q11.2. This can be identified in a number of ways, but the most common way is a fluorescent in situ hybridization (FISH) analysis. Use of a FISH analysis test has made the diagnosis of the DiGeorge syndrome more precise.

Therapy

Therapy for DiGeorge syndrome is aimed at correcting the defects in the organs or tissues that are affected. Therefore, therapy depends on the nature of the defect and its severity. Treatment of the low calcium and hypoparathyroidism may involve calcium supplementation and replacement of the missing parathyroid hormone. A heart (or cardiac) defect may require medications to improve the function of the heart or corrective surgery. If surgery is required, the exact nature of the surgery depends on the heart defect. Surgery can be performed before any immune defects are corrected. However, all the precautions that are usually taken with children with T-cell immunodeficiencies need to be observed, such as irradiating all blood products to prevent graft-vs-host disease.

The immunologic defect in T-lymphocyte function varies from child to child. Therefore, the need for therapy of the T-lymphocyte defect varies from child to child. Many children with the DiGeorge syndrome have perfectly normal T-lymphocyte function and require no therapy for immunodeficiency. Other children initially have mild defects in T-lymphocyte function which improve as they grow older. This spontaneous improvement and increase in T-lymphocyte immunity is related to growth of a tiny but otherwise normal thymus gland. In most cases of the DiGeorge syndrome, the tiny thymus ultimately grows enough to provide adequate T-lymphocyte function. In the remaining children (approximately 25%), the thymus is either completely absent or never grows enough to develop adequate numbers of T-lymphocytes. The severity of the defect depends upon how much thymus tissue the child develops. In some children with the DiGeorge syndrome, the T-lymphocyte defect is significant enough to cause the B-lymphocytes to fail to make sufficient antibodies. This occurs because antibodies are produced by B-lymphocytes under the direction of a specific subset of T-lymphocytes.

Not all children with the DiGeorge syndrome require therapy for their immune deficiency. In children who do require therapy for their immunodeficiency, some form of transplantation of normal immune system tissue may help. The immune defect in the DiGeorge syndrome involves the thymus and T-lymphocytes. Therefore, thymus transplants have been used in children with the DiGeorge syndrome. In fact, fetal thymuses were successfully transplanted for the DiGeorge syndrome as early as 1968. The overall success rate is difficult to determine because of different techniques and because some children who received the transplant may have improved spontaneously without the transplant. Recently, bone marrow transplants from matched sibling donors have been performed in patients with severe T- and B-lymphocytes defects with successful outcomes. Also, newer methods of thymus transplantation have improved long term outcomes.

Expectations

The outlook for a child with the DiGeorge syndrome depends on the degree to which the child is affected. The severity of the heart disease is usually the most important determining factor. Most children have no immune defect or only a transient problem with their immune system. If the immunodeficiency is severe and persistent, correction is necessary.

Additional Information

Immune Deficiency Foundation
40 W. Chesapeake Ave., Suite 308
Towson, MD 21204
Toll-Free: 800-296-4433
Website: http://www.primaryimmune.org
E-mail: idf@primaryimmune.org

Chapter 19

Familial Mediterranean Fever

Alternative names: Familial paroxysmal polyserositis; periodic peritonitis; recurrent polyserositis; benign paroxysmal peritonitis; periodic disease; periodic fever.

Definition: Familial Mediterranean fever is an inherited disorder characterized by recurrent fever and inflammation, often involving the abdomen or the lung.

Causes, Incidence, and Risk Factors

The cause of familial Mediterranean fever is unknown. It usually affects people of Mediterranean ancestry, especially non-Ashkenazi (Sephardic) Jews, Armenians, and Arabs, although people from other ethnic groups may also be affected.

Symptoms usually begin between age 5 and 15. Inflammation in the lining of the abdominal cavity, chest cavity, skin, or joints occurs along with high fevers that usually peak in 12 to 24 hours. Attacks may vary in severity of symptoms, and people are usually symptom free between attacks.

This disease is very rare. Risk factors include a family history of familial Mediterranean fever or having Mediterranean ancestry.

"Familial Mediterranean Fever," © 2005 A.D.A.M., Inc. Reprinted with permission.

Symptoms

- Fever or alternating chills and fever (relapsing)
- Abdominal pain
- Chest pain that occurs repeatedly (recurrent)
- Recurrent abdominal pain
- Recurrent joint pain
  - Pain in hip, knee, ankle, shoulder, elbow, or wrist
  - Pain over the small joints of the foot or hand
  - Pain in other joints
- Skin lesions that are red and swollen and range from 5–20 cm in diameter

Signs and Tests

There is no specific test to diagnose this disease. Sometimes analysis of the chromosomes can help. Elimination of other possible diseases by laboratory tests or x-rays will help determine the diagnosis.

Patients with familial Mediterranean fever may have any of the following during an attack:

- Elevated white blood cell count
- Elevated erythrocyte sedimentation rate (ESR)
- Elevated plasma fibrinogen
- Elevated serum haptoglobin
- Elevated ceruloplasmin
- Elevated C-reactive protein (CRP)

Treatment

The treatment for familial Mediterranean fever is treatment of symptoms. Colchicine, a medicine that reduces inflammation, may help during an attack and may prevent further attacks.

Expectations (Prognosis)

There is no known cure for familial Mediterranean fever. Most people continue to have attacks, but the number and severity of attacks is different from person to person.

Complications

- Discomfort is the primary complication.

- Narcotic addiction may sometimes occur, but addiction rates are not higher than for the general population if the pain associated with the condition is recognized and treated appropriately.

- Gallbladder disease may also occur.

- Amyloidosis (deposits of protein in different organs) is more common in patients with familial Mediterranean fever.

Calling Your Health Care Provider

Call your health care provider if symptoms develop, to rule out other possible causes and get appropriate treatment. See a pain specialist if there is chronic pain.

Chapter 20

Hyper-Immunoglobulin M (IgM) Syndrome

Patients with the X-linked hyper IgM (XHIGM) syndrome have a defect or deficiency of a protein that is found on the surface of T-lymphocytes. The affected protein is called CD40 ligand and is made by a gene on the X chromosome. Thus, this primary immunodeficiency disease is inherited as an X-linked recessive trait and usually found only in boys.

As a consequence of their deficiency in CD40 ligand, affected patients' T-lymphocytes are unable to instruct B-lymphocytes to switch their production of gamma globulins from IgM to IgG and IgA. As a result, patients with this primary immunodeficiency disease have decreased levels of serum IgG and IgA and normal or elevated levels of IgM. In addition, since CD40 ligand is important to other functions of T-lymphocytes, they also have a defect in some of the protective functions of their T-lymphocytes.

A disease resembling the XHIGM syndrome has also been observed in females and in some males in whom the CD40 ligand gene is normal. The precise molecular basis for these other forms of the hyper IgM syndrome is being studied and several defects have recently been identified.

Clinical Presentation

Most patients with the X-linked hyper IgM (XHIGM) syndrome develop clinical symptoms during their first year or second year of life. Their most common problem is an increased susceptibility to infection.

The most common infections are recurrent upper and lower respiratory tract infections. The most frequent infective agents are bacteria. However, a variety of other microorganisms can also cause serious infections. For example, *Pneumocystis carinii* pneumonia is relatively common during the first few months of life and its presence may be the first clue that the child has XHIGM syndrome. Lung infections may also be caused by viruses such as Cytomegalovirus (CMV) and fungi such as *Cryptococcus*.

Gastrointestinal complaints, most commonly diarrhea and malabsorption, have also been reported in some patients. One of the major organisms causing gastrointestinal symptoms is *Cryptosporidium* that may cause sclerosing cholangitis, a severe disease of the liver.

Approximately half of the patients with the XHIGM syndrome develop neutropenia (low white blood cell count), either transient or persistent. The cause of the neutropenia is unknown, although most patients respond to treatment with the colony stimulating factor, G-CSF. Neutropenia is often associated with oral ulcers, proctitis (inflammation of the rectum), and skin infections.

Enlargement of the lymph nodes is seen more frequently in patients with the XHIGM syndrome than most of the other primary immunodeficiency diseases. As a result, patients often have enlarged tonsils, a big spleen and liver, and enlarged lymph nodes.

Autoimmune disorders may also occur in patients with the XHIGM syndrome. Their manifestations may include chronic arthritis, low platelet counts (thrombocytopenia), hemolytic anemia, hypothyroidism, and kidney disease.

Diagnosis

The diagnosis of the X-linked hyper IgM (XHIGM) syndrome should be considered in any boy presenting with hypogammaglobulinemia characterized by low or absent IgG and IgA and normal or elevated IgM levels. Failure to express CD40 ligand on activated T-cells is a characteristic finding. However, some patients with common variable immunodeficiency may have a markedly depressed expression of CD40 ligand while their CD40 ligand gene is perfectly normal. Therefore, the final diagnosis of the XHIGM syndrome depends on the identification of a mutation affecting the CD40 ligand gene. This type of DNA analysis can be done in several specialized laboratories.

Inheritance

The X-linked hyper IgM (XHIGM) syndrome is inherited as an X-linked recessive disorder. Therefore, only boys are affected. Since this is an inherited disease, transmitted as an X-linked recessive trait, there may be brothers or maternal uncles (mother's brothers) who have similar clinical findings. However, as in other X-linked disorders, there may also be no other affected members of the family. If the precise mutation in the gene for CD40 ligand is known in a given family, and if the fetus is male, it is possible to make a prenatal diagnosis. Similarly, women in the family can be tested to see if they carry the mutation and are at risk for having an affected son.

Treatment

Because patients with the X-linked hyper IgM (XHIGM) syndrome have a severe deficiency in IgG, regular infusions of IVIG every 3 to 4 weeks are effective in decreasing the number of infections. Regular IVIG infusions replace the missing IgG, and they also often result in a reduction or normalization of the serum IgM level.

Because patients with the XHIGM syndrome also have a marked susceptibility to *Pneumocystis carinii* pneumonia, it is important to initiate prophylactic treatment for *Pneumocystis carinii* pneumonia by starting affected infants on trimethoprim-sulfamethoxazole (Bactrim, Septra) prophylaxis as soon as the diagnosis of XHIGM syndrome is made.

Sometimes, neutropenia may improve during treatment with IVIG. Patients with persistent neutropenia may also respond to granulocyte colony stimulating factor (G-CSF) therapy. However, G-CSF treatment is only necessary in selected patients and long-term treatment with G-CSF is not recommended.

Boys with XHIGM, similar to other patients with primary immunodeficiency diseases, should not receive live virus vaccines since there is a remote possibility that the vaccine strain of the virus may cause disease.

It is also important to reduce the possibility of drinking water that is contaminated with *Cryptosporidium* because exposure to this organism may cause severe gastrointestinal symptoms, and chronic liver disease. The family should be proactive and contact the authorities responsible for the local water supply and ask if the water is safe and tested for *Cryptosporidium*.

Since patients with the XHIGM syndrome have defects in T-lymphocyte function in addition to their hypogammaglobulinemia, treatment with IVIG may not fully protect them against all infections. Therefore, bone marrow transplantation or cord blood stem cell transplantation has been advocated in recent years. If healthy siblings who have the same parents are available, the entire family, including the patient and potential donors, should be tissue typed to determine whether there is an HLA identical sibling available who could serve as bone marrow transplant donor. More than a dozen patients with XHIGM have received an HLA identical sibling bone marrow transplant with excellent success. Thus, a permanent cure for this disorder is possible. Cord blood stem cell transplants, fully or partially matched, have also been successfully performed, resulting in complete immune reconstitution. This strategy is especially promising if a matched sibling donor is not available. Matched unrelated donor (MUD) transplants are nearly as successful as matched sibling transplants, especially if performed when the recipient is young (under 8 years). Because patients with the XHIGM syndrome have strong T-cell responses against organ transplants, including bone marrow transplants, immunosuppressive drugs or low dose radiation are required.

Expectations

Although patients with the X-linked hyper IgM syndrome have defects in both the production of IgG and IgM and some aspects of their T-lymphocyte function, a number of effective therapies exist which allow these children to grow into happy and successful adults.

Additional Information

Immune Deficiency Foundation
40 W. Chesapeake Ave., Suite 308
Towson, MD 21204
Toll-Free: 800-296-4433
Website: http://www.primaryimmune.org
E-mail: idf@primaryimmune.org

Chapter 21

Selective Immunoglobulin A (IgA) Deficiency

Selective IgA deficiency is the severe deficiency or total absence of the IgA class of immunoglobulins in the blood serum and secretions. There are five types (classes) of immunoglobulins or antibodies in the blood: IgG, IgA, IgM, IgD, and IgE. The immunoglobulin class present in the largest amount in blood is IgG, followed by IgM and IgA. IgD and IgE are present in very small amounts in the blood.

Of these immunoglobulin classes, it is primarily IgM and IgG that protect the bloodstream, body tissues, and internal organs from infection. It is also important that the body is protected at surfaces that come in close contact with the environment. These sites are the mucosal surfaces: the mouth and nose, the throat, the airways within the lung, the gastrointestinal tract, the eyes, and the genitalia. The IgA antibodies (which are transported in secretions to mucosal surfaces) play a major role in protecting mucosal surfaces from infection. IgG, IgM, and IgE antibodies are also found in secretions at mucosal surfaces, but not in the same amount as the IgA antibody. This is why IgA is known as the secretory antibody. If the mucosal surfaces were spread out, they would cover any area equal to one and one half tennis courts, so the importance of IgA in protecting a person's mucosal surfaces cannot be overstated.

IgA has some special chemical characteristics. It is present in secretions as two antibody molecules attached by a component called the J chain (J for joining). In order for these antibodies to be secreted, they must also be attached to another molecule called the secretory piece. The IgA unit that protects the mucosal surfaces is actually composed of two IgA molecules joined by the J chain and attached to the secretory piece.

Individuals with selective IgA deficiency do not produce IgA. They do, however, produce all the other immunoglobulin classes. In addition, the function of their T-lymphocytes, phagocytic cells, and complement system are normal or near normal. Hence, this condition is known as selective IgA deficiency.

The cause or causes of selective IgA deficiency are unknown. It is likely that there are a variety of causes for selective IgA deficiency and that the cause may differ from patient to patient. Individuals with selective IgA deficiency have B-lymphocytes that appear to be normal, but do not mature into IgA producing plasma cells.

Clinical Features

Selective IgA deficiency is the most common primary immunodeficiency disease. Studies have indicated that as many as one in every five hundred people have selective IgA deficiency. Many of these individuals have relatively mild illnesses and are generally not sick enough to be seen by a doctor. Therefore, they are never discovered to have IgA deficiency. In fact, the majority of individuals with selective IgA deficiency are relatively healthy and free of symptoms. In contrast, there are also individuals with selective IgA deficiency who have significant illnesses. Currently, it is not understood why some individuals with IgA deficiency have almost no illness while others are very sick. Studies have suggested that some patients with IgA deficiency may be missing a fraction of their IgG (the IgG2 subclass), and that may be one explanation of why some patients with IgA deficiency are more susceptible to infection than others.

A common problem in IgA deficiency is susceptibility to infections. Recurrent ear infections, sinusitis, bronchitis, and pneumonia are the most common infections seen in patients with selective IgA deficiency. This is easy to understand because IgA protects mucosal surfaces from infections. These infections may become chronic. Furthermore, the infection may not completely clear with treatment, and patients may have to remain on antibiotics for longer than usual.

A second major problem in IgA deficiency is the occurrence of autoimmune diseases. In autoimmune diseases an individual produces antibodies or T-lymphocytes which react with his/her own tissues with resulting damage to these tissues. Some of the more frequent autoimmune diseases associated with IgA deficiency are:

- Rheumatoid arthritis
- Systemic lupus erythematosus
- Immune thrombocytopenic purpura (ITP).

These autoimmune diseases may cause sore and swollen joints of the hands or knees, a rash on the face, anemia (a low red blood cell count), or thrombocytopenia (a low platelet count). Other kinds of autoimmune disease may affect the endocrine system and/or the gastrointestinal system.

Allergies may also be more common among individuals with selective IgA deficiency than among the general population. The types of allergies vary. Asthma is one of the common allergic diseases that occur with selective IgA deficiency. It has been suggested that asthma may be more severe and less responsive to therapy in individuals with IgA deficiency than it is in normal individuals. Another type of allergy associated with IgA deficiency is food allergy, in which patients have reactions to certain foods. Symptoms associated with food allergies are diarrhea or abdominal cramping. It is not certain whether there is an increased incidence of allergic rhinitis (hay fever) or eczema in selective IgA deficiency.

Another unusual, but important form of allergy may also occur in IgA deficiency. In people whose blood contains no IgA, IgA from other individuals may be recognized by the immune system as a foreign protein. Because antibodies are normally made against foreign proteins, some people with selective IgA deficiency make an IgG or IgE antibody against IgA. In this situation, if an IgA deficient person who has antibodies against IgA receives a blood product that contains IgA, an allergic reaction may result. Although allergic reactions to IgA are very uncommon, it is important that every patient with selective IgA deficiency is aware of the potential risk of transfusion reactions if they receive blood or blood products.

Diagnosis

The diagnosis of selective IgA deficiency is usually suspected because of either chronic or recurrent infections, allergies, autoimmune diseases, or chronic diarrhea. The diagnosis is established when tests of the patient's blood serum demonstrate a marked reduction or near absence of IgA with normal levels of the other major classes of immunoglobulins (IgG and IgM). Most patients make antibodies normally. An occasional patient may also have IgG2 subclass deficiency and associated antibody deficiency. The numbers and functions of T-lymphocytes are normal.

Several other tests that may be important include a complete blood count, measurement of lung function, and a urinalysis. Other tests that may be obtained in specific patients include measurement of thyroid function, measurement of kidney function, measurements of absorption of nutrients by the gastrointestinal (GI) tract, and the test for antibodies directed against the body's own tissues (autoantibodies).

Treatment

The currently available preparations of gamma globulin do not contain significant amounts of IgA. Even if such products could be prepared, there is no way to cause IgA administered by injection to find its way to the mucous membranes that lack this immunoglobulin. Therefore, it is not currently possible to replace IgA in IgA deficient patients. However, an occasional patient who has IgA deficiency also has IgG2 subclass deficiency with a deficiency of antibody production. In these individuals, the use of replacement gamma globulin may be helpful in diminishing the frequency of infections.

Treatment of the problems associated with selective IgA deficiency should be directed toward the particular problem. For example, patients with chronic or recurrent infections need appropriate antibiotics. Ideally, antibiotic therapy should be directed at the specific organism causing the infection. It is not always possible to identify these organisms, however, and the use of broad-spectrum antibiotics may be necessary. Certain patients who have chronic sinusitis or chronic bronchitis may need to stay on long-term antibiotic therapy. It is important that the doctor and the patient communicate closely so that appropriate decisions can be reached for therapy.

There are a variety of therapies for the treatment of autoimmune diseases.

- Anti-inflammatory drugs, such as aspirin or ibuprofen, are used in diseases that cause joint inflammation.

- Steroids may be helpful in a variety of autoimmune diseases.

- If autoimmune disease results in an abnormality of the endocrine system, replacement therapy with hormones may be necessary.

- Treatment of the allergies associated with IgA deficiency is similar to treatment of allergies in general. It is not known whether immunotherapy (allergy shots) is helpful in the allergies associated with selective IgA deficiency.

- As a matter of precaution, it may also be desirable to test the blood of a patient with selective IgA deficiency for antibodies against IgA in order to prepare for the possibility that the patient may need a blood transfusion.

The most important aspect of therapy in IgA deficiency is close communication between the patient (and/or the patient's family) and the physician so that problems can be recognized and treated as soon as they arise.

Expectations

Although selective IgA deficiency is one of the milder forms of immunodeficiency, it may result in severe disease in some people. Therefore, it is difficult to predict the long-term outcome in a given patient with selective IgA deficiency. In general, the prognosis in selective IgA deficiency depends on the prognosis of the associated diseases. It is important for physicians to continually assess and reevaluate patients with selective IgA deficiency for the existence of associated diseases and the development of more extensive immunodeficiency. For example, rarely, IgA deficiency will progress to become common variable immunodeficiency with its deficiencies of IgG and IgM. The physician should be notified of anything unusual especially fever, productive cough, skin rash, or sore joints. The key to a good prognosis is adequate communication with the physician and the development of effective therapeutic strategies as soon as disease processes are recognized.

Additional Information

Immune Deficiency Foundation
40 W. Chesapeake Ave., Suite 308
Towson, MD 21204
Toll-Free: 800-296-4433
Website: http://www.primaryimmune.org
E-mail: idf@primaryimmune.org

Chapter 22

Severe Combined
Immunodeficiency (SCID)

In the time following birth, newborns are protected by immunity transmitted to them by their mothers. Within the next few months, though, their immune systems develop and begin to assume responsibility for fighting off infections. But it doesn't take long to determine that a few babies don't have the ability to fight off routine infections on their own.

Severe combined immunodeficiency (SCID) is a rare immune deficiency. There are many other immune deficiencies that may result in recurrent infections, but some children are born with an incomplete, or deficient, immune system. The symptoms of immune deficiency depend on what part of the immune system is affected and can range from mild to life-threatening. SCID is a primary immune deficiency that can be successfully treated if it's identified early. Otherwise, it's often fatal within the first year.

What Is SCID?

SCID is actually a group of inherited disorders characterized by a lack of immune response. It occurs when a child lacks lymphocytes, the specialized white blood cells that the body uses to fight infection.

This information was provided by KidsHealth, one of the largest resources online for medically reviewed health information written for parents, kids, and teens. For more articles like this one, visit www.KidsHealth.org, or www.TeensHealth .org. © 2002 The Nemours Center for Children's Health Media, a division of The Nemours Foundation. Also, "Rapid, New Test Developed for Inherited Immune Deficiency," NIH News, National Institutes of Health (NIH), February 22, 2005.

Lymphocytes are made in the bone marrow. Some lymphocytes move to the thymus gland, where they become T cells. B cells remain in the bone marrow to mature. Each specialized type of cell is responsible for a particular immune response. T cells attack antigens (usually invading germs) directly and help the body reject foreign tissue. T cells are also needed to activate the B cells that produce immunoglobulins (antibodies) to fight specific invaders.

If a child's immune system isn't functioning properly, it can be difficult or impossible to fight off viruses, bacteria, and fungi that cause infections. Sometimes called "bubble boy disease," SCID became more widely known in the 1970s when the world learned of David Vetter, a boy with SCID who lived for 12 years in a plastic, germ-free bubble.

There are several forms of SCID. The most common type is linked to the X chromosome, which makes it more common among males. Another form is linked to a deficiency of the enzyme adenosine deaminase (ADA). Other cases of SCID are caused by a variety of other genetic defects. Children with untreated SCID rarely live to age 2.

Signs and Symptoms

An increased susceptibility to infection and failure to thrive (failure to grow and gain weight as expected) as a result of infections are classic signs of SCID. A baby with SCID may have recurrent infections, such as ear infections (acute otitis media), sinus infections (sinusitis), bronchitis, oral thrush (a type of yeast that multiplies rapidly, creating white, sore areas in the mouth), and pneumonia. Infants with SCID may also have chronic diarrhea.

Your child's doctor may test for SCID or other types of immune deficiency if your baby exhibits any of these signs within the first year of life:

- eight or more ear infections
- two or more serious sinus infections
- two or more cases of pneumonia
- ineffective treatment with antibiotics for 2 or more months
- infections that require intravenous antibiotic treatment
- two or more deep-seated infections, such as pneumonia that affects an entire lung or an abscess in the liver

Because SCID is an inherited condition, be sure your child's doctor knows whether you have a history of primary immune deficiencies in your family.

164

Diagnosing SCID

The average age at which babies are diagnosed with SCID is just over 6 months. Blood tests can help your child's doctor diagnose SCID. If your child has any infections at the time of the testing, it may affect the results, making it necessary to test again. Also, babies gain some immunity from their mothers during pregnancy or breast feeding, which may also affect results. Blood tests that indicate SCID reveal:

- lymphocyte counts significantly below normal
- lower-than-normal levels of B cells and T cells
- deficiency of the immunoglobulins produced by B cells.

If you have a child with SCID or have a family history of immunodeficiency, you might want to consider genetic counseling and early blood testing. Although some doctors believe that high-risk babies should be tested before birth, other specialists note that babies born with SCID can have a healthy immune system if they receive a bone marrow transplant within 3 months of birth.

"Although early diagnosis and treatment are critical, SCID is a rare disease and it's important to evaluate the risks and costs associated with testing and somewhat experimental procedures done before birth," says Michael Trigg, M.D.

Treating SCID

If your child has SCID, your child's doctor can refer you to someone in your area who specializes in treating immune deficiencies—usually a pediatric immunologist or pediatric infectious disease expert.

The most effective treatment for SCID is a hematopoietic stem cell transplant. This is when blood-forming (hematopoietic) stem cells—primitive (early) cells found primarily in the bone marrow from which all types of blood cells develop—are introduced into the body in the hopes that these new cells will rebuild the immune system.

To provide the best chances of a match, a transplant is usually done using the bone marrow of a sister or brother. However, if a transplant is done within the first 3 months of the baby's life, a parent's marrow is acceptable. Transplants done this early have a high success rate and help the baby avoid the pretransplant chemotherapy that's often necessary to prevent rejection of the donor bone marrow cells in an older child.

The use of pretransplant chemotherapy depends on the severity of the child's immune deficiency. Children with complete immune deficiency and with severe SCID usually have little ability to reject new stem cells and do not require therapy to allow new, healthy cells to grow. But children whose immune systems are not as suppressed may be able to reject the new stem cells, so before transplant they may need to undergo chemotherapy to suppress their immune systems.

Although there have been a few successful cases of gene therapy to treat SCID, Dr. Trigg and other specialists caution that much of this work is still in the experimental stages. Researchers at the National Institutes of Health performed the first gene therapy surgery for SCID in 1990 on two girls who went on to lead fairly normal lives. The treatments consisted of removing some of the girls' few remaining T cells, exposing them to the ADA gene for 10 days and returning them to the girls' bodies through a vein. After a similar treatment a month later, the girls' bodies began to produce healthy T cells. Within a year, the number of T cells in their blood was within the normal range.

Another new technique was used to help four children in Paris, France. In this case, a portion of bone marrow was removed and infected with a harmless virus that had some of its genes replaced with correct versions of the defective gene. The virus was used to introduce the gene because viruses are able to break into cells and incorporate their genes into the cells' DNA. Doctors are still observing these children's levels of immunity to evaluate the success of the procedure.

Caring for Your Child

If your child has SCID, your child should not be immunized with live viruses, like the chicken pox (varicella) or measles, mumps, and rubella (MMR) vaccine. A child with SCID lacks the normal defense of developing antibodies to the viruses, so introducing a virus, even a weakened vaccine virus, can be dangerous.

Babies who have had bone marrow transplants may need supplemental therapy with antibiotics or immunoglobulins. Your child's doctor will advise you about these treatments.

You can help reduce your child's risk of contracting an infection following a bone marrow transplant by having him wear a mask. A mask can also serve as a signal to others that your child is trying to avoid becoming infected.

Until his immune system offers adequate protection, call your child's doctor if your child gets sick.

166

When to Call Your Child's Doctor

If you are concerned that your child has more frequent infections than usual, discuss the possibility of immune deficiency with your doctor. If your child has a serious infection, contact your child's doctor immediately. Because early treatment is more successful, you can improve your child's chances of developing a healthy immune system by acting quickly.

If your child has SCID, any illness merits close medical attention.

Rapid, New Test Developed for Inherited Immune Deficiency Newborn Screening Could Detect Bubble Boy Illness Early, Save Lives

Researchers at the National Human Genome Research Institute (NHGRI), part of the National Institutes of Health (NIH), have developed a new laboratory method that rapidly identifies babies born with inherited forms of severe immune deficiency. The new genetic test, which still must be validated before widespread use, could someday be added to the panel of tests that already screen newborns for a variety of disorders.

The test identifies babies born with severe combined immunodeficiency, or SCID, an illness in which the infant fails to develop a normal immune system. SCID babies can be infected by a wide range of viruses, bacteria, and fungi that are normally controlled by a healthy baby's immune system. If undetected and untreated, SCID typically leads to death before the baby's first birthday.

Developed in the National Human Genome Research Institute (NHGRI) Division of Intramural Research (DIR), the new test can use the same dried blood samples already collected from newborns and would provide the first accurate, high-throughput screen for immune deficiencies. Prior efforts to identify this disorder by counting white blood cells in newborns proved unreliable and expensive.

"This new laboratory technique is an excellent example of how increasingly sophisticated genetic tools can be applied to important public health problems," said NHGRI Scientific Director Eric D. Green, M.D., Ph.D. "Here we have a chance to catch an illness early when treatment is most effective. This new approach provides a rapid, accurate indication of a possible immune problem immediately after birth while the infant is protected by the mother's antibodies still circulating in the baby's blood."

If SCID is diagnosed in time, there are effective treatments. One form of the disease can be treated with an injectable medication. All

167

forms of the disorder can be cured through the transplantation of bone marrow if a matching donor can be identified. And finally, SCID may be treated through human gene therapy in which a normal copy of the defective gene may be inserted into the patient's own blood-forming cells. The first gene therapy experiments in history were carried out at NIH in 1990 in two young Ohio girls with SCID. The patients are alive, continue to do well and are involved in ongoing research at NHGRI. The sooner a child is diagnosed, the sooner treatment can begin and the more likely it is to be effective.

"Too many babies are diagnosed too late," said Jennifer M. Puck, M.D., chief of NHGRI's Genetics and Molecular Biology Branch. "And some babies develop fatal infections before their condition is recognized. Recent research shows that bone marrow transplants in the first three months of life work better than transplants at a later age. So it is critical to identify affected children immediately after birth. Since the babies lack overt clinical symptoms for some time, a molecular test is a good approach."

The newly developed screening tool exploits a detailed understanding of the maturation of T cells, one of the essential types of white blood cells that make up the immune system. Without a sufficient number of normal T cells, the immune system does not work. During normal development, an individual T cell rearranges the gene that produces a so-called antigen receptor on the surface of the cell. The antigen receptor allows the T cell to identify an infectious agent and launch a defensive attack to kill the invader. While rearranging the receptor gene, the maturing T cell produces a bit of leftover genetic material that forms a ring structure within the cell. Using a quantitative laboratory technique that measures the number of these rings within a blood sample, Dr. Puck's group was able to differentiate normal infants from those with SCID. In dried blood samples from healthy babies, the team was able to detect an average of 1,000 of these genetic rings; children with SCID had 30 or fewer. "That's a big difference," she said.

The development of the new test was described in the February 2005 issue of *The Journal of Allergy and Clinical Immunology.* Although the availability of the test raises the question of whether states should begin using it on all newborns, Dr. Puck concluded that the new test is not quite ready for widespread use. It must first be validated. "Our false positive rate was about 1.5 percent, which is too high to be practical for screening," Dr. Puck said. A baby with a positive test would need to be evaluated to see if he or she was actually sick; a false positive rate of 1.5 percent would mean three out of every 200 newborns would need further testing. "That would be a lot of babies going back to the doctor and a lot of worried parents. We are now working on ways to decrease the number of false positives."

To validate the test, Dr. Puck's group is collaborating with the newborn screening laboratory of the Maryland Department of Health and Mental Hygiene in Baltimore. The Maryland state lab is supplying some 5,000 blood samples already collected on newborns for the NHGRI lab to test. Although these samples are likely to be normal, they will be used to refine the laboratory procedures and establish quality control. Once the high-throughput screening approach has been validated with this large set of existing samples from Maryland, the NHGRI lab plans to begin prospectively testing newborns from the state. Other state testing laboratories also have expressed interest in participating in the prospective studies.

Although considered a rare disease, SCID is best known to the public from media accounts—and a made-for-TV movie starring John Travolta—about David, the Bubble Boy, a Texas boy who spent his entire life in a germ-free environment, ultimately dying after a failed bone marrow transplant in early adolescence. No one knows exactly how many babies are born with SCID. Current estimates suggest that 1 in every 50,000 to 100,000 births may be affected, indicating SCID may be about as common as some of the inherited illnesses for which states currently screen all newborns. Experts suspect that many children with SCID die from infections before being diagnosed, so the true incidence of the disease may be even higher. Newborn screening may reveal the true incidence.

Chapter 23

Wiskott-Aldrich Syndrome

In 1937, Dr. Wiskott described three brothers with low platelet counts (thrombocytopenia), bloody diarrhea, eczema, and recurrent ear infections. Seventeen years later, in 1954, Dr. Aldrich demonstrated that this syndrome was inherited as an X-linked recessive trait. In the 1960s, the features of the underlying immunodeficiency were identified and the Wiskott-Aldrich syndrome joined the list of primary immune deficiency diseases.

The Wiskott-Aldrich syndrome (WAS) is a primary immune deficiency disease involving both T- and B-lymphocytes. In addition, another type of blood cell called platelets, which helps control bleeding, is also affected. In its classic form, the WAS has a characteristic pattern of findings that include:

1. an increased tendency to bleed caused by a reduced number of platelets,

2. recurrent bacterial, viral, and fungal infections, and

3. eczema of the skin.

In addition, long-term observations of patients with WAS have revealed an increased incidence of malignancies, including lymphoma

---

and leukemia, and an increased incidence of autoimmune diseases in some patients.

WAS is caused by mutations (or mistakes) in the gene which produces a protein named in honor of the disorder, the Wiskott-Aldrich syndrome protein (WASP). The WASP gene is located on the short arm of the X chromosome. The majority of these mutations are unique. This means that almost every family has its own characteristic mutation of the WASP gene. If the mutation is severe and interferes almost completely with the gene's ability to produce the WAS protein, the patient has the classic, more severe form of WAS. In contrast, if there is some production of mutated WAS protein, a milder form of the disorder may result.

Clinical Presentations

The clinical presentation of the Wiskott-Aldrich syndrome (WAS) varies from patient to patient. Some patients present with all three classic manifestations, including low platelets and bleeding, immunodeficiency and infection, and eczema. Other patients present just with low platelet counts (thrombocytopenia) and bleeding. In fact, in past years the patients who presented with just low platelet counts were felt to have a different disease called X-linked thrombocytopenia (XLT). However, after the identification of the WAS gene, it was realized that both WAS and X-linked thrombocytopenia are due to mutations of the same gene, and thus are different clinical forms of the same disorder.

The initial clinical manifestations of WAS may be present soon after birth or develop in the first year of life. They usually are due to the low platelet count or the underlying immunodeficiency.

Bleeding Tendency

A reduced number of platelets is a characteristic hallmark of all patients with WAS. In addition, the platelets are smaller than normal. The precise mechanism for the thrombocytopenia (low platelet count) is unknown, but may include inefficient production of platelets by the bone marrow or increased removal of platelets by the spleen. Hemorrhage following circumcision may be an early clue to the presence of the disease. The bleeding into the skin caused by the thrombocytopenia may cause pinhead sized red spots, called petechiae, or may be larger and resemble bruises. Affected boys may also have bloody bowel movements (especially during infancy), bleeding gums, prolonged nose bleeds, and bleeding into the joints. Hemorrhage into the brain is a dangerous complication; toddlers may benefit from wearing a helmet to prevent head injuries until treatment is able to raise their platelet count.

Infections

Because of the profound deficiency of T- and B-lymphocytes, infections are common in classic WAS. These infections may include upper and lower respiratory infections such as otitis media, sinusitis, and pneumonia. More severe infections such as sepsis (blood stream infection or blood poisoning), meningitis, and severe viral infections are less frequent. Some patients with classic WAS develop recurrent herpes simplex infections (cold sores) and some have *Pneumocystis carinii* pneumonia.

Eczema

Eczema is a very common finding in patients with classic WAS. In infants, the eczema may resemble cradle cap, a severe diaper rash, or be generalized. In older boys, eczema is usually limited to the skin creases around the front of the elbow, around the wrist and neck, and behind the knees. Because the eczema is extremely pruritic or itchy, affected boys often scratch until they bleed, even while asleep. Eczema may be absent or mild in some patients.

Autoimmune Manifestations

A problem observed frequently in older boys and adults with WAS is a high incidence of autoimmune-like symptoms. The word autoimmune describes conditions that appear to be the result of a deregulated immune system reacting against part of the patient's own body. The most common autoimmune manifestation observed in WAS patients is a form of anemia caused by antibodies which destroy red blood cells. Some patients have a more generalized disorder in which there may be fevers in the absence of infection associated with swollen joints, kidney inflammation, and gastrointestinal symptoms such as diarrhea. Occasionally, inflammation of arteries (vasculitis) in the skin, heart, brain, or other internal organs develops and causes a wide range of symptoms. These autoimmune episodes may last only a few days or may occur in waves over a period of many years.

Malignancies

Malignancies can occur in young children with WAS, but are more frequent in adolescents and young adults. Most of these malignancies involve the lymphocytes (e.g., lymphoma and leukemia).

Diagnosis

Because of the wide spectrum of findings, the diagnosis of Wiskott-Aldrich syndrome (WAS) should be considered in any boy presenting with unusual bleeding and bruises, congenital or early onset thrombocytopenia, and small platelets. In fact, the characteristic platelet abnormalities—low numbers and small size—are already present in the cord blood of newborns.

The simplest and most useful test to diagnose WAS is to obtain a platelet count and to carefully determine the platelet size. WAS platelets are significantly smaller than normal platelets. In older children, over the age of two years, a variety of immunologic abnormalities can also be identified and used to support the diagnosis. Certain types of serum antibodies are characteristically low or absent in boys with WAS. They often have low levels of antibodies to blood group antigens (antibodies against type A or B red cells), and fail to produce antibodies against certain vaccines that contain polysaccharides or complex sugars. Skin tests to test T-lymphocyte function may show a negative response and laboratory tests of T-lymphocytes function may be abnormal.

The diagnosis is confirmed by demonstrating a decrease or absence of the WAS protein in blood cells or by the presence of a mutation within the WASP gene. These tests are done in a few specialized laboratories and require blood or other tissue.

Inheritance

The Wiskott-Aldrich syndrome (WAS) is inherited as an X-linked recessive disorder. Therefore, only boys are affected with this disease. Since this is an inherited disease transmitted as an X-linked recessive trait, there may be brothers or maternal uncles (the patient's mother's brother) with similar findings. However, the family history may be entirely negative because of small family size or because of the occurrence of a new mutation. If the precise mutation of WASP is known in a given family, it is possible to perform prenatal diagnosis.

Treatment

All children with serious chronic illness need the support of the parents and family. The demands on the parents of boys with Wiskott-Aldrich Syndrome (WAS) and the decisions they have to make may

174

be overwhelming. Progress in nutrition and antimicrobial therapy, prophylactic use of IVIG, and bone marrow transplantation have improved the life expectancy of patients with WAS.

Because of increased blood loss, iron deficiency anemia is common and iron supplementation may be necessary. When there are symptoms of infection, a thorough search for bacterial, viral, and fungal infections is necessary to determine the most effective antimicrobial treatment. Because patients with WAS have abnormal antibody responses to vaccines and to invading microorganisms, the prophylactic infusion of intravenous immunoglobulin may be indicated for those patients who suffer from frequent bacterial infections.

Eczema can be severe and persistent, requiring constant care. Excessive bathing should be avoided because frequent baths cause drying of the skin and make the eczema worse. Bath oils should be used during the bath and a moisturizing cream should be applied after bathing, and several times daily to areas of dry skin/eczema. Steroid creams applied sparingly to areas of chronic inflammation are often helpful, but their overuse should be avoided. Do not use strong steroid creams (e.g., fluorinated steroids) on the face. If certain foods make the eczema worse, and if known food allergies exist, attempts should be made to remove the offending food items. Systemic antibiotics may also improve the eczema in some cases.

Platelet transfusions may be used in some situations to treat the low platelet count and bleeding. For example, if serious bleeding occurs that cannot be stopped by conservative measures, platelet transfusions are usually indicated. Hemorrhages into the brain usually require immediate platelet transfusions. Surgical removal of the spleen (a lymphoid organ in the abdomen that filters the blood) has been performed in WAS patients and has been shown to correct the low platelet count, or thrombocytopenia, in over 90% of the cases. However, removal of the spleen increases the susceptibility of WAS patients to bacterial infections, especially infections of the blood stream and meningitis.

The symptoms of autoimmune diseases may require treatment with drugs that further suppress the patient's immune system. High dose IVIG and systemic steroids may correct the problem; if possible, the steroid dose should be reduced to the lowest level that will control symptoms.

As with all children with primary immune deficiency diseases involving T-lymphocytes and/or B-lymphocytes, boys with WAS should

175

not receive live virus vaccines because there is a possibility that a vaccine strain of the virus may cause disease.

Chicken pox complications occur frequently and may require treatment with antiviral drugs, high dose IVIG or herpes zoster hyper immune serum.

The only permanent cure for WAS is a bone marrow transplantation or cord blood stem cell transplantation. Because patients with WAS have some residual T-lymphocyte function in spite of their immune deficiency, immunosuppressive drugs and/or total body irradiation are required to condition the patient before transplantation. If the affected boy has healthy siblings with the same parents, the entire family should be tissue typed to determine whether there is an HLA-identical sibling (a good tissue match) who could serve as bone marrow transplant donor. The results with HLA-identical sibling donor bone marrow transplantation in WAS are excellent with an overall success (cure) rate of 80–90%. This procedure is therefore the treatment of choice for boys with significant clinical findings of the WAS. The decision to perform an HLA-matched sibling bone marrow transplant in patients with milder clinical forms, such as isolated thrombocytopenia, is more difficult, and should be discussed with an experienced immunologist.

Matched, unrelated donor (MUD) transplants are nearly as successful as matched sibling transplants if performed in younger children (up to 5–6 years of age). The success rate of MUD transplants decreases with age and the decision to transplant teenagers or adults with WAS may be difficult.

Cord blood stem cells, fully or partially matched, have successfully been used for immune reconstitution and the correction of platelet abnormalities. This strategy is especially promising if a matched sibling donor is not available.

In contrast to the excellent outcome of matched transplants, haploidentical bone marrow transplantation (the use of a parent) has not been as successful as HLA-matched transplants.

Expectations

Three decades ago, the classic Wiskott-Aldrich syndrome was one of the most severe primary immunodeficiency disorders with a life expectancy of only 2–3 years. Although it remains a serious disease in which life-threatening complications may occur, many affected males go through puberty, enter adulthood, live productive lives, and have families of their own. The oldest bone marrow transplanted patients are now in their twenties and thirties and seem to be cured, without developing malignancies or autoimmune diseases.

Additional Information

Immune Deficiency Foundation
40 W. Chesapeake Ave., Suite 308
Towson, MD 21204
Toll-Free: 800-296-4433
Website: http://www.primaryimmune.org
E-mail: idf@primaryimmune.org

Chapter 24

X-Linked
Agammaglobulinemia

X-linked agammaglobulinemia (XLA) was first described in 1952 by Dr. Ogden Bruton. This disease, sometimes called Bruton agammaglobulinemia or congenital agammaglobulinemia, was one of the first immunodeficiency diseases to be identified. XLA is an inherited immunodeficiency disease in which patients lack the ability to produce antibodies, proteins that make up the gamma globulin or immunoglobulin fraction of blood plasma.

Antibodies are an integral part of the body's defense mechanism against certain microorganisms (e.g., bacteria, viruses). Antibodies are important in the recovery from infections, and also protect against getting certain infections more than once. There are antibodies specifically designed to combine with each and every microorganism— much like a lock and key. When microorganisms, such as bacteria, land on a mucus membrane or enter the body, antibody molecules specific for that microorganism stick to the surface of the microorganism. Antibody bound to the surface of a microorganism can have one or more effects that are beneficial to the person. For example, some microorganisms must attach to body cells before they can cause an infection, and antibody prevents the microorganism from sticking to the cells. Antibody attached to the surface of some microorganisms will also cause the activation of other body defenses (such as a group of blood proteins called serum complement) which can directly kill the bacteria or viruses. Finally, antibody coated bacteria are much easier for white blood cells (phagocytes) to ingest and kill than bacteria which are not coated with antibody. All of these actions prevent microorganisms from invading body tissues where they may cause serious infections.

The basic defect in XLA is an inability of the patient to produce antibodies. Antibodies are proteins that are produced by specialized cells in the body, the plasma cells. The development of plasma cells proceeds in an orderly fashion from stem cells located in the bone marrow. The stem cells give rise to immature lymphocytes called pro-B lymphocytes. Pro-B lymphocytes give rise to pre-B lymphocytes, which in turn give rise to B lymphocytes. On contact with a foreign substance called an antigen (such as a microorganism) B lymphocytes mature into the plasma cells that produce and secrete antibodies.

Most patients with XLA have B lymphocyte precursors, but very few of these go on to become B lymphocytes. Thus, the underlying defect in XLA is a failure of B lymphocyte precursors to mature into B cells. Patients with XLA have mutations in a gene that is necessary for the normal development of B lymphocytes. This gene, discovered in 1993, is named *BTK* or Bruton's tyrosine kinase, in honor of the discoverer of the disorder, Colonel Ogden Bruton, M.D. As the name of the disorder suggests, the *BTK* gene is located on the X chromosome.

Clinical Presentation

Patients with X-linked agammaglobulinemia (XLA) are prone to develop infections because they lack antibodies. The infections frequently occur at or near the surfaces of mucus membranes, such as the middle ear, sinuses, and lungs, but in some instances can also involve the bloodstream or internal organs. Thus patients with XLA may have infections that involve the sinuses (sinusitis), the eyes (conjunctivitis), the ears (otitis), the nose (rhinitis), the airways to the lung, (bronchitis), or the lung itself (pneumonia). They also may have recurrent gastrointestinal tract infections that can cause diarrhea (gastroenteritis). In patients without antibodies, any of these infections may also penetrate the mucosal surface, invade the bloodstream, and spread to other organs deep within the body, such as the bones, joints, or brain. Infections in XLA patients are usually caused by microorganisms that are killed or inactivated very effectively by antibodies in normal people.

180

The most common bacteria that cause infection are the *pneumo-coccus*, the *streptococcus*, the *staphylococcus* and *Haemophilus influen-zae*. Some specific kinds of viruses may also cause serious infections in these patients.

Diagnosis

When a patient is suspected of having X-linked agammaglobuline-mia (XLA), the diagnosis is established by several tests. In XLA, all of the immunoglobulins (IgG, IgM, and IgA) are markedly reduced or absent in the blood. It is difficult to provide exact numbers for nor-mal immunoglobulin levels because they vary with the age of the child. Since normal babies make only small quantities of immunoglobulins in the first few months of life, it is important to remember that it may be difficult to distinguish a very young baby (less than 6 months old) with XLA from a normal baby by only testing blood levels of immu-noglobulins.

In some cases, tests may also be performed to see how well the patient's immunoglobulins function as antibodies. For example, the patient's blood may be tested to determine if he has responded with specific antibodies to the usual childhood immunizations (for example, tetanus and/or diphtheria), or the child may be immunized with these killed vaccines and then tested.

The most characteristic laboratory feature of XLA is the absence of B lymphocytes in the blood. Blood may be tested to determine if the patient has B lymphocytes in many laboratories. This is the most reliable test, since it is not influenced by age, previous immunizations, or the IgG that the baby received across the placenta from the mother.

Finally, it is now possible to test the *BTK* gene for errors or muta-tions.

Inheritance

X-linked agammaglobulinemia (XLA) is a genetic disease and as such can be inherited or passed on in a family. It is inherited as an X-linked recessive trait. It is important to understand the type of in-heritance so that families can understand why a child has been affected, the risk that subsequent children may be affected, and the implications for other members of the family.

Now that the precise gene that causes XLA has been identified, it is possible to test the female siblings (sisters) of a patient with XLA, and other female relatives such as the child's maternal aunts, to determine if they are carriers of the disease. Carriers of XLA have no symptoms, but have a 50% chance of transmitting the disease to each of their sons. In some instances, it is also possible to determine if a fetus of a carrier female will be born with XLA. At the present time, these genetic tests are being performed in only a few laboratories.

Treatment

At the present time, there is no way to cure patients who have X-linked agammaglobulinemia (XLA). The defective gene cannot be repaired or replaced, nor can the maturation of B lymphocyte precursors to B lymphocytes and plasma cells be induced.

However, patients with XLA can be given some of the antibodies that they are lacking. The antibodies are supplied in the form of gamma globulins (or immunoglobulins) and can be given directly into the blood stream intravenously.

The gamma globulin preparations contain antibodies that substitute for the antibodies that the XLA patient cannot make himself. They contain antibodies to a wide variety of microorganisms. Gamma globulin is particularly effective in preventing the spread of infections into the bloodstream and to deep body tissues or organs. Recurrent or chronic infections of the mucus membranes, such as sinusitis, occur in some patients with XLA despite the use of gamma globulin. In these patients, it may be necessary to obtain specimens of infected secretions such as sputum, stool, or occasionally the infected tissue itself. These specimens are cultured in the laboratory in order to identify exactly which microorganisms are responsible for causing the infection. The culture results will guide the specific course of therapy, which may include antibiotics.

Finally patients with XLA should not receive any live viral vaccines, such as live polio or the measles, mumps, rubella (MMR) vaccine. Although uncommon, it is possible that live vaccines (particularly the oral polio vaccine) in agammaglobulinemia patients can transmit the diseases that they were designed to prevent.

Expectations

Most X-linked agammaglobulinemia (XLA) patients who are receiving gamma globulin on a regular basis will be able to lead relatively normal lives. They do not need to be isolated or limited in their activities. Infections may require some extra attention from time to time, but children with XLA can participate in all regular school and extracurricular activities, and adults can have productive careers and families. A full active lifestyle is to be encouraged and expected.

Additional Information

Immune Deficiency Foundation
40 W. Chesapeake Ave., Suite 308
Towson, MD 21204
Toll-Free: 800-296-4433
Website: http://www.primaryimmune.org
E-mail: idf@primaryimmune.org

Chapter 25

Rare Primary Immunodeficiency Diseases

When people are born with a faulty immune system, they are said to have a primary immune deficiency or immunodeficiency. Unlike people with acquired immunodeficiency syndrome (AIDS), caused by the human immunodeficiency virus (HIV), people with primary immunodeficiency (PI) diseases have inherited abnormal changes in the cells of their immune systems. Between 25,000 and 50,000 people suffer from the most serious forms of PI diseases in the United States, but experts believe that many more have milder disease that is not yet diagnosed.

Each type of immune system cell has its own special function and must work together with other types to fight disease effectively. Because there are many different types of cells that make up the immune system, an error in any one of them can disrupt our immune defenses. Depending on the cell and the type of error that occurs, more than 80 different forms of PI diseases are possible. Some are severe, while others cause few or no symptoms. Having any of them makes it easier to get infections and other medical conditions. More boys than girls have PI, and first symptoms often begin in infancy or later in childhood.

Primary care doctors who suspect a patient has a problem with the immune system will run screening tests. If those tests indicate the person's immune system is not functioning normally, the doctor will consult with a special kind of doctor called a clinical immunologist. The immunologist can run special blood tests to find out the exact type

Excerpts from "Primary Immune Deficiency," Fact Sheet, National Institute of Allergy and Infectious Diseases (NIAID), March 2003.

of PI disease and how best to treat it. Other experts the doctor may consult include pulmonologists, rheumatologists, gastroenterologists, and hematologists.

This chapter describes some of the rare primary immunodeficiency diseases.

Common Variable Immunodeficiency (CVI)

CVI is relatively common. Infants sometimes have symptoms of CVI. In most cases, however, symptoms do not show up until the teen years or early adulthood. CVI is also called:

- hypogammaglobulinemia
- adult-onset agammaglobulinemia
- late-onset hypogammaglobulinemia
- acquired agammaglobulinemia.

What causes CVI?

No one knows the cause. Experts cannot trace a clear pattern showing that this PI is inherited.

What are the signs and symptoms of CVI?

Most people with CVI have:

- Frequent bacterial infections of the ears, sinuses, bronchi, and lungs
- Painful swollen joints in the knee, ankle, elbow, or wrist
- Problems involving the digestive tract
- An enlarged spleen and swollen glands or lymph nodes.

Along with other autoimmune problems, some develop autoantibodies that attack their own blood cells. People with CVI also have an increased risk of developing some cancers.

How is CVI diagnosed?

To diagnose CVI, doctors look for:

- Below-normal levels of IgG and IgA
- Zero-to-slightly-low levels of IgG

- Low-to-normal IgM levels
- Whether B cells produce antibodies following a common vaccination like a tetanus shot
- How well the T cells are working
- Gastrointestinal infections if there are digestive symptoms.

How is CVI treated?

CVI patients receive intravenous immunoglobulin (IVIG) every 3 to 4 weeks to restore normal antibody levels. Bacterial infections are treated with antibiotics. Physical therapy and daily postural drainage may help clear clogged lungs.

Interferon-Gamma Receptor (IFNGR) Deficiency

This very rare inherited disorder causes individuals to be more susceptible to mycobacteria that cause tuberculosis, as well as other types of mycobacteria, and infections caused by salmonella bacteria. Patients have either partial or complete IFNGR deficiency.

What causes IFNGR deficiency?

IFNGR deficiency is caused by an inherited mutation in a gene. The affected gene is found on cells called granulocytes. These granulocytes have protein receptors on their surfaces that reject interferon gamma, a chemical needed to fight off tuberculosis and other infections caused by mycobacteria as well as salmonella infections.

What are the symptoms of IFNGR deficiency?

Mycobacteria cause the most serious problems for people with IFNGR deficiency. Infections may involve the lungs, lymph nodes, blood, and bone marrow. People with complete IFNGR deficiency have more serious infections than those with partial IFNGR deficiency. The disease occurs early in infancy in those with complete IFNGR deficiency. Those with partial deficiency are more likely to develop illness later in childhood.

How is IFNGR deficiency diagnosed?

A doctor suspects IFNGR deficiency in a patient with a history of severe or repeated mycobacterial infections. Sophisticated laboratory tests measure the amount of interferon gamma in the blood and show

187

the patient's white blood cells respond poorly, or not at all, to interferon gamma. Depending on whether the patient has complete or partial IFNGR deficiency, the blood will have either very high or very low levels of interferon gamma. Genetic testing can determine whether the patient has one of four mutations that cause either partial or complete IFNGR deficiency.

How is IFNGR deficiency treated?

Patients with complete IFNGR deficiency have a poorer outlook than those with partial IFNGR deficiency. They need aggressive and long-term treatment with antibiotics. Patients with partial IFNGR deficiency have milder disease that is easier to treat with antibiotics. Bone marrow transplantation has cured a small number of patients.

NIAID scientists are developing methods to add a corrective gene to bone marrow cells that will become granulocytes. They are also working to improve the multi-drug treatment that is the mainstay for IFNGR-deficient patients. Patients with complete IFNGR deficiency may especially benefit from treatment that includes immune boosters or cytokines, including interleukin-2 (IL-2), IL-12, interferon gamma, and granulocyte-macrophage colony-stimulating factor (GM-CSF).

Hyper-IgE (HIE) Syndrome

This rare condition is also called Job syndrome. Health care experts have reported only 200 cases of HIE. People with HIE have very high levels of the IgE antibody. HIE causes recurring bacterial infections and other complications.

What causes HIE?

HIE is caused by an inherited abnormality in a gene. In about half of the cases, the flawed gene is linked to chromosome 4. In most known cases, it is autosomal dominant. This means that to be born with this disease, a person needs to inherit the affected gene from only one parent. Scientists suspect that the affected gene (or genes) may prevent T cells from properly regulating the immune response to germs.

What are the symptoms of HIE?

People with HIE have repeated bacterial infections of the skin, sinuses, and lungs. These infections are often caused by *Staphylococcus aureus* (staph). HIE patients may also have scoliosis (curvature of the spine), weak bones and recurrent bone fractures, strokes or other brain problems, severe itching, and inflamed skin. They may fail to lose baby teeth.

How is HIE diagnosed?

Doctors will suspect HIE in a person who has a red, itchy, skin rash and recurring staph infections of the skin, sinuses, lungs, or joints. Patients with HIE often have distinctive facial characteristics including:

- Asymmetry or uneven facial features
- Prominent forehead
- Deep-set eyes
- Broad nasal bridge
- Wide, fleshy nasal tip
- Protruding lower jaw.

Blood tests show normal levels of IgG, IgA, and IgM, but very high levels of IgE and a high number of white blood cells called eosinophils. Tests also show poor immune response to immunizations.

How is HIE treated?

There is no specific treatment for HIE. Patients receive lifelong antibiotics to fight the recurring infections. People with HIE who lack other types of antibodies may find intravenous immunoglobulin injections (IVIG) helpful.

NIAID scientists are evaluating HIE patients and their relatives to better understand the medical problems associated with this disease to identify and treat complications. Finding the gene or genes involved in HIE will be critically important to developing better therapies for HIE, especially gene therapy.

Leukocyte Adhesion Deficiency (LAD)

LAD is a rare PI disease, found in one out of every million people. This disease causes recurrent, life-threatening infections. Phagocytes cannot find their way to the site of infection to fight off invading germs. LAD is autosomal recessive disease, meaning that to be born with this disease, both parents must have the affected gene.

What causes LAD?

LAD is caused by a lack of beta 2 integrin, also called CD18, molecules. These molecules are normally found on the outer surface of phagocytes. Without them, the phagocytes cannot attach to blood vessel walls and enter infected tissues where they help fight infection. Mutations in the gene that instructs, or codes for, the production of CD18 cause LAD.

What are the symptoms of LAD?

Children with LAD cannot fight off infection properly. They may have:

- Severe infections of the soft tissue
- Eroding skin sores without pus
- Severe infections of the gums with tooth loss
- Infections of the gastrointestinal tract
- Wounds that heal slowly and may leave scars.

There are at least two forms of LAD.

- A severe form, called LAD type 1, which commonly causes death from infections in early infancy.
- A more moderate form in which children may survive into young adulthood.

How is LAD diagnosed?

Blood tests to diagnose patients with LAD show a very high number of white blood cells and very low levels of CD18, a protein. Doctors may suspect LAD if an infant's umbilical cord does not fall off and heal properly after birth. They also will suspect the disease in children who develop severe infections caused by bacteria and fungi, and whose wounds are slow to heal.

How is LAD treated?

Doctors treat patients with bacterial infections early and aggressively with antibiotics. Some patients have been treated successfully with bone marrow transplants.

Interferon gamma increases CD18 and improves the ability of white blood cells to move about. NIAID researchers are using interferon gamma in people with LAD type 1 to see if it can help reduce the number and severity of their recurrent infections. Researchers are also investigating gene therapy as a potential cure for LAD.

Additional Information

National Institute of Allergy and Infectious Diseases
Office of Communications
6610 Rockledge Dr., MSC 6612
Bethesda, MD 20892-6612
Phone: 301-496-5717
Website: http://www.niaid.nih.gov/publications
Clinical Trials Information: http://www.niaid.nih.gov/clintrials/default.htm

Immune Deficiency Foundation
40 W. Chesapeake Ave., Suite 308
Towson, MD 21204
Toll-Free: 800-296-4433
Website: http://www.primaryimmune.org
E-mail: idf@primaryimmune.org

Jeffrey Modell Foundation
National Primary Immunodeficiency Resource Center
747 Third Ave.
New York, NY 10017
Phone: 212-819-0200
Fax: 212-764-4180
Website: http://www.jmfworld.org/index.cfm
E-mail: info@jmfworld.org

Part Four

Acquired Immune Deficiency Diseases

Chapter 26

Acquired Immunodeficiency Syndrome (AIDS) and Human Immunodeficiency Virus (HIV)

Overview

AIDS (acquired immunodeficiency syndrome) was first reported in the United States in 1981 and has since become a major worldwide epidemic. AIDS is caused by the human immunodeficiency virus (HIV). By killing or damaging cells of the body's immune system, HIV progressively destroys the body's ability to fight infections and certain cancers. People diagnosed with AIDS may get life-threatening diseases called opportunistic infections, which are caused by microbes such as viruses or bacteria that usually do not make healthy people sick. More than 830,000 cases of AIDS have been reported in the United States since 1981. As many as 950,000 Americans may be infected with HIV, one-quarter of who are unaware of their infection. The epidemic is growing most rapidly among minority populations and is a leading killer of African-American males ages 25 to 44. According to the U.S. Centers for Disease Control and Prevention (CDC), AIDS affects nearly seven times more African-Americans and three times more Hispanics than whites.

How Is HIV Transmitted?

HIV is spread most commonly by having unprotected sex with an infected partner. The virus can enter the body through the lining of the vagina, vulva, penis, rectum, or mouth during sex.

"HIV Infection and AIDS: An Overview," National Institute of Allergy and Infectious Diseases (NIAID), October 2003.

HIV also is spread through contact with infected blood. Before donated blood was screened for evidence of HIV infection and before heat-treating techniques to destroy HIV in blood products were introduced, HIV was transmitted through transfusions of contaminated blood or blood components. Today, because of blood screening and heat treatment, the risk of getting HIV from such transfusions is extremely small.

HIV frequently is spread among injection drug users by the sharing of needles or syringes contaminated with very small quantities of blood from someone infected with the virus. It is rare, however, for a patient to give HIV to a health care worker or vice-versa by accidental sticks with contaminated needles or other medical instruments.

Women can transmit HIV to their babies during pregnancy or birth. Approximately one-quarter to one-third of all untreated pregnant women infected with HIV will pass the infection to their babies. HIV also can be spread to babies through the breast milk of mothers infected with the virus. If the mother takes the drug azidothymidine (AZT) during pregnancy, she can significantly reduce the chances that her baby will get infected with HIV. If health care providers treat mothers with AZT and deliver their babies by cesarean section, the chances of the baby being infected can be reduced to a rate of 1 percent.

A study sponsored by the National Institute of Allergy and Infectious Diseases (NIAID) in Uganda found a highly effective and safe drug for preventing transmission of HIV from an infected mother to her newborn. This regimen is more affordable and practical than any other examined to date. Results from the study show that a single oral dose of the antiretroviral drug nevirapine (NVP) given to an HIV-infected woman in labor and another to her baby within three days of birth reduces the transmission rate of HIV by half compared with a similar short course of AZT.

Although researchers have found HIV in the saliva of infected people, there is no evidence that the virus is spread by contact with saliva. Laboratory studies reveal that saliva has natural properties that limit the power of HIV to infect. Research studies of people infected with HIV have found no evidence that the virus is spread to others through saliva by kissing. No one knows, however, whether so-called deep kissing, involving the exchange of large amounts of saliva, or oral intercourse increase the risk of infection. Scientists also have found no evidence that HIV is spread through sweat, tears, urine, or feces.

Studies of families of HIV-infected people have shown clearly that HIV is not spread through casual contact such as the sharing of food utensils, towels and bedding, swimming pools, telephones, or toilet seats. HIV is not spread by biting insects such as mosquitoes or bedbugs. HIV can infect anyone who practices risky behaviors such as:

- Sharing drug needles or syringes.
- Having sexual contact with an infected person without using a condom.
- Having sexual contact with someone whose HIV status is unknown.

Having a sexually transmitted disease such as syphilis, genital herpes, chlamydial infection, gonorrhea, or bacterial vaginosis appears to make people more susceptible to getting HIV infection during sex with infected partners.

Symptoms of HIV Infection

Many people do not have any symptoms when they first become infected with HIV. Some people, however, have a flu-like illness within a month or two after exposure to the virus. This illness may include:

- Fever
- Headache
- Tiredness
- Enlarged lymph nodes (glands of the immune system easily felt in the neck and groin).

These symptoms usually disappear within a week to a month and are often mistaken for those of another viral infection. During this period, people are very infectious, and HIV is present in large quantities in genital fluids.

More persistent or severe symptoms may not appear for 10 years or more after HIV first enters the body in adults, or within two years in children born with HIV infection. This period of asymptomatic infection is highly individual. Some people may begin to have symptoms within a few months, while others may be symptom-free for more than 10 years.

Even during the asymptomatic period, the virus is actively multiplying, infecting, and killing cells of the immune system. The most obvious effect of HIV infection is a decline in the number of CD4 positive T cells (also called T4 cells) found in the blood—the immune system's key infection fighters. At the beginning of its life in the human body, the virus disables or destroys these cells without causing symptoms.

As the immune system worsens, a variety of complications start to take over. For many people, the first signs of infection are large lymph nodes or swollen glands that may be enlarged for more than three months. Other symptoms often experienced months to years before the onset of AIDS include:

- Lack of energy

- Weight loss

- Frequent fevers and sweats

- Persistent or frequent yeast infections (oral or vaginal)

- Persistent skin rashes or flaky skin

- Pelvic inflammatory disease in women that does not respond to treatment

- Short-term memory loss

- Some people develop frequent and severe herpes infections that cause mouth, genital, or anal sores, or a painful nerve disease called shingles.

- Children may grow slowly or be sick a lot.

AIDS

The term AIDS applies to the most advanced stages of HIV infection. The CDC developed official criteria for the definition of AIDS and is responsible for tracking the spread of AIDS in the United States.

The CDC definition of AIDS includes all HIV-infected people who have fewer than 200 CD4 positive T cells (abbreviated CD4+ T cells) per cubic millimeter of blood. (Healthy adults usually have CD4 positive T-cell counts of 1,000 or more.) In addition, the definition includes 26 clinical conditions that affect people with advanced HIV disease. Most of these conditions are opportunistic infections that generally do not affect healthy people. In people with AIDS, these infections are often severe and sometimes fatal because the immune system is so ravaged by HIV that the body cannot fight off certain bacteria, viruses, fungi, parasites, and other microbes.

Symptoms of opportunistic infections common in people with AIDS include:

- Coughing and shortness of breath

- Seizures and lack of coordination
- Difficult or painful swallowing
- Mental symptoms such as confusion and forgetfulness
- Severe and persistent diarrhea
- Fever
- Vision loss
- Nausea, abdominal cramps, and vomiting
- Weight loss and extreme fatigue
- Severe headaches
- Coma.

Children with AIDS may get the same opportunistic infections as do adults with the disease. In addition, they also have severe forms of the bacterial infections all children may get, such as conjunctivitis (pink eye), ear infections, and tonsillitis.

People with AIDS are particularly prone to developing various cancers, especially those caused by viruses such as Kaposi sarcoma and cervical cancer, or cancers of the immune system known as lymphomas. These cancers are usually more aggressive and difficult to treat in people with AIDS. Signs of Kaposi sarcoma in light-skinned people are round brown, reddish, or purple spots that develop in the skin or in the mouth. In dark-skinned people, the spots are more pigmented.

During the course of HIV infection, most people experience a gradual decline in the number of CD4 positive T cells; although some may have abrupt and dramatic drops in their CD4 positive T-cell counts. A person with CD4 positive T cells above 200 may experience some of the early symptoms of HIV disease. Others may have no symptoms even though their CD4 positive T-cell count is below 200.

Many people are so debilitated by the symptoms of AIDS that they cannot hold steady employment nor do household chores. Other people with AIDS may experience phases of intense life-threatening illness followed by phases in which they function normally.

A small number of people first infected with HIV ten or more years ago have not developed symptoms of AIDS. Scientists are trying to determine what factors may account for their lack of progression to AIDS, such as particular characteristics of their immune systems, whether they were infected with a less aggressive strain of the virus, or if their genes may protect them from the effects of HIV. Scientists hope that understanding the body's natural method of control may lead to ideas for protective HIV vaccines and use of vaccines to prevent the disease from progressing.

Diagnosis

Because early HIV infection often causes no symptoms, a doctor or other health care provider usually can diagnose it by testing a person's blood for the presence of antibodies (disease-fighting proteins) to HIV. HIV antibodies generally do not reach detectable levels in the blood for one to three months following infection. It may take the antibodies as long as six months to be produced in quantities large enough to show up in standard blood tests.

People exposed to the virus should get an HIV test as soon as they are likely to develop antibodies to the virus—within 6 weeks to 12 months after possible exposure to the virus. By getting tested early, people with HIV infection can discuss with a health care provider when they should start treatment to help their immune systems combat HIV and help prevent the emergence of certain opportunistic infections. Early testing also alerts HIV-infected people to avoid high-risk behaviors that could spread the virus to others.

Most health care providers can do HIV testing and will usually offer counseling to the patient at the same time. Of course, individuals can be tested anonymously at many sites if they are concerned about confidentiality.

Health care providers diagnose HIV infection by using two different types of antibody tests, enzyme-linked immunosorbent assay (ELISA) and Western blot. If a person is highly likely to be infected with HIV and yet both tests are negative, the health care provider may request additional tests. The person also may be told to repeat antibody testing at a later date, when antibodies to HIV are more likely to have developed.

Babies born to mothers infected with HIV may or may not be infected with the virus, but all carry their mothers' antibodies to HIV for several months. If these babies lack symptoms, a doctor cannot make a definitive diagnosis of HIV infection using standard antibody tests until after 15 months of age. By then, babies are unlikely to still carry their mother's antibodies and will have produced their own, if they are infected. Health care experts are using new technologies to detect HIV itself to more accurately determine HIV infection in infants between ages 3 months and 15 months. They are evaluating a number of blood tests to determine if they can diagnose HIV infection in babies younger than 3 months.

Treatment

When AIDS first surfaced in the United States, there were no medicines to combat the underlying immune deficiency and few treatments existed for the opportunistic diseases that resulted. During the past 10 years, however, researchers have developed drugs to fight both HIV infection and its associated infections and cancers.

The U.S. Food and Drug Administration (FDA) has approved a number of drugs for treating HIV infection. The first group of drugs used to treat HIV infection, called nucleoside reverse transcriptase (RT) inhibitors, interrupts an early stage of the virus making copies of itself. Included in this class of drugs (called nucleoside analogs) are AZT, ddC (zalcitabine), ddI (dideoxyinosine), d4T (stavudine), 3TC (lamivudine), abacavir (Ziagen), and tenofovir (Viread). These drugs may slow the spread of HIV in the body and delay the start of opportunistic infections.

Health care providers can prescribe non-nucleoside reverse transcriptase inhibitors (NNRTI), such as delavirdine (Rescriptor), nevirapine (Viramune), and efavirenz (Sustiva), in combination with other antiretroviral drugs.

FDA also has approved a second class of drugs for treating HIV infection. These drugs, called protease inhibitors, interrupt virus replication at a later step in its life cycle. They include:

- Ritonavir (Norvir)
- Saquinavir (Invirase)
- Indinavir (Crixivan)
- Amprenavir (Agenerase)
- Nelfinavir (Viracept)
- Lopinavir (Kaletra).

Because HIV can become resistant to any of these drugs, health care providers must use a combination treatment to effectively suppress the virus. When RT inhibitors and protease inhibitors are used in combination, it is referred to as highly active antiretroviral therapy, or HAART, and can be used by people who are newly infected with HIV as well as people with AIDS.

Researchers have credited HAART as being a major factor in significantly reducing the number of deaths from AIDS in this country. While HAART is not a cure for AIDS, it has greatly improved the health of many people with AIDS, and it reduces the amount of virus circulating in the blood to nearly undetectable levels. Researchers, however, have shown that HIV remains present in hiding places, such as the lymph nodes, brain, testes, and retina of the eye, even in patients who have been treated.

Despite the beneficial effects of HAART, there are side effects associated with the use of antiviral drugs that can be severe. Some of the nucleoside RT inhibitors may cause a decrease of red or white blood cells, especially when taken in the later stages of the disease. Some may also cause inflammation of the pancreas and painful nerve damage. There have been reports of complications and other severe reactions, including death, to some of the antiretroviral nucleoside analogs when used alone or in combination. Therefore, health care experts recommend that people on antiretroviral therapy be routinely seen and followed by their health care providers. The most common side effects associated with protease inhibitors include nausea, diarrhea, and other gastrointestinal symptoms. In addition, protease inhibitors can interact with other drugs resulting in serious side effects.

A number of drugs are available to help treat opportunistic infections to which people with HIV are especially prone. These drugs include:

- Foscarnet and ganciclovir to treat cytomegalovirus (CMV) eye infections

- Fluconazole to treat yeast and other fungal infections

- Trimethoprim/sulfamethoxazole (TMP/SMX) or pentamidine to treat *Pneumocystis carinii* pneumonia (PCP).

In addition to antiretroviral therapy, health care providers treat adults with HIV, whose CD4+ T-cell counts drop below 200, to prevent the occurrence of PCP, which is one of the most common and deadly opportunistic infections associated with HIV. They give children PCP preventive therapy when their CD4+ T-cell counts drop to levels considered below normal for their age group. Regardless of their CD4+ T-cell counts, HIV-infected children and adults who have survived an episode of PCP take drugs for the rest of their lives to prevent a recurrence of the pneumonia.

HIV-infected individuals who develop Kaposi sarcoma or other cancers are treated with radiation, chemotherapy, or injections of alpha interferon, a genetically engineered protein that occurs naturally in the human body.

Prevention

Because no vaccine for HIV is available, the only way to prevent infection by the virus is to avoid behaviors that put a person at risk of infection, such as sharing needles and having unprotected sex. Many people infected with HIV have no symptoms. Therefore, there is no way of knowing with certainty whether a sexual partner is infected unless he or she has repeatedly tested negative for the virus and has not engaged in any risky behavior.

People should either abstain from having sex or use male latex condoms or female polyurethane condoms, which may offer partial protection, during oral, anal, or vaginal sex. Only water-based lubricants should be used with male latex condoms. Although some laboratory evidence shows that spermicides can kill HIV, researchers have not found that these products can prevent a person from getting HIV. The risk of HIV transmission from a pregnant woman to her baby is significantly reduced if she takes AZT during pregnancy, labor, and delivery, and if her baby takes it for the first six weeks of life.

Additional Information

AIDSinfo
P.O. Box 6303
Rockville, MD 20849-6303
Toll-Free: 800-448-0440
Toll-Free TTY: 888-480-3739
Fax: 301-519-6616
Live, Online Assistance: http://aidsinfo.nih.gov/live_help (Mon.–Fri., 12:00 p.m.–4:00 p.m. ET)
Website: http://aidsinfo.nih.gov
E-mail: ContactUs@aidsinfo.nih.gov

Chapter 27

Graft Versus Host Disease

What Is Graft Versus Host Disease (GVHD)?

The immune system is the body's tool to fight infection. It works by seeing harmful cells as foreign and attacking them. When you receive a donor's stem cells (the graft), their job is to recreate the donor's immune system in your body (the host). Graft versus host disease (GVHD) is the term used when this new immune system attacks your body. Your donor's cells see your body as foreign and attack it—causing damage.

GVHD most commonly affects the:

- skin
- liver
- gastrointestinal (GI) tract.

How Long Can GVHD Last?

GVHD can be acute or chronic. Acute GVHD usually occurs within the first 100 days after a transplant. Chronic GVHD develops after the first 100 days of transplant. Chronic GVHD can reoccur for several years after transplant.

"Graft Versus Host Disease (GVHD): A Guide for Patients and Families after Stem Cell Transplant," National Institutes of Health, NIH Clinical Center, 2004.

Can I Prevent GVHD?

There is nothing you can do to prevent GVHD. However, skin GVHD can be triggered and worsened by sun exposure. Wearing a hat, long sleeves, long pants, and sunscreen will help to control skin GVHD caused by sun damage. Avoiding sun exposure is the best prevention.

GVHD cannot be predicted, but depending on the type of stem cell transplant received, the doctor may use immunosuppressive medications (medications that decrease the immune system's ability to fight infections) to lessen GVHD.

Medications such as cyclosporine, tacrolimus, and sirolimus, suppress the immune system to lessen harmful GVHD. It may be necessary to take these medications for several months after a transplant. It is important to take these medications as prescribed and to report any side effects.

Signs and Symptoms of GVHD

Skin GVHD

- red rash
- itching
- darkening of skin

Liver GVHD

- elevated liver tests
- yellow color to the skin and whites of the eyes
- abdominal pain (later symptom)

Gastrointestinal (GI) GVHD

- watery diarrhea
- stomach cramping (especially before and during bowel movements, and after eating)
- persistent nausea

Report all new or worsening symptoms to your doctor.

How Is GVHD Diagnosed?

Diagnosis is based on symptoms, laboratory results, and tissue biopsies. Diagnosis of GVHD is difficult because early symptoms are often the same as other side effects and complications after transplant. It is important that you report any changes in your skin or bowel patterns to your health care provider.

Treatment for GVHD

Treatment aims at decreasing the donor's immune reaction against the host's body. Immunosuppressive medication will be given to decrease this reaction. Steroids, such as prednisone and methylprednisolone, are first-line treatments for GVHD. But steroids weaken the immune system and the ability to fight infection. So, depending on how severe the GVHD is, the doctor may admit the patient to the hospital for treatment.

Manage Symptoms of GVHD

Skin Care

- Avoid scratching.
- Use moisturizing lotion. Avoid perfumed lotions.
- Avoid hot showers.
- Use sunscreen with SPF 30 or greater.
- Avoid prolonged sun exposure.
- Wear long sleeves and pants.

Diarrhea

- Follow the prescribed diet to prevent worsening diarrhea.
- Avoid spicy foods.
- To avoid skin problems (such as irritation) around your rectal area, it is very important to keep this area clean. Cleanse this area well after each episode of diarrhea. Tell your health care provider if this area gets red, cracked, painful, or infected.

Preventing Infection

- Wash your hands often.
- Stay away from sick family members and friends.
- Your doctor may ask you to wear a mask.
- Notify your doctor if you have fevers, chills, or redness/pain at your catheter site.

Chapter 28

Idiopathic Environmental Intolerance (IEI) [Formerly Multiple Chemical Sensitivities Syndrome (MCSS)]

What Is MCSS and What Is Known about It?

The preferred medical term is idiopathic environmental intolerance (IEI), which can be defined as a chronic, recurring disease caused by a person's inability to tolerate an environmental chemical or class of foreign chemicals.

IEI thus represents a complex gene/environment interaction, the true cause of which is currently unknown. There is almost always a precipitating event, usually associated with the smell of a chemical, and a response involving one or more organ systems. Once the imitating event has passed, the same response or even an exaggerated response occurs each time the stimulus is encountered again. Often the initiating stimulus is a higher dose or an overwhelming dose, but subsequently much lower doses can trigger the symptoms. A number of unrelated chemicals (e.g., insecticides, antiseptic cleaning agents) might precipitate the same response. Because the syndrome is similar to certain allergic conditions and to certain organ/system responses caused by emotional disturbances, IEI has often been confused with allergy (atopy) or psychiatric illness. Disagreement among physicians and medical researchers—as to what IEI really is—has, of course, made research funding difficult. (Is this a real syndrome, a mental

"Multiple Chemical Sensitivities Syndrome (MCSS): What Is It, and What is Known about It?" by Daniel W. Nebert, M.D., Editor, *Interface: Genes and the Environment*, Fall/Winter 2001, Issue 22, 1-3. © 2001 University of Cincinnati Center for Environmental Genetics. Reprinted with permission.

problem, or a simple allergy?) In fact, in an environmental health sciences meeting in Brisbane, Australia, several years ago, there was an old-fashioned debate on MCSS, and the proponents who believed that it was simply a psychiatric disorder won the debate.

Six Criteria of IEI

Several years ago a committee of experts in their field decided upon a consensus as to what qualifies the patient as truly having IEI [*Arch Environ Health* 1999; 54: 147]. Six criteria were decided upon:

- Symptoms are reproducible with repeated (chemical) exposures.

- The condition is chronic.

- Low levels of exposure (lower than previously or commonly tolerated) result in manifestations of the syndrome (i.e., increased sensitivity).

- The symptoms improve, or resolve completely, when the triggering chemicals are removed.

- Responses often occur to multiple, chemically-unrelated substances.

- Symptoms involve multiple-organ symptoms (runny nose, itchy eyes, headache, scratchy throat, ear ache, scalp pain, mental confusion or sleepiness, palpitations of the heart, upset stomach, nausea and/or diarrhea, abdominal cramping, aching joints).

Several medical conditions appear to be related to, or overlap with, IEI—such as sick-building syndrome (SBS), food intolerance syndrome (FIS), and perhaps the Gulf War illness (GWI). In each of these, a chemical (smell usually, or taste) appears to precipitate one or more organ/system responses. The initiating culprit might be: chemicals in a new rug, cockroach dander, or Freon circulating in a closed-ventilation building (SBS); chemicals in wine, processed corn products, or sulfites consumed (FIS); nerve gas, organophosphates, or pesticides to which soldiers were exposed during the 1991 war in the Middle East (GWI). Additional conditions (of discomfort, pain, or dysfunction) that might have a genetic component, but also seem to have an environmental stimulus include: chronic fatigue syndrome, fibromyalgia, irritable bowel syndrome, atypical connective tissue disease after silicone breast implants, chronic hypoglycemia (low blood sugar), drug-induced autoantibodies/hepatitis (liver toxicity), illness while living near a toxic waste dump site, dental amalgam disease, and MTBE (methyl-tert-butyl ether, a gasoline additive). Inflammation of the lungs caused by diesel exhaust particles (DEP) is of particular interest, since it illustrates the potential for the drug-biotransformation and immune systems (which protect us from small and large foreign compounds, respectively) to interact and contribute to the disease process. In this situation, cellular processes regulated by the aryl hydrocarbon receptor (AHR) apparently activate an inflammatory response involving TH2 helper cells, subsequently increasing immunoglobulin E (IgE) production.

How might we dissect this complex disease?

Frequently, individuals with IEI present with symptoms of rhinitis (runny nose), along with other diffuse systemic complaints. First, the physician must determine whether the patient has a runny nose due to an allergy problem (allergic rhinitis) or not (nonallergic rhinitis).

Seasonal allergic rhinitis refers to patients with allergy symptoms triggered by pollen or mold allergens. Triggering stimuli occur when the patient is outdoors during the pollen seasons. Symptoms can include sneezing fits (i.e., 5–10 sneezes in succession), itching of the eyes/ears/nose/throat/roof of the mouth, runny nose, watery/puffy eyes, nasal stuffiness, post-nasal drip, sinus pressure, and fatigue. Perennial allergic rhinitis refers to year-round hay fever symptoms that are triggered by indoor allergens such as dust mites, cockroaches, mold, feathers, and animal dander. Perennial allergens may be difficult to identify by history alone; skin testing is necessary to confirm sensitization to these allergens, but it does not indicate that the individual is currently being exposed.

A patient with nonallergic rhinitis is one who has had an allergic component ruled out by skin tests. Nonallergic rhinitis can be further divided into inflammatory (nonallergic rhinitis with eosinophilic syndrome, NARES) and noninflammatory (vasomotor rhinitis, VMR) subtypes. Nonallergic rhinitis is an organ-specific disorder of unknown etiology (cause not understood) that is aggravated by strange chemical smells and weather changes. The noninflammatory form of nonallergic rhinitis, VMR, satisfies the first five of the above criteria, suggesting that this disorder is a potential model (*Ann Allergy Asthma Immunol* 2001: 86;494] for investigating the genetic etiology of the more global disease, IEI.

Nonallergic VMR can mimic allergic rhinitis. Patients with nonallergic VMR experience nasal congestion, postnasal drip, headaches/

sinus pressure, and ear-plugging. Skin testing of seasonal and perennial allergens is negative (i.e., non-atopic). Triggering stimuli for nonallergic VMR include weather changes (temperature or barometric pressure changes), postural changes, and irritants such as smoke, perfumes, potpourris, solvents, cleaning agents, incense, and soaps and detergents (to name a few).

Is IEI associated with mutations in olfactory receptor (OR) genes?

The field of olfaction (ability to smell distinct classes of things) has recently exploded with the advent of genomics and the Human Genome Project. A superfamily of ~1000 odorant receptor (OR) genes has been discovered, located in multiple clusters on all but two of the 24 human chromosomes (22 autosomes, X Y chromosome). These OR clusters comprise 17 gene families, four of which contain more than 100 members each [*Genome Res* 2001; 11;685]. Interestingly, 64% of the human's OR genes are nonfunctional (pseudogenes). The fact that apes have a greater percentage of functional OR genes is strong evidence that the evolving human species has lost its need for maintaining a very keen sense of smell. The OR gene superfamily comprises 1–3% of the entire genomic complement of genes, and is likely to be the largest gene superfamily in the genome of any species.

Other clusters of human chemosensory genes include the vomeronasal receptors, related to an accessory olfactory organ thought to be largely inactive in primates. The OR genes are members of the 7-transmembrane domain G-protein-coupled receptor (GPCR) superfamily. In situ hybridization studies indicate that each OR gene is expressed in ~1 per 1000 olfactory epithelial (OE) neurons, suggesting that each OE neuron expresses only one OR gene [*Cell* 2000;100:611]. People clearly have very different abilities to sense smells. Polymorphisms in many of these genes have been reported, implying a mechanism for interindividual variation in olfactory responses [*Gene* 2000; 260:87]— and perhaps to diseases triggered by olfactory stimuli.

Conclusions

IEI is a complex disease involving gene/environment interactions [*Environ Health Perspect* 2000; 108:1219]. Perhaps one place to begin, in dissecting this complex disease, would be to study nonallergic VMR because it can be more precisely defined. Would polymorphisms, in particular functional OR genes, be responsible for nonallergic VMR?

Could nonallergic VMR be a sufficient phenotypic end-point such that it could be examined in a phenotype-genotype association study involving a candidate-gene approach, a candidate-gene-region approach, or a total genome scan?

It seems tempting to postulate that nonallergic VMR might be a sufficiently quantitative trait that it can be used first in attempting to dissect the very complex disease syndromes associated with IEI, SBS, FIS, and GWI. Anyway, this is the approach that is being taken by three University of Cincinnati CEG researchers—Jonathan Bernstein, Dan Nebert, and Li (Felix) Jin. Given the exploding advances in our knowledge about the human genome, it seems that the time to tackle this complicated (and very common) environmental disease is now.

Part Five

Autoimmune Diseases

Chapter 29

How Autoimmune Diseases Are Related

Disease Classification

When medicine grew up in the middle ages, physicians had to divide diseases into various kinds and various categories. The only way they could classify diseases was anatomically, that is, where does the disease occur? Physicians later divided themselves into doctors who were interested in diseases of the lungs, and other doctors who were interested in diseases of the skin, and other doctors were interested in disease of the intestinal tract, the reproductive tract, or the urinary tract. Most medicine is still organized on the basis of the anatomy of the disease, on where the disease occurs. You go to a heart specialist (a cardiologist) if you have heart disease, to a neurologist if you have nervous system disease, to a dermatologist if you have a skin disease, and on and on. The medical community organized itself that way because that was all the doctors knew. They did not know what caused disease, but they knew where it occurred. But starting with Louis Pasteur about a hundred years ago, a change occurred. For the very first time, we began to understand why disease occurs—not where it occurs, but why it occurs. When we speak of why disease occurs, we speak of something else, etiology.

Etiology means cause, why the disease occurs. If we are concerned with curing disease and possibly even preventing disease, the etiology

Excerpted from "Autoimmune Diseases: How Are They Related?" by Noel R. Rose, M.D., Ph.D., *InFocus* Newsletter, January 2004. © 2004 American Autoimmune Related Diseases Association, Inc. Reprinted with permission.

is the most important information. Why have we been able to control so many infectious diseases? Because we now know the bacteria, viruses, and parasites that cause these diseases, and we can develop antibiotics and other drugs that will specifically attack that organism. Discovering the etiology has allowed medicine to progress to its present state where we can successfully treat and even cure many diseases.

Within the lifetime of most of us, we have found ways of effectively treating infectious disease. Until World War II, until antibiotics were introduced, we did not have methods that cured disease. We had treatments that alleviated the symptoms of disease, but we really did not cure disease. With the introduction of antibiotics—penicillin, streptomycin, and other substances—we now have a way of treating diseases. And that is why it is so important to understand etiology.

For example, allergies are now defined by their etiology. If you have an allergy, it does not matter whether it is an allergy of the nose (hay fever), the lungs (asthma), or atopic dermatitis (a skin disease). You may go to an allergist because all of these diseases have the same etiology. They have different anatomies, but they have the same etiology. That is the way progress is being made by bringing together diseases with the same etiology.

Autoimmunity: A Cause of Disease

Autoimmunity is an etiology: it is a cause of disease. Anatomically, autoimmune disease is very diverse; and that is why we see specialists in so many areas of medicine studying autoimmunity. They may be rheumatologists who are interested in joints; dermatologists who are interested in skin; cardiologists who are interested in the heart; or gastroenterologists who are interested in the gastrointestinal tract. But the common etiology for all of these diseases—for Crohn disease of the gut; for lupus of the skin; for rheumatoid arthritis of the joint— is autoimmunity.

A major aim of the American Autoimmune Related Diseases Association (AARDA) is to help us to understand that all of these diseases, diverse as they are in their anatomical location and in their clinical manifestation, are related because they have the same etiology—they are all caused by autoimmunity. In my opinion, the only way we are going to develop really effective treatments will be to treat the cause of the disease, not the symptoms. The symptoms are late; the symptoms are at the end of the train of events. We want to get on the train at the very beginning.

Etiology of Autoimmune Disease

Unlike some diseases, autoimmune diseases do not generally have a simple, single cause. There are usually two major categories of factors that are involved in causing autoimmune diseases: genetics and environment. Virtually every autoimmune disease combines these two.

Genetics

Genetics is involved in the development of autoimmune disease, but autoimmune diseases are not typical genetic diseases. What is a typical genetic disease? Most of us have heard of sickle cell anemia, and that is a genetic disease. That is a disease in which the victims of the disease have a specific genetic mutation. If you inherit this mutation from one parent, you have sickle cell trait; and if you inherit it from both parents, you have sickle cell disease. We know what the gene is, and we even know a great deal of how that works; so we know the etiology of that disease.

That is not the way genetics works in autoimmune disease. In autoimmune disease, multiple genes are involved; we have genes that collectively increase the vulnerability or susceptibility to autoimmune disease. What is inherited is not a specific gene that causes a specific defect in metabolism; several genes increase vulnerability or susceptibility to autoimmune disease.

How do we know that there is a genetic basis of autoimmune disease? I can cite three kinds of evidence.

Autoimmune disease in families. The first is autoimmune diseases tend to occur in families. If there is one case of autoimmune disease in the family, there's likely to be another case. However, it is not a particular autoimmune disease; it is generally a tendency to autoimmunity. One family member may have lupus, another family member may have Sjögren disease, a third member of the family may have rheumatoid arthritis. That's one bit of evidence for genetic involvement, and we have known this for a number of years. If we ask patients when they come to us, "Is there other autoimmune disease in your family?"—and we actually have to mention them because people do not know these are all autoimmune diseases—they will usually say, "Yes, my aunt had thyroid trouble...my grandmother had that disease...my grandmother had Crohn disease...." But we call this soft data in science because families share genes and that is some indication of genetics; but families share other things.

Twin studies. The second thing we do is to look at twins. We compare two kinds of twins. There are twins that are genetically identical, and there are twins that are non-genetically identical. If something is caused by an environmental factor, there should be no difference between identical twins and non-identical twins. If there is a difference, it suggests that genetics plays a role. These studies have been done for a number of autoimmune diseases, and the answer has always come up about the same. Genetic components represent something in the order of half of the risks. In other words, if you have a genetic predisposition to autoimmunity, you may have twice or five times as much chance of developing autoimmunity as someone else—not 100 times, but not zero, so genetics plays an important role.

One group of genetic factors is particularly important. One of the things that immunology has taught us through the years is obvious, but needed some kind of physical basis—it is simply that every human being is different from every other human being (unless you have a genetically identical twin). Every person is a little different from everybody else; we know that for certain when we try to transplant tissues, like kidneys or hearts. In general you cannot accept a kidney or heart from someone else unless we dampen your immune response.

There clearly are significant physical differences between different people. And we call the substance that causes that difference histocompatibility complex. We call the genes that provide that difference major histocompatibility complex (MHC) genes. In a human we call it human leukocyte antigen (HLA).

HLA is the major group of genes that distinguishes one human being from another. It is important in transplantation, and we do HLA typing regularly. It's important to us in autoimmunity because susceptibility to autoimmunity is associated with the HLA type. It represents the most important single genetic trait in estimating susceptibility to autoimmune disease.

There are three kinds of information that tell us if autoimmune diseases are genetic. I've mentioned two. One is family clustering; the second is the association with HLA.

Autoimmune disease in animals. The third is that autoimmune diseases occur in animals as well as in human beings. With animals we can do the breeding that is necessary for investigation.

We can infer the same must be true in humans. In animals the equivalent of HLA determines susceptibility. In animals this trait is actually predictive. In humans we are not yet at that point because we do not have enough information from humans to say, "Because of your

HLA factor you are going to develop an autoimmune disease." We can, however, say that you have a greater likelihood of this happening.

So we are getting to a point where we can almost predict who is more likely or less likely to develop autoimmune disease. Now this, again, is an example of how very basic research on a molecular level or on a genetic molecular level is beginning to pay off in human medicine.

Environmental Triggers

Genetics accounts for about half of the risk that you develop an autoimmune disease. The other half is the agent in the environment which triggers the process. Unfortunately, we do not know very many of the triggers. We know there are certain drugs that can induce lupus. We know there are certain environmental substances like silica that can induce scleroderma. We suspect that there are certain dietary substances, such as iodine, that can exacerbate thyroid disease. So we are beginning to define the other half of the story, the environmental half. It is going to be, I think, an equally fascinating chapter in the saga of autoimmune disease in the next decade.

In summary, that is what autoimmune diseases have in common. That is why there should be a society like the American Autoimmune Related Diseases Association that brings together all of the research, all of the investigators, and all of the physicians, as well as all of the patients interested in autoimmune diseases. Let us begin to get to questions of etiology, to get at the root causes of these diseases, rather than being left at the superficial level, that is, treating the symptoms after the disease has had its destructive effects.

—by Noel R. Rose, M.D., Ph.D.

Dr. Rose is Chairman Emeritus, AARDA Scientific Advisory Board; Chair, National Institutes of Health Autoimmune Diseases Coordinating Committee; Director, Johns Hopkins University Autoimmune Disease Center; and Professor of Pathology, Molecular Microbiology, and Immunology, Johns Hopkins University Bloomberg School of Public Health.

Additional Information

American Autoimmune Related Diseases Association
22100 Gratiot Ave.
East Detroit, MI 48021
Toll-Free for Literature Requests: 800-598-4668
Phone: 586-776-3900
Website: http://www.aarda.org

Chapter 30

Questions and Answers about Autoimmunity

What Is Autoimmunity?

When your body is attacked—perhaps by a virus or germs on a nail you stepped on—your immune system defends you. It sees and kills the germs that might hurt you. But when the system does not work right, this process can cause harm. Immune cells can mistake your body's own cells as invaders and attack them. This friendly fire can affect almost any part of the body. It can sometimes affect many parts of the body at once. This is called autoimmunity (meaning self-immunity).

What Causes Autoimmunity?

No one knows why the immune system treats some body parts like germs. We do know that you cannot catch autoimmune diseases from another person. Most scientists think that our genes and things in the environment are involved. If you have a certain gene or combination of genes, you may be at higher risk for autoimmune disease. But you will not get the disease until something around you turns on your immune system. This may include the sun, infections, drugs, or, in some women, pregnancy.

Excerpted from "Questions and Answers about Autoimmunity," National Institute of Arthritis and Musculoskeletal and Skin Diseases (NIAMS), NIH Publication No. 02–4858, January 2002.

Problems Caused by Autoimmunity

Autoimmunity can affect almost any organ or body system. The exact problem one has with autoimmunity (or its diseases) depends on which tissues are targeted. If the skin is the target, you may have skin rashes, blisters, or color changes. If it is the thyroid gland, you may be tired, gain weight, be more sensitive to cold, and have muscle aches. If it is the joints, you may have joint pain, stiffness, and loss of function.

You may know which organ or system is affected from the start. But you may not know the site of the attack. In many people, the first symptoms are fatigue, muscle aches, and low fever.

Because autoimmune diseases can affect almost any organ or system of the body, one way to group them is by the body system(s) they attack. The following is a list (not inclusive) of body systems and the autoimmune diseases that can affect them.

Blood and Blood Vessels

- Autoimmune hemolytic anemia
- Pernicious anemia
- Polyarteritis nodosa
- Systemic lupus erythematosus
- Wegener granulomatosis

Digestive Tract (Including the Mouth)

- Autoimmune hepatitis
- Behçet disease
- Crohn disease
- Primary biliary cirrhosis
- Scleroderma
- Ulcerative colitis

Eyes

- Sjögren syndrome
- Type 1 diabetes mellitus
- Uveitis

Glands

- Graves disease
- Thyroiditis
- Type 1 diabetes mellitus

Heart

- Myocarditis
- Rheumatic fever
- Scleroderma
- Systemic lupus erythematosus

Joints

- Ankylosing spondylitis
- Rheumatoid arthritis
- Systemic lupus erythematosus

Kidneys

- Glomerulonephritis
- Systemic lupus erythematosus
- Type 1 diabetes mellitus

Lungs

- Rheumatoid arthritis
- Sarcoidosis
- Scleroderma
- Systemic lupus erythematosus

Muscles

- Dermatomyositis
- Myasthenia gravis
- Polymyositis

Nerves and Brain

- Guillain-Barré syndrome

- Multiple sclerosis
- Systemic lupus erythematosus

Skin

- Alopecia areata
- Pemphigus/pemphigoid
- Psoriasis
- Scleroderma
- Systemic lupus erythematosus
- Vitiligo

How Are Autoimmune Diseases Diagnosed?

Autoimmune diseases often do not show a clear pattern of symptoms at first. So diagnosing them can be hard. But with time, a diagnosis can usually be made by using:

- **Medical history**—The doctor will ask about your symptoms and how long you have had them. Your symptoms may not point to one disease. But they can be a starting point for your doctor. You should tell your doctor if you have a family member with autoimmune disease. You may not have the same disease as your family member. But having a family history of any autoimmune disease makes you more likely to have one.

- **Physical exam**—During the exam, the doctor will check for any signs. Inflamed joints, swollen lymph nodes, or discolored skin might give clues.

- **Medical tests**—No one test will show that you have an autoimmune disease. But doctors may find clues in a blood sample. For example, people with lupus or rheumatoid arthritis often have certain autoantibodies in their blood. Autoantibodies are blood proteins formed against the body's own parts. Not all people with these diseases have these autoantibodies. And some people without autoimmune disease do have them. So blood tests alone may not always help.

The key is patience. Your doctor may be able to diagnose your condition quickly based on your history, exam, and test results. But the process often takes time. It may take several visits to find out exactly what is wrong and the best way to treat it.

Treatment of Autoimmune Diseases

Autoimmunity takes many forms. There are also many treatments for it. Treatment depends on the type of disease, how severe it is, and its symptoms. Generally, treatments have one of three goals:

- **Relieving symptoms**—If your symptoms bother you, your doctor may suggest treatments that give some relief. Relieving symptoms may be as simple as taking a drug for pain relief. It may also be as involved as having surgery.

- **Preserving organ function**—When autoimmune diseases threaten organs, treatment may be needed to prevent damage. Such treatments may include drugs to control an inflamed kidney in people with lupus. Insulin injections can regulate blood sugar in people with diabetes. These treatments do not stop the disease. But they can save organ function. They can also help people live with disease complications.

- **Targeting disease mechanisms**—Some drugs may also be used to target how the disease works. In other words, they can suppress the immune system. These drugs include cyclophosphamide (Cytoxan) and cyclosporine (Neoral and Sandimmune). The same immune-suppressing drug may be used for many diseases.

Your doctor may not prescribe a treatment. If your symptoms are mild, the risks of treatment may be worse than the symptoms. You may choose to put off treatment for now. But you should watch for signs that your disease is progressing. Visit your doctor regularly. You need to catch changes before they lead to serious damage.

Doctors That Treat Autoimmune Diseases

Treatments for autoimmune diseases vary. So do the types of doctors who provide them. For some people, one doctor will be enough to manage their disease. Others may require a team approach. One doctor might coordinate and give care, and others would treat specific organ problems. For example, a person with lupus might be seen by a rheumatologist. But that person might also see a nephrologist for related kidney problems and a dermatologist for skin problems.

Specialists you may need to see include:

- A rheumatologist, who treats arthritis and other rheumatic diseases including scleroderma and systemic lupus erythematosus (lupus or SLE).

- An endocrinologist, who treats gland and hormone problems including diabetes and thyroid disease.

- A neurologist, who treats nerve problems including multiple sclerosis and myasthenia gravis.

- A hematologist, who treats diseases that affect the blood including pernicious anemia and autoimmune hemolytic anemia.

- A gastroenterologist, who treats problems with the digestive system including Crohn disease and ulcerative colitis.

- A dermatologist, who treats problems of the skin, hair, and nails including psoriasis, pemphigus/pemphigoid, and alopecia areata.

- A nephrologist, who treats kidney problems including glomerulonephritis and inflamed kidneys associated with lupus.

Other Problems Related to Autoimmune Diseases

Having a chronic disease can affect almost every part of your life. The problems you might have with an autoimmune disease vary. They may include:

- **How you look and your self-esteem**—Depending on your disease, you may have discolored or damaged skin or hair loss. Your joints may look different. These can all affect how you look and your self-esteem. Such problems cannot always be prevented, but their effects can be reduced with treatment. Cosmetics, for example, can hide a skin rash. Surgery can correct a malformed joint.

- **Caring for yourself**—Painful joints or weak muscles can make it hard to do simple tasks. You may have trouble climbing stairs, making your bed, or brushing your hair. If doing daily tasks is hard, talk with a physical therapist. The therapist can teach you exercises to improve strength and function. An occupational therapist can show you new ways to do things or tools to make tasks easier. Sometimes regular exercise or simple devices can help you do more things on your own.

- **Family relationships**—Family members may not understand why you do not have energy to do things you used to do. They may even think you are just being lazy. But they may also be overly concerned and eager to help you. They may not let you do the things you can do. They may even give up their own interests to be with you. Learn as much as you can about your disease. Share what you learn with your family. Involve them in counseling or a support group. It may help them better understand the disease and how they can help.

- **Sexual relations**—Sexual relationships can also be affected. For men, diseases that affect blood vessels can lead to problems with erection. In women, damage to glands that produce moisture can lead to vaginal dryness. This makes intercourse painful. In both men and women, pain, weakness, or stiff joints may make it hard for them to move the way they once did. They may not be sure about how they look. Or they may be afraid that their partner will no longer find them attractive. With communication, good medical care, and perhaps counseling, many of these issues can be overcome or at least worked around.

- **Pregnancy and childbearing**—In the past, women with some autoimmune diseases were told not to have children. But better treatments and understanding have changed that advice. Autoimmune diseases can affect pregnancy, and pregnancy can affect autoimmune diseases. But women with many such diseases can safely have children. How a pregnancy turns out can vary by disease and disease severity. If you have an autoimmune disease, you should consult your doctor about having children.

Additional Information

National Institute of Arthritis and Musculoskeletal and Skin Diseases
Information Clearinghouse/NIH
1 AMS Circle
Bethesda, MD 20892-3675
Toll-Free: 877-22-NIAMS (64267)
Phone: 301-495-4484
TTY: 301-565-2966
Fast Facts: 301-881-2731 (to receive information by fax)
Website: http://www.nih.gov/niams/healthinfo
E-mail: niamsinfo@mail.nih.gov

American Autoimmune-Related Diseases Association, Inc. (AARDA)
22100 Gratiot Ave.
East Detroit, MI 48021
(AARDA contact information continued on next page)

Toll-Free: 800-598-4668 (for literature requests)
Phone: 586-776-3900
Fax: 586-776-3903
Website: http://www.aarda.org
E-mail: aarda@aarda.org

Chapter 31

Autoimmune Disease in Women

Autoimmune Disease

The term autoimmune disease refers to a varied group of more than 80 serious, chronic illnesses that involve almost every human organ system. It includes diseases of the nervous, gastrointestinal, and endocrine systems as well as skin and other connective tissues, eyes, blood, and blood vessels. In all of these diseases, the underlying problem is similar—the body's immune system becomes misdirected, attacking the very organs it was designed to protect.

A Women's Issue

For reasons we do not understand, about 75 percent of autoimmune diseases occur in women, most frequently during the childbearing years. Table 31.1 lists the female-to-male ratios in autoimmune diseases. Hormones are thought to play a role, because some autoimmune illnesses occur more frequently after menopause, others suddenly improve during pregnancy with flare-ups occurring after delivery, while still others will get worse during pregnancy.

Autoimmune diseases also seem to have a genetic component, but mysteriously, they can cluster in families as different illnesses. For example, a mother may have lupus erythematosus; her daughter,

231

diabetes; her grandmother, rheumatoid arthritis. Research is shedding light on genetic as well as hormonal and environmental risk factors that contribute to the causes of these diseases.

Individually, autoimmune diseases are not very common, with the exception of thyroid disease, diabetes, and systemic lupus erythematosus (SLE). However, taken as a whole, they represent the fourth largest cause of disability among women in the United States.

A Need for Knowledge

Autoimmune diseases remain among the most poorly understood and poorly recognized of any category of illnesses. Individual diseases range from the benign to the severe. Symptoms vary widely, notably from one illness to another, but even within the same disease. And because the diseases affect multiple body systems, their symptoms are often misleading which hinders accurate diagnosis. To help women live longer, healthier lives, a better understanding of these diseases is needed, as well as providing early diagnosis and treatment.

Table 31.1. Female to Male Ratios in Autoimmune Diseases

Autoimmune Disease	Female to Male Ratio
Hashimoto disease/hypothyroiditis	50:1
Systemic lupus erythematosus	9:1
Sjögren syndrome	9:1
Antiphospholipid syndrome	9:1
Primary biliary cirrhosis	9:1
Mixed connective tissue disease	8:1
Chronic active hepatitis	8:1
Graves disease/hyperthyroiditis	7:1
Rheumatoid arthritis	4:1
Scleroderma	3:1
Myasthenia gravis	2:1
Multiple sclerosis	2:1
Chronic idiopathic thrombocytopenic purpura	2:1

Major Autoimmune Diseases: Connective Tissue Diseases

Systemic Lupus Erythematosus (SLE)

An inflammation of the connective tissues, SLE can afflict every organ system. It is up to nine times more common in women than men, and strikes black women three times as often as white women. The condition is aggravated by sunlight.

Symptoms: Fever, weight loss, hair loss, mouth and nose sores, malaise, fatigue, seizures, and symptoms of mental illness. Ninety percent of patients experience joint inflammation similar to rheumatoid arthritis. Fifty percent develop a classic butterfly rash on the nose and cheeks. Raynaud phenomenon (extreme sensitivity to cold in the hands and feet) appears in about 20 percent of people with SLE.

Treatment: Anti-inflammatory drugs can help control arthritis symptoms; skin lesions may respond to topical treatment such as corticosteroid creams. Oral steroids, such as prednisone, are used for the systemic symptoms. Wearing protective clothing and sunscreen when outdoors is recommended.

Rheumatoid Arthritis

Rheumatoid arthritis is a systemic disorder in which immune cells attack and inflame the membrane around joints. It also can affect the heart, lungs, and eyes. Of the estimated 2.1 million Americans with rheumatoid arthritis, approximately 1.5 million (71 percent) are women.

Symptoms: Inflamed and/or deformed joints, loss of strength, swelling, pain.

Treatment: Rest and exercise; anti-inflammatory drugs when necessary.

Systemic Sclerosus (Scleroderma)

Scleroderma is an activation of immune cells which produces scar tissue in the skin, internal organs, and small blood vessels. It affects women three times more often than men overall, but increases to a rate 15 times greater for women during childbearing years, and appears to be more common among black women.

233

Symptoms: In most patients, the first symptoms are Raynaud phenomenon and swelling and puffiness of the fingers or hands. Skin thickening follows a few months later. Other symptoms include skin ulcers on the fingers, joint stiffness in the hands, pain, sore throat, and diarrhea.

Treatment: The drug D-penicillamine has been shown to decrease skin thickening. Symptoms involving other organs such as the kidneys, esophagus, intestines, and blood vessels are treated individually.

Sjögren Syndrome

Sjögren syndrome (also called Sjögren disease) is a chronic, slowly progressing inability to secrete saliva and tears. It can occur alone or with rheumatoid arthritis, scleroderma, or systemic lupus erythematosus. Nine out of 10 cases occur in women, most often at or around mid-life.

Symptoms: Dryness of the eyes and mouth, swollen neck glands, difficulty swallowing or talking, unusual tastes or smells, thirst, tongue ulcers, and severe dental caries.

Treatment: Interventions to keep the mouth and eyes moist include drinking a lot of fluids and using eye drops, as well as good oral hygiene and eye care.

Major Autoimmune Diseases: Neuromuscular Diseases

Multiple Sclerosis (MS)

A disease of the central nervous system that usually first appears between the ages of 20 and 40, and affects women twice as often as men. MS is the leading cause of disability among young adults.

Symptoms: Numbness, weakness, tingling or paralysis in one or more limbs, impaired vision and eye pain, tremor, lack of coordination or unsteady gait, and rapid involuntary eye movement. A history of at least two episodes of a cluster of symptoms is necessary for a diagnosis of MS. Because MS affects the central nervous system, symptoms may be misdiagnosed as mental illness.

Treatment: The drug baclofen is used to suppress muscle spasticity, and corticosteroids help reduce inflammation. Interferons also are being used to treat this disease.

Myasthenia Gravis

This is a chronic autoimmune disorder characterized by gradual muscle weakness, often appearing first in the face.

Symptoms: Drooping eyelids, double vision, and difficulty breathing, talking, chewing, and swallowing.

Treatment: The drug edrophonium along with daily rest periods can improve muscle strength.

Guillain-Barré Syndrome

Guillain-Barré syndrome is an acute illness that causes severe nerve damage. Two-thirds of all cases occur after a viral infection.

Symptoms: Tingling in the fingers and toes, general muscle weakness, difficulty breathing, and in severe cases, paralysis.

Treatment: Supportive care until the condition is stabilized, then rehabilitation therapy combined with whirlpool baths to relieve pain and facilitate retraining of movements. A process called plasmapheresis, which removes plasma and nerve-damaging antibodies from the blood, is used during the first few weeks after a severe attack and may improve the chance of a full recovery.

Major Autoimmune Disease: Endocrine Diseases

Hashimoto Thyroiditis

Hashimoto thyroiditis is a type of autoimmune disease in which the immune system destroys the thyroid, the gland that helps set the rate of metabolism. It attacks women 50 times more often than men.

Symptoms: Low levels of thyroid hormone cause mental and physical slowing, greater sensitivity to cold, weight gain, coarsening of the skin, and goiter (a swelling of the neck due to an enlarged thyroid gland).

Treatment: Thyroid hormone replacement therapy.

Graves Disease

Graves disease is one of the most common autoimmune diseases, affecting 13 million people and targeting women seven times as often as men. Patients with Graves disease produce an excessive amount of thyroid hormone.

Symptoms: Weight loss due to increased energy expenditure; increased appetite, heart rate, and blood pressure; tremors, nervousness and sweating; frequent bowel movements.

Treatment: Antithyroid drug therapy or removal of the thyroid gland surgically or by radioiodine.

Insulin-Dependent (Type 1) Diabetes

Type 1 diabetes is caused by too little insulin production in the pancreas, and usually occurs in children and young adults, but it can occur at any age.

Symptoms: Increased thirst, increased urination, weight loss, fatigue, nausea and vomiting, frequent infections.

Treatment: Monitoring of diet and insulin.

Major Autoimmune Disease: Gastrointestinal Diseases

Inflammatory Bowel Disease

Inflammatory bowel disease describes two autoimmune disorder of the small intestine—Crohn disease and ulcerative colitis.

Symptoms of Crohn disease: Persistent diarrhea, abdominal pain, fever, and general fatigue.

Symptoms of ulcerative colitis: Bloody diarrhea, pain, urgent bowel movements, joint pains, and skin lesions. In both diseases, there is a risk of significant weight loss and malnutrition.

Treatment: Antidiarrheal pills or increased fiber for mild cases. For more serious cases, anti-inflammatory drugs are effective. Corticosteroids are reserved for acute flare-ups of these diseases. In some cases, surgery may be required to remove obstructions or repair perforation of the colon.

Major Autoimmune Disease: Other Autoimmune Diseases

Vasculitis Syndromes

This is a broad and heterogeneous group of diseases characterized by inflammation and damage to the blood vessels, thought to be brought on by an autoimmune response. Any type, size, and location of blood vessel may be involved. Vasculitis may occur alone or in combination with other diseases, and may be confined to one organ or involve several organ systems.

Hematologic Autoimmune Diseases

Blood also can be affected by autoimmune disorder. In autoimmune hemolytic anemia, red blood cells are prematurely destroyed by antibodies. Other autoimmune diseases of the blood include autoimmune thrombocytopenic purpura and autoimmune neutropenia.

Autoimmune Skin Diseases

The skin frequently gives the first sign that an autoimmune disease is present. In many of the diseases mentioned, the skin is only peripherally involved, but in others the skin is the primary site of the disease. One of the foremost is psoriasis, a common skin disease that results from a malfunction in the life cycle of skin cells. The process of skin cell production that normally takes about a month is speeded up to several days, resulting in a build-up of thick scales.

Summary

Autoimmune diseases run the gamut from mild to disabling and potentially life-threatening. Nearly all affect women at far greater rates than men. The question before the scientific community is why? We have come a long way in the diagnosis and treatment of autoimmune disease. But more work is needed, especially in the areas of discovering the causes and developing more effective treatments and prevention strategies.

The U.S. Public Health Service's (PHS) Office on Women's Health in the Department of Health and Human Services was established to redress the inequities in research, health services, and education that have placed the health of American women at risk. Its mission is to direct, stimulate, and coordinate women's health research, health care services, and public and health care professional education and training across the Public Health Service agencies and to collaborate with other government organizations, foundations, private industry, consumer, and health care professional groups to advance women's health. The focal point for women's health activities in the Department of Health and Human Services, the PHS Office on Women's Health is working to improve the health of American women in this decade and beyond, into the 21st century.

The programs and activities in autoimmune diseases of the PHS Office on Women's Health, joined with initiatives and programs across the agencies and Office of the Department of Health and Human Services, are providing a solid foundation from which to increase knowledge about autoimmune disorders in women.

Additional Information

American Autoimmune-Related Diseases Association, Inc. (AARDA)

22100 Gratiot Ave.
East Detroit, MI 48021
Toll-Free: 800-598-4668 (for literature requests)
Phone: 586-776-3900
Fax: 586-776-3903
Website: http://www.aarda.org
E-mail: aarda@aarda.org

Chapter 32

Addison Disease

Addison disease is an endocrine or hormonal disorder that occurs in all age groups and afflicts men and women equally. The disease is characterized by weight loss, muscle weakness, fatigue, low blood pressure, and sometimes darkening of the skin in both exposed and unexposed parts of the body.

Addison disease occurs when the adrenal glands do not produce enough of the hormone cortisol and, in some cases, the hormone aldosterone. The disease is also called adrenal insufficiency.

Cortisol

Cortisol is normally produced by the adrenal glands, located just above the kidneys. It belongs to a class of hormones called glucocorticoids, which affect almost every organ and tissue in the body. Scientists think that cortisol has possibly hundreds of effects in the body. The most important job of cortisol is to help the body respond to stress. Among its other vital tasks, cortisol:

* helps maintain blood pressure and cardiovascular function.

* helps slow the immune system's inflammatory response.

* helps balance the effects of insulin in breaking down sugar for energy.

"Addison's Disease: Adrenal Insufficiency," National Institute of Diabetes and Digestive and Kidney Diseases (NIDDK), NIH Publication No. 04–3054, June 2004.

- helps regulate the metabolism of proteins, carbohydrates, and fats.

- helps maintain proper arousal and sense of well-being.

Because cortisol is so vital to health, the amount of cortisol produced by the adrenals is precisely balanced. Like many other hormones, cortisol is regulated by the brain's hypothalamus and the pituitary gland, a bean-sized organ at the base of the brain. First, the hypothalamus sends releasing hormones to the pituitary gland. The pituitary responds by secreting hormones that regulate growth and thyroid and adrenal function, and sex hormones such as estrogen and testosterone. One of the pituitary's main functions is to secrete adrenocorticotropic hormone (ACTH), a hormone that stimulates the adrenal glands. When the adrenals receive the pituitary's signal in the form of ACTH, they respond by producing cortisol. Completing the cycle, cortisol then signals the pituitary to lower secretion of ACTH.

Aldosterone

Aldosterone belongs to a class of hormones called mineralocorticoids, also produced by the adrenal glands. It helps maintain blood pressure and water and salt balance in the body by helping the kidney retain sodium and excrete potassium. When aldosterone production falls too low, the kidneys are not able to regulate salt and water balance, causing blood volume and blood pressure to drop.

Addison Disease Caused by Autoimmune Disorder

Failure to produce adequate levels of cortisol can occur for different reasons. The problem may be due to a disorder of the adrenal glands themselves (primary adrenal insufficiency) or to inadequate secretion of ACTH by the pituitary gland (secondary adrenal insufficiency).

Primary Adrenal Insufficiency

Addison disease affects about 1 in 100,000 people. Most cases are caused by the gradual destruction of the adrenal cortex, the outer layer of the adrenal glands, by the body's own immune system. About 70 percent of reported cases of Addison disease are caused by autoimmune disorders, in which the immune system makes antibodies that attack the body's own tissues or organs and slowly destroy them. Adrenal insufficiency occurs when at least 90 percent of the adrenal cortex has been destroyed. As a result, often both glucocorticoid (cortisol) and mineralocorticoid (aldosterone) hormones are lacking. Sometimes only the adrenal gland is affected, as in idiopathic adrenal insufficiency; sometimes other glands also are affected, as in the polyendocrine deficiency syndrome.

Symptoms

The symptoms of adrenal insufficiency usually begin gradually. Characteristics of the disease are:

* chronic, worsening fatigue,
* muscle weakness,
* loss of appetite, and
* weight loss.

About 50 percent of the time, one will notice:

* nausea,
* vomiting, and
* diarrhea.

Other symptoms include:

* low blood pressure that falls further when standing, causing dizziness or fainting.
* skin changes in Addison disease, with areas of hyperpigmentation, or dark tanning, covering exposed and unexposed parts of the body; this darkening of the skin is most visible on scars; skin folds; pressure points such as the elbows, knees, knuckles, and toes; lips; and mucous membranes.

Addison disease can cause irritability and depression. Because of salt loss, a craving for salty foods also is common. Hypoglycemia, or low blood glucose, is more severe in children than in adults. In women, menstrual periods may become irregular or stop.

Because the symptoms progress slowly, they are usually ignored until a stressful event like an illness or an accident causes them to become worse. This is called an addisonian crisis, or acute adrenal insufficiency. In most cases, symptoms are severe enough that patients seek medical treatment before a crisis occurs. However, in about 25 percent of patients, symptoms first appear during an addisonian crisis.

Symptoms of an addisonian crisis include the following:

- sudden penetrating pain in the lower back, abdomen, or legs
- severe vomiting and diarrhea
- dehydration
- low blood pressure
- loss of consciousness

Left untreated, an addisonian crisis can be fatal.

Diagnosis

In its early stages, adrenal insufficiency can be difficult to diagnose. A review of a patient's medical history based on the symptoms, especially the dark tanning of the skin, will lead a doctor to suspect Addison disease.

A diagnosis of Addison disease is made by laboratory tests. The aim of these tests is first to determine whether levels of cortisol are insufficient and then to establish the cause. X-ray exams of the adrenal and pituitary glands also are useful in helping to establish the cause.

ACTH Stimulation Test

This is the most specific test for diagnosing Addison disease. In this test, blood cortisol, urine cortisol, or both are measured before and after a synthetic form of ACTH is given by injection. In the so-called short, or rapid, ACTH test, measurement of cortisol in blood is repeated 30 to 60 minutes after an intravenous ACTH injection. The normal response after an injection of ACTH is a rise in blood and urine cortisol levels. Patients with either form of adrenal insufficiency respond poorly or do not respond at all.

Corticotropin-Releasing Hormone (CRH) Stimulation Test

When the response to the short ACTH test is abnormal, a long CRH stimulation test is required to determine the cause of adrenal insufficiency. In this test, synthetic CRH is injected intravenously and blood cortisol is measured before and 30, 60, 90, and 120 minutes after the injection. Patients with primary adrenal insufficiency have high ACTH, but do not produce cortisol. Patients with secondary adrenal insufficiency have deficient cortisol responses, but absent or delayed

ACTH responses. Absent ACTH response points to the pituitary as the cause; a delayed ACTH response points to the hypothalamus as the cause.

In patients suspected of having an addisonian crisis, the doctor must begin treatment with injections of salt, fluids, and glucocorticoid hormones immediately. Although a reliable diagnosis is not possible while the patient is being treated for the crisis, measurement of blood ACTH and cortisol during the crisis and before glucocorticoids are given is enough to make the diagnosis. Once the crisis is controlled and medication has been stopped, the doctor will delay further testing for up to 1 month to obtain an accurate diagnosis.

Other Tests

Once a diagnosis of primary adrenal insufficiency has been made, x-ray exams of the abdomen may be taken to see if the adrenals have any signs of calcium deposits. Calcium deposits may indicate TB. A tuberculin skin test also may be used.

If secondary adrenal insufficiency is the cause, doctors may use different imaging tools to reveal the size and shape of the pituitary gland. The most common is the CT scan, which produces a series of x-ray pictures giving a cross-sectional image of a body part. The function of the pituitary and its ability to produce other hormones also are tested.

Treatment

Treatment of Addison disease involves replacing, or substituting, the hormones that the adrenal glands are not making. Cortisol is replaced orally with hydrocortisone tablets, a synthetic glucocorticoid, taken once or twice a day. If aldosterone is also deficient, it is replaced with oral doses of a mineralocorticoid called fludrocortisone acetate (Florinef), which is taken once a day. Patients receiving aldosterone replacement therapy are usually advised by a doctor to increase their salt intake. Because patients with secondary adrenal insufficiency normally maintain aldosterone production, they do not require aldosterone replacement therapy. The doses of each of these medications are adjusted to meet the needs of individual patients.

During an addisonian crisis, low blood pressure, low blood glucose, and high levels of potassium can be life-threatening. Standard therapy involves intravenous injections of hydrocortisone, saline (salt water), and dextrose (sugar). This treatment usually brings rapid improvement. When the patient can take fluids and medications by mouth, the amount of hydrocortisone is decreased until a maintenance dose is achieved. If aldosterone is deficient, maintenance therapy also includes oral doses of fludrocortisone acetate.

Special Problems

Surgery

Patients with chronic adrenal insufficiency who need surgery with general anesthesia are treated with injections of hydrocortisone and saline. Injections begin on the evening before surgery and continue until the patient is fully awake and able to take medication by mouth. The dosage is adjusted until the maintenance dosage given before surgery is reached.

Pregnancy

Women with primary adrenal insufficiency who become pregnant are treated with standard replacement therapy. If nausea and vomiting in early pregnancy interfere with oral medication, injections of the hormone may be necessary. During delivery, treatment is similar to that of patients needing surgery; following delivery, the dose is gradually tapered and the usual maintenance doses of hydrocortisone and fludrocortisone acetate by mouth are reached by about 10 days after childbirth.

Patient Education

A person who has adrenal insufficiency should always carry identification stating his or her condition in case of an emergency. The card should alert emergency personnel about the need to inject 100 milligrams (mg) of cortisol if its bearer is found severely injured or unable to answer questions. The card should also include the doctor's name and telephone number, and the name and telephone number of the nearest relative to be notified. When traveling, a needle, syringe, and an injectable form of cortisol should be carried for emergencies. A person with Addison disease also should know how to increase medication during periods of stress or mild upper respiratory infections. Immediate medical attention is needed when severe infections, vomiting, or diarrhea occur. These conditions can precipitate an addisonian crisis. A patient who is vomiting may require injections of hydrocortisone.

People with medical problems may wish to wear a descriptive warning bracelet or neck chain to alert emergency personnel. A number of companies manufacture medical identification products.

Suggested Reading

The following materials can be found in medical libraries, many college and university libraries, and through interlibrary loan in most public libraries.

Stewart PM. The adrenal cortex. In: Larsen P, ed. *Williams Textbook of Endocrinology. 10ᵗʰ ed.* Philadelphia: Saunders; 2003: 491-551.

Chrousos GP. Glucocorticoid therapy. In: Felig P, Frohman L, eds. *Endocrinology and Metabolism. 4ᵗʰ ed.* New York: McGraw-Hill; 2001: 609-632.

Miller W, Chrousos GP. The adrenal cortex. In: Felig P, Frohman L, eds. *Endocrinology and Metabolism. 4ᵗʰ ed.* New York: McGraw-Hill; 2001: 387-524.

Ten S, New M, Maclaren N. Clinical Review 130: Addison's disease 2001. *Journal of Clinical Endocrinology & Metabolism.* 2001;86(7): 2909-2922.

Williams GH, Dluhy, RC. Disorders of the adrenal cortex. In: Braunwald E, ed. *Harrison's Principles of Internal Medicine. 15ᵗʰ ed.* New York: McGraw-Hill Professional; 2001: 2084-2105.

Additional Information

American Autoimmune-Related Diseases Association, Inc. (AARDA)
22100 Gratiot Ave.
East Detroit, MI 48021
Toll-Free: 800-598-4668 (for literature requests)
Phone: 586-776-3900
Fax: 586-776-3903
Website: http://www.aarda.org
E-mail: aarda@aarda.org

National Adrenal Diseases Foundation
505 Northern Blvd.
Great Neck, NY 11021
Phone: 516-487-4992
Website: http://www.medhelp.org/nadf
E-mail: nadfmail@aol.com

National Institute of Diabetes and Digestive and Kidney Diseases (NIDDK)

Information Clearinghouse
5 Information Way
Bethesda, MD 20892-3560
Toll-Free: 800-860-8747
Phone: 301-654-3810
Website: http://www.niddk.nih.gov

Chapter 33

Alopecia Areata

Alopecia areata is considered an autoimmune disease, in which the immune system, which is designed to protect the body from foreign invaders such as viruses and bacteria, mistakenly attacks the hair follicles, the tiny cup-shaped structures from which hairs grow. This can lead to hair loss on the scalp and elsewhere.

In most cases, hair falls out in small, round patches about the size of a quarter. In many cases, the disease does not extend beyond a few bare patches. In some people, hair loss is more extensive. Although uncommon, the disease can progress to cause total loss of hair on the head (referred to as alopecia areata totalis), or complete loss of hair on the head, face, and body (alopecia areata universalis).

Causes

In alopecia areata, immune system cells called white blood cells attack the rapidly growing cells in the hair follicles that make the hair. The affected hair follicles become small and drastically slow down hair production. Fortunately, the stem cells that continually supply the follicle with new cells do not seem to be targeted. So the follicle always has the potential to regrow hair.

Scientists do not know exactly why the hair follicles undergo these changes, but they suspect that a combination of genes may predispose

Excerpted from "Questions and Answers about Alopecia Areata," National Institute of Arthritis and Musculoskeletal and Skin Diseases (NIAMS), February 2003.

some people to the disease. In those who are genetically predisposed, some type of trigger—perhaps a virus or something in the person's environment—brings on the attack against the hair follicles.

Who Is Affected?

Alopecia areata affects an estimated four million Americans of both sexes and of all ages and ethnic backgrounds. It often begins in childhood.

If you have a close family member with the disease, your risk of developing it is slightly increased. If your family member lost his or her first patch of hair before age 30, the risk to other family members is greater. Overall, one in five people with the disease have a family member who has it as well.

Is my hair loss a symptom of a serious disease?

Alopecia areata is not a life-threatening disease. It does not cause any physical pain, and people with the condition are generally healthy otherwise. But for most people, a disease that unpredictably affects their appearance the way alopecia areata does is a serious matter.

The effects of alopecia areata are primarily socially and emotionally disturbing. In alopecia universalis, however, loss of eyelashes and eyebrows and hair in the nose and ears can make the person more vulnerable to dust, germs, and foreign particles entering the eyes, nose, and ears.

Alopecia areata often occurs in people whose family members have other autoimmune diseases, such as diabetes, rheumatoid arthritis, thyroid disease, systemic lupus erythematosus, pernicious anemia, or Addison disease. People who have alopecia areata do not usually have other autoimmune diseases, but they do have a higher occurrence of thyroid disease, atopic eczema, nasal allergies, and asthma.

Can I pass it on to my children?

It is possible, but not likely, for alopecia areata to be inherited. Most children with alopecia areata do not have a parent with the disease, and the vast majority of parents with alopecia areata do not pass it along to their children.

Will my hair ever grow back?

There is every chance that your hair will regrow, but it may also fall out again. No one can predict when it might regrow or fall out.

The course of the disease varies from person to person. Some people lose just a few patches of hair, then the hair regrows, and the condition never recurs. Other people continue to lose and regrow hair for many years. A few lose all the hair on their head; some lose all the hair on their head, face, and body. Even in those who lose all their hair, the possibility for full regrowth remains. In some, the initial hair regrowth is white, with a gradual return of the original hair color. In most, the regrown hair is ultimately the same color and texture as the original hair.

Prognosis

The course of alopecia areata is highly unpredictable, and the uncertainty of what will happen next is probably the most difficult and frustrating aspect of the disease. You may continue to lose hair, or your hair loss may stop. The hair you have lost may or may not grow back, and you may or may not continue to develop new bare patches.

Treatment

While there is neither a cure for alopecia areata nor drugs approved for its treatment, some people find that medications approved for other purposes can help hair grow back, at least temporarily. The following are some treatments for alopecia areata. Keep in mind that while these treatments may promote hair growth, none of them prevent new patches or actually cure the underlying disease. Consult your health care professional about the best option for you.

- **Corticosteroids**—Corticosteroids are powerful anti-inflammatory drugs similar to a hormone called cortisol produced in the body. Because these drugs suppress the immune system if given orally, they are often used in the treatment of various autoimmune diseases, including alopecia areata. Corticosteroids may be administered in three ways for alopecia areata:
  - **Local injections**—Injections of steroids directly into hairless patches on the scalp and sometimes the brow and beard areas are effective in increasing hair growth in most people. It usually takes about 4 weeks for new hair growth to become visible. Injections deliver small amounts of cortisone to affected areas, avoiding the more serious side effects encountered with long-term oral use. The main side effects of injections are transient pain, mild swelling, and sometimes changes in

pigmentation, as well as small indentations in the skin that go away when injections are stopped. Because injections can be painful, they may not be the preferred treatment for children. After 1 or 2 months, new hair growth usually becomes visible, and the injections usually have to be repeated monthly. The cortisone removes the confused immune cells and allows the hair to grow. Large areas cannot be treated, however, because the discomfort and the amount of medicine become too great and can result in side effects similar to those of the oral regimen.

- **Oral corticosteroids**—Corticosteroids taken by mouth are a mainstay of treatment for many autoimmune diseases and may be used in more extensive alopecia areata. But because of the risk of side effects of oral corticosteroids, such as hypertension and cataracts, they are used only occasionally for alopecia areata and for shorter periods of time.

- **Topical ointments**—Ointments or creams containing steroids rubbed directly onto the affected area are less traumatic than injections, and therefore, are sometimes preferred for children. However, corticosteroid ointments and creams alone are less effective than injections; they work best when combined with other topical treatments, such as minoxidil or anthralin.

- **Minoxidil (5%)** (Rogaine*)—Topical minoxidil solution promotes hair growth in several conditions in which the hair follicle is small and not growing to its full potential. Minoxidil is FDA-approved for treating male and female pattern hair loss. It may also be useful in promoting hair growth in alopecia areata. The solution, applied twice daily, has been shown to promote hair growth in both adults and children, and may be used on the scalp, brow, and beard areas. With regular and proper use of the solution, new hair growth appears in about 12 weeks.

- **Anthralin** (Psoriatic)—Anthralin, a synthetic tar-like substance that alters immune function in the affected skin, is an approved treatment for psoriasis. Anthralin is also commonly used to treat alopecia areata. Anthralin is applied for 20 to 60 minutes (short contact therapy) to avoid skin irritation, which is not needed for the drug to work. When it works, new hair growth is usually evident in 8 to 12 weeks. Anthralin is often used in combination with other treatments, such as corticosteroid injections or minoxidil, for improved results.

- **Sulfasalazine**—A sulfa drug, sulfasalazine has been used as a treatment for different autoimmune disorders, including psoriasis. It acts on the immune system and has been used to some effect in patients with severe alopecia areata.

- **Topical sensitizers**—Topical sensitizers are medications that, when applied to the scalp, provoke an allergic reaction that leads to itching, scaling, and eventually hair growth. If the medication works, new hair growth is usually established in 3 to 12 months. Two topical sensitizers are used in alopecia areata: squaric acid dibutyl ester (SADBE) and diphenylcyclopropenone (DPCP). Their safety and consistency of formula are currently under review.

- **Oral cyclosporine**—Originally developed to keep people's immune systems from rejecting transplanted organs, oral cyclosporine is sometimes used to suppress the immune system response in psoriasis and other immune-mediated skin conditions. But suppressing the immune system can also cause problems, including an increased risk of serious infection and possibly skin cancer. Although oral cyclosporine may regrow hair in alopecia areata, it does not turn the disease off. Most doctors feel the dangers of the drug outweigh its benefits for alopecia areata.

- **Photochemotherapy**—In photochemotherapy, a treatment used most commonly for psoriasis, a person is given a light-sensitive drug called a psoralen either orally or topically and then exposed to an ultraviolet light source. This combined treatment is called PUVA. In clinical trials, approximately 55 percent of people achieve cosmetically acceptable hair growth using photochemotherapy. However, the relapse rate is high, and patients must go to a treatment center where the equipment is available at least two to three times per week. Furthermore, the treatment carries the risk of developing skin cancer.

- **Alternative therapies**—When drug treatments fail to bring sufficient hair regrowth, some people turn to alternative therapies. Alternatives purported to help alopecia areata include acupuncture, aroma therapy, evening primrose oil, zinc and vitamin supplements, and Chinese herbs. Because many alternative therapies are not backed by clinical trials, they may or may not be effective for regrowing hair. In fact, some may actually make hair loss worse. Furthermore, just because these therapies are natural does not mean that they are safe. As with any therapy, it is best to discuss these treatments with your doctor before you try them.

*Brand names included in this chapter are provided as examples only, and their inclusion does not mean that these products are endorsed by the National Institutes of Health or any other Government agency. Also, if a particular brand name is not mentioned, this does not mean or imply that the product is unsatisfactory.

In addition to treatments to help hair grow, there are measures that can be taken to minimize the physical dangers or discomforts of lost hair.

- Sunscreens are important for the scalp, face, and all exposed areas.

- Eyeglasses (or sunglasses) protect the eyes from excessive sun, and from dust and debris, when eyebrows or eyelashes are missing.

- Wigs, caps, or scarves protect the scalp from the sun and keep the head warm.

- Antibiotic ointment applied inside the nostrils helps to protect against organisms invading the nose when nostril hair is missing.

Living with Alopecia Areata

The comforting news is that alopecia areata is not a painful disease and does not make people feel sick physically. It is not contagious, and people who have the disease are generally healthy otherwise. It does not reduce life expectancy, and it should not interfere with the ability to achieve such life goals as going to school, working, marrying, raising a family, playing sports, and exercising.

The emotional aspects of living with hair loss, however, can be challenging. Many people cope by learning as much as they can about the disease; speaking with others who are facing the same problem; and, if necessary, seeking counseling to help build a positive self-image.

Many people learning to cope with alopecia areata find it helpful to talk with other people who are dealing with the same problems by joining a support group or online discussion. More than four million people nationwide have this disease at some point in their lives.

Additional Information

American Academy of Dermatology (AAD)
P.O. Box 4014
Schaumberg, IL 60168-4014
Toll-Free: 888-462-3376

Phone: 847-330-0230
Fax: 847-330-0050
Website: http://www.aad.org

American Hair Loss Council
125 Seventh St., Suite 625
Pittsburgh, PA 15222
Phone: 412-765-3666
Fax: 412-765-3669
Website: http://www.ahlc.org
E-mail: ahlc@e-zign.com

National Alopecia Areata Foundation (NAAF)
P.O. Box 150760
San Rafael, CA 94915-0760
Phone: 415-472-3780
Fax: 415-472-5343
Website: http://www.naaf.org
E-mail: info@naaf.org

The National Alopecia Areata Foundation (NAAF) has a pen pal program, message boards, annual conference, and support groups that meet in various locations nationwide.

National Alopecia Areata Registry
Alopecia Areata Study
University of Texas
M.D. Anderson Cancer Center
1515 Holcombe Blvd.
Houston, TX 77030
Phone: 713-792-5999
Website: http://www.mdanderson.org/departments/alopecia
E-mail: alopeciaregistry@mdanderson.org

The registry is seeking U.S. residents with alopecia areata, alopecia totalis, or alopecia universalis diagnosed by a dermatologist. Although the registry itself will not be involved in any kind of treatment for alopecia areata, people who register will be made aware of studies for which they may qualify. To take part in the registry, people do not have to live near or travel to one of the five centers; however, they do have to meet some requirements to participate. The registry, a network of five centers, will identify and register patients with the disease and collect information and blood samples (containing genes).

Data, including genetic information, will be made available to researchers studying the genetic basis and other aspects of the disease and disease risk.

National Institute of Arthritis and Musculoskeletal and Skin Diseases
Information Clearinghouse/NIH
1 AMS Circle
Bethesda, MD 20892-3675
Toll-Free: 877-22-NIAMS (64267)
Phone: 301-495-4484
TTY: 301-565-2966
Fast Facts: 301-881-2731 (to receive information by fax)
Website: http://www.nih.gov/niams/healthinfo
E-mail: niamsinfo@mail.nih.gov

Chapter 34

Autoimmune-Related Anemias

Chapter Contents

255

Section 34.1

Autoimmune Hemolytic Anemia

"Idiopathic Autoimmune Hemolytic Anemia," © 2005 A.D.A.M., Inc.
Reprinted with permission.

Definition: This disorder results from an abnormality of the immune system that destroys red blood cells prematurely. The cause is unknown.

Causes, Incidence, and Risk Factors

Autoimmune hemolytic anemia is an acquired disease that occurs when antibodies form against the person's own red blood cells. In the idiopathic form of this disease, the cause is unknown.

There are other types of immune hemolytic anemias where the cause may result from an underlying disease or medication. Idiopathic autoimmune hemolytic anemia accounts for one-half of all immune hemolytic anemias. The onset of the disease may be quite rapid and very serious. Risk factors are not known.

Symptoms

- Fatigue
- Pale color
- Shortness of breath
- Rapid heartbeat
- Yellow skin color
- Dark urine
- Enlarged spleen

Signs and Tests

- Positive direct Coombs test
- Indirect Coombs test

- Elevated bilirubin levels
- Low serum haptoglobin
- Hemoglobin in the urine
- Elevated reticulocyte count
- Low red blood cell count and low serum hemoglobin

Treatment

The first therapy tried is usually treatment with prednisone. If prednisone does not improve the condition, a splenectomy (removal of the spleen) may be considered.

Immunosuppressive therapy is given if the person does not respond to prednisone and splenectomy. Imuran and Cytoxan have both been used.

Blood transfusions are given with caution, if indicated for severe anemia, because of the potential that blood may not be compatible and precipitate a reaction.

Expectations (Prognosis)

Adults may have chronic, relapsing disease, but in children the anemia is usually short-lived.

Complications

- Infection (from treatment)
- Severe anemia

Calling Your Health Care Provider

Call your health care provider if you notice symptoms of anemia.

Prevention

There is no known prevention for autoimmune hemolytic anemia, because the cause is unknown.

Section 34.2

Pernicious Anemia

"Pernicious Anemia," © 2005 A.D.A.M., Inc. Reprinted with permission.

Alternative names: Macrocytic achylic anemia; congenital pernicious anemia; juvenile pernicious anemia; vitamin B_{12} deficiency (malabsorption).

Definition: Pernicious anemia is caused by a lack of intrinsic factor, a substance needed to absorb vitamin B_{12} from the gastrointestinal tract. Vitamin B_{12}, in turn, is necessary for the formation of red blood cells. Anemia is a condition where red blood cells are not providing adequate oxygen to body tissues. There are many types and causes of anemia. Pernicious anemia is a type of megaloblastic anemia.

Causes, Incidence, and Risk Factors

Intrinsic factor is a protein the body uses to absorb vitamin B_{12}. When gastric secretions do not have enough intrinsic factor, vitamin B_{12} is not adequately absorbed, resulting in pernicious anemia and other problems related to low levels of vitamin B_{12}.

Because vitamin B_{12} is needed by nerve cells and blood cells for them to function properly, deficiency can cause a wide variety of symptoms, including fatigue, shortness of breath, tingling sensations, difficulty walking, and diarrhea.

Other causes of low levels of intrinsic factor (and thus of pernicious anemia) include atrophic gastric mucosa, autoimmunity against gastric parietal cells, and autoimmunity against intrinsic factor.

Absence of intrinsic factor itself is the most common cause of vitamin B_{12} deficiency. Intrinsic factor is produced by cells within the stomach. In adults, the inability to make intrinsic factor can be the result of chronic gastritis or the result of surgery to remove the stomach. The onset of the disease is slow and may span decades.

Very rarely, infants and children are found to have been born lacking the ability to produce effective intrinsic factor. This form of congenital pernicious anemia is inherited as an autosomal recessive disorder. (You need a defective gene from both parents to get it.) However, most often, pernicious anemia and other forms of megaloblastic anemia in children results from other causes of vitamin B_{12} deficiency or other vitamin deficiencies.

Although a juvenile form of the disease can occur in children, pernicious anemia usually does not appear before the age of 30. The average age at diagnosis is 60 years. In fact, one recent study revealed that nearly 2 percent of individuals over 60 years old suffer from pernicious anemia. Furthermore, slightly more women than men are affected. The disease can affect all racial groups, but occurs more often among people of Scandinavian or Northern European descent.

Risk factors include a family history of pernicious anemia, Scandinavian or Northern European descent, and a history of autoimmune endocrine disorders. Pernicious anemia is seen in association with some autoimmune endocrine diseases such as type 1 diabetes, hypoparathyroidism, Addison disease, hypopituitarism, testicular dysfunction, Graves disease, chronic thyroiditis, myasthenia gravis, secondary amenorrhea, and vitiligo.

In addition to pernicious anemia, other causes of vitamin B_{12} deficiency include:

- Nutrition (strict vegetarians without B_{12} supplementation, poor diet in infant, or poor maternal nutrition during pregnancy).

- Infection (intestinal parasites, bacterial overgrowth).

- Gastrointestinal disease (stomach removal surgery, celiac disease (sprue), Crohn disease).

- Drugs (colchicine, neomycin, tuberculosis treatment with para amino salicylic acid).

- Metabolic disorders (methylmalonic aciduria, homocystinuria).

Symptoms

Many cells in our body need vitamin B_{12}, including nerve cells and blood cells. Inadequate vitamin B_{12} gradually affects sensory and motor nerves, causing neurological problems to develop over time. It is important to know that the neurological effects of vitamin B_{12} deficiency may be seen before anemia is diagnosed.

The anemia also affects the gastrointestinal system and the cardiovascular system. The following symptoms may indicate pernicious anemia:

- shortness of breath

- fatigue
- pallor
- rapid heart rate
- loss of appetite
- diarrhea
- tingling and numbness of hands and feet
- sore mouth
- unsteady gait, especially in the dark
- tongue problems
- smell, impaired
- gums, bleeding
- positive Babinski reflex
- loss of deep tendon reflexes
- personality changes, "megaloblastic madness"

Signs and Tests

Tests that may indicate pernicious anemia include:

- CBC results that show low hematocrit and hemoglobin with elevated MCV (low red blood cell count with large-sized red blood cells).
- CBC showing low white blood count and low platelets.
- low reticulocyte count.
- bone marrow examination (only needed if diagnosis is unclear).
- serum lactate dehydrogenase (LDH).
- below normal serum vitamin B_{12} level.
- Schilling test.
- measurement of serum holotranscobalamin II.
- measurement of methylmalonic acid (MMA).

This disease may also alter the results of the following tests:

- Total iron binding capacity (TIBC)
- peripheral smear
- leukocyte alkaline phosphatase
- gastrin

- cholesterol test
- bilirubin

Treatment

Monthly vitamin B_{12} injections are the definitive treatment to correct the vitamin B_{12} deficiency. This therapy corrects the anemia and may correct the neurological complications if given soon enough. Since about 1% of vitamin B_{12} is absorbed (even in the absence of intrinsic factor), some doctors recommend that elderly patients with gastric atrophy take oral vitamin B_{12} supplements in addition to monthly injections.

There is also a preparation of vitamin B_{12} that may be given intranasally (in the nose). A well-balanced diet is essential to provide other elements such as folic acid, iron, and vitamin C for healthy blood cell development.

Expectations (Prognosis)

The outcome is usually excellent with treatment.

Complications

- People with pernicious anemia may have gastric polyps and have twice the incidence of gastric cancer and gastric carcinoid tumors than the normal population.
- Persistent neurological defects may be present if treatment is delayed.
- Vitamin B_{12} deficiency affects the appearance of all epithelial cells, therefore an untreated woman may obtain a false positive pap smear.

Calling Your Health Care Provider

Call your health care provider if symptoms suggestive of vitamin B_{12} deficiency develop.

Prevention

Pernicious anemia is not preventable, but with early detection and treatment of vitamin B_{12} deficiency, complications are readily controlled.

261

Chapter 35

Arthritis

Chapter Contents

Section 35.1

Ankylosing Spondylitis

Fast Facts about Ankylosing Spondylitis (AS)

- AS (ankylosing spondylitis) is arthritis of the spine that strikes young people. The typical age of onset is between 17 and 35.

- Nearly one million Americans have spondylitis. AS is more prevalent than multiple sclerosis, cystic fibrosis, and Lou Gehrig disease combined.

- Difficult to diagnose in the early stages, it is the most overlooked cause of persistent back pain in young adults.

- AS can also damage other joints such as the hips and shoulders, as well as other areas of the body including the eyes, heart, and lungs.

- AS causes pain and spinal stiffness, and, in severe cases, the spine fuses solidly in a forward-stooped posture.

About Ankylosing Spondylitis (AS)

AS is the primary disease in the group of diseases known as spondylitis, spondyloarthropathy, or spondyloarthritis. Ankylosis means fusion, which may be fibrous, or bony. Spondylitis means inflammation of the spine.

Ankylosing spondylitis (pronounced ank-kih-low-sing spon-dill-eye-tiss), or AS, is a form of arthritis that primarily affects the spine. It causes inflammation of the spinal joints (vertebrae) that can lead to severe back pain and discomfort. In the most advanced cases (but not in all cases), this inflammation can lead to new bone formation on the spine, causing the spine to fuse in a fixed, immobile position, sometimes creating a forward-stooped posture.

AS can also cause inflammation, pain, and stiffness in other areas of the body such as the shoulders, hips, ribs, heels, and small joints of the hands and feet. Sometimes the eyes can become involved (known as Iritis or Uveitis), and rarely, the lungs and heart can be affected.

The hallmark feature of ankylosing spondylitis is the involvement of the sacroiliac (SI) joints during the progression of the disease, which are the joints at the base of the spine, where the spine joins the pelvis.

Is There a Cure?

Currently, there is no known cure for AS, but there are treatments and medications available to reduce symptoms, manage the pain, and recent studies show that the new biologic medications can potentially slow or halt the disease progression in some people.

Causes of Ankylosing Spondylitis

Although the exact cause of AS is unknown, we do know that genetics play a key role in AS. Most individuals who have AS also have a gene that produces a genetic marker—in this case, a protein—called HLA-B27. This marker is found in over 95% of people with AS. It is important to note, however, that you do not have to be HLA-B27 positive to have AS. Also, a majority of the people with this marker never contract ankylosing spondylitis. HLA-B27 is found in about 7% of the unaffected population.

Scientists know that other genes, along with a triggering environmental factor, such as a bacterial infection, are needed to trigger AS in susceptible people. HLA-B27 probably accounts for about 40% of the overall risk, but then there are other genes working in concert with B27. There are probably five or six genes involved in susceptibility toward AS. It is thought that perhaps AS starts when the defenses of the intestines start breaking down and bacteria from the intestines pass into the bloodstream directly into the region where the sacroiliac joints are located.

Who Is At Risk?

The risk factors that predispose a person to ankylosing spondylitis include the following:

- Testing positive for the HLA-B27 marker
- A family history of AS
- Frequent gastrointestinal infections

Unlike other forms of arthritis and rheumatic diseases, general onset of AS commonly occurs in younger people, between the ages of 17–35. However, it can affect children and those who are much older. AS is more common in men, but occurs in women as well.

Prevalence of AS

There are at least half a million people with AS in the United States, but likely more because the disease is under-recognized. AS is more prevalent than multiple sclerosis, cystic fibrosis, and Lou Gehrig disease combined.

Disease Course/Prognosis

The severity of AS varies greatly from person to person, and not everyone will experience the most serious complications or have spinal fusion. Some will experience only intermittent back pain and discomfort, but others will experience severe pain and stiffness over multiple areas of the body for long periods of time. AS can be very debilitating, and in some cases, lead to disability.

Almost all cases of AS are characterized by acute, painful episodes (also known as flares) followed by temporary periods of remission where symptoms subside. It is important to know that ankylosing spondylitis is a chronic, or life-long disease and that the severity of AS has nothing to do with age or gender. It can be just as severe in women and children as it is in men. Remember that even if you have AS and are experiencing only mild symptoms, which you are able to manage quite well, it is important to see your rheumatologist once a year in order to detect and treat any underlying complications.

Frequently Asked Questions

How is spondylitis diagnosed?

Although x-ray findings of sacroiliitis are necessary to the diagnosis, these may not show up in very early disease on a plain x-ray. Magnetic resonance imaging (MRI) screening is sometimes used. However, this type of testing may not be available in all cases for a variety of reasons, which include its high cost. And even when it is available, many rheumatologists do not believe that MRI testing is that useful, because interpretation of the results is not yet properly fine tuned. Interestingly, several recent studies actually suggest the reintroduction of an old tool—ultrasonography—that can potentially detect early inflammation in the joints—particularly in the lower peripheral joints (for example, the knees).

The work-up should also include a detailed clinical history of your symptoms and physical examination. And according to David Yu, M.D., researcher and rheumatologist at UCLA, it is the doctor's duty to determine during the initial consultation what the prognosis (the natural course of the disease) is likely to be in each patient. That way, those who have a more serious prognosis can be treated aggressively with more powerful medications, and those with a milder prognosis can avoid unnecessary treatment with medications that potentially have more serious side-effects. According to Dr. Yu, a rheumatologist can use a point count system tool to help make this critical decision when seeing a newly diagnosed person with ankylosing spondylitis.

Is there a cure?

While there is not yet a cure, much is being discovered about AS. Researchers have begun to identify markers of disease activity, and develop better measurements of function in AS in order to better follow patients. Also, problems associated with AS (such as osteoporosis) are being studied to find out whether some of the promising new drugs to combat osteoporosis are helpful for people with AS. All of this contributes to a better understanding of AS, and is leading to better patient care.

How is it treated?

Treatment consists of medicines to alleviate the pain and stiffness, special daily exercises that incorporate stretching and strengthening, good posture habits, a healthy diet, and a supportive social environment of family and friends. Peer networking through Spondylitis Association of America (SAA) can be very helpful. There is much that can be done to reduce the affects of AS. Initial medication for AS includes the use of non-steroidal anti-inflammatory drugs (NSAIDs). If the response to NSAIDs is unsatisfactory, new medications can be prescribed including: Enbrel®, Remicade®, and Humira®, but only after specific conditions are met.

Additional Information

Spondylitis Association of America (SAA)
P.O. Box 5872
Sherman Oaks, CA 91413
Toll-Free: 800-777-8189
Phone: 818-981-1616
Website: http://www.spondylitis.org
E-mail: info@spondylitis.org

Section 35.2

Juvenile Rheumatoid Arthritis

Excerpted from "Questions and Answers about Juvenile Rheumatoid Arthritis," National Institute of Arthritis and Musculoskeletal and Skin Diseases (NIAMS), NIH Publication No. 01–4942, July 2001.

Arthritis means joint inflammation, and refers to a group of diseases that cause pain, swelling, stiffness, and loss of motion in the joints. Arthritis is often used as a more general term to refer to the more than 100 rheumatic diseases that may affect the joints, but can also cause pain, swelling, and stiffness in other supporting structures of the body such as muscles, tendons, ligaments, and bones. Some rheumatic diseases can affect other parts of the body, including various internal organs. Children can develop almost all types of arthritis that affect adults, but the most common type that affects children is juvenile rheumatoid arthritis (JRA).

Juvenile Rheumatoid Arthritis

Juvenile rheumatoid arthritis is arthritis that causes joint inflammation and stiffness for more than 6 weeks in a child of 16 years of age or less. Inflammation causes redness, swelling, warmth, and soreness in the joints, although many children with JRA do not complain of joint pain. Any joint can be affected and inflammation may limit the mobility of affected joints. One type of JRA can also affect the internal

268

organs. Doctors classify JRA into three types by the number of joints involved, the symptoms, and the presence or absence of certain antibodies found by a blood test. (Antibodies are special proteins made by the immune system.) These classifications help the doctor determine how the disease will progress and whether the internal organs or skin are affected.

- **Pauciarticular** (PAW-see-are-TICK-you-lar)—Pauciarticular means that four or fewer joints are affected. Pauciarticular is the most common form of JRA; about half of all children with JRA have this type. Pauciarticular disease typically affects large joints, such as the knees. Girls under age 8 are most likely to develop this type of JRA. Some children have special kinds of antibodies in the blood. One is called antinuclear antibody (ANA) and one is called rheumatoid factor. Eye disease affects about 20 to 30 percent of children with pauciarticular JRA. Up to 80 percent of those with eye disease also test positive for ANA and the disease tends to develop at a particularly early age in these children. Regular examinations by an ophthalmologist (a doctor who specializes in eye diseases) are necessary to prevent serious eye problems such as iritis (inflammation of the iris, the colored part of the eye) or uveitis (inflammation of the uvea, or the inner eye). Some children with pauciarticular disease outgrow arthritis by adulthood, although eye problems can continue and joint symptoms may recur in some people.

- **Polyarticular**—About 30 percent of all children with JRA have polyarticular disease. In polyarticular disease, five or more joints are affected. The small joints, such as those in the hands and feet, are most commonly involved, but the disease may also affect large joints. Polyarticular JRA often is symmetrical; that is, it affects the same joint on both sides of the body. Some children with polyarticular disease have an antibody in their blood called immunoglobulin M (IgM) rheumatoid factor (RF). These children often have a more severe form of the disease, which doctors consider to be similar in many ways to adult rheumatoid arthritis.

- **Systemic**—Besides joint swelling, the systemic form of JRA is characterized by fever and a light skin rash, and may also affect internal organs such as the heart, liver, spleen, and lymph nodes. Doctors sometimes call it Still disease. Almost all children with this type of JRA test negative for both RF and ANA. The systemic form affects 20 percent of all children with JRA. A small percentage of these children develop arthritis in many joints and can have severe arthritis that continues into adulthood.

Causes of Juvenile Rheumatoid Arthritis

JRA is an autoimmune disorder, which means that the body mistakenly identifies some of its own cells and tissues as foreign. The immune system, which normally helps to fight off harmful, foreign substances such as bacteria or viruses, begins to attack healthy cells and tissues. The result is inflammation—marked by redness, heat, pain, and swelling. Doctors do not know why the immune system goes awry in children who develop JRA. Scientists suspect that it is a two-step process. First, something in a child's genetic makeup gives them a tendency to develop JRA; then an environmental factor, such as a virus, triggers the development of JRA.

Symptoms and Signs of Juvenile Rheumatoid Arthritis

The most common symptom of all types of JRA is persistent joint swelling, pain, and stiffness that typically is worse in the morning or after a nap. The pain may limit movement of the affected joint although many children, especially younger ones, will not complain of pain. JRA commonly affects the knees and joints in the hands and feet. One of the earliest signs of JRA may be limping in the morning because of an affected knee. Besides joint symptoms, children with systemic JRA have a high fever and a light skin rash. The rash and fever may appear and disappear very quickly. Systemic JRA also may cause the lymph nodes located in the neck and other parts of the body to swell. In some cases (less than half), internal organs including the heart, and very rarely, the lungs may be involved.

Eye inflammation is a potentially severe complication that sometimes occurs in children with pauciarticular JRA. Eye diseases such as iritis and uveitis often are not present until some time after a child first develops JRA.

Typically, there are periods when the symptoms of JRA are better or disappear (remissions) and times when symptoms are worse (flare-ups). JRA is different in each child—some may have just one or two flare-ups and never have symptoms again, while others experience many flare-ups or even have symptoms that never go away.

Some children with JRA may have growth problems. Depending on the severity of the disease and the joints involved, growth in affected joints may be too fast or too slow, causing one leg or arm to be longer than the other. Overall growth may also be slowed. Doctors are exploring the use of growth hormones to treat this problem. JRA also may cause joints to grow unevenly or to one side.

Diagnosing Juvenile Rheumatoid Arthritis

Doctors usually suspect JRA, along with several other possible conditions, when they see children with persistent joint pain or swelling, unexplained skin rashes and fever, swelling of lymph nodes, or inflammation of internal organs. A diagnosis of JRA also is considered in children with an unexplained limp or excessive clumsiness.

No single test can be used to diagnose JRA. A doctor diagnoses JRA by carefully examining the patient and considering the patient's medical history, the results of laboratory tests, and x-rays that help rule out other conditions.

- **Symptoms**—One important consideration in diagnosing JRA is the length of time that symptoms have been present. Joint swelling or pain must last for at least 6 weeks for the doctor to consider a diagnosis of JRA. Because this factor is so important, it may be useful to keep a record of the symptoms, when they first appear, and when they are worse or better.

- **Laboratory tests**—Laboratory tests, usually blood tests, cannot by themselves provide the doctor with a clear diagnosis. But these tests can be used to help rule out other conditions and to help classify the type of JRA that a patient has. Blood may be taken to test for RF and ANA, and to determine the erythrocyte sedimentation rate (ESR).

  - ANA is found in the blood more often than RF, and both are found in only a small portion of JRA patients. The RF test helps the doctor tell the difference among the three types of JRA.

  - ESR is a test that measures how quickly red blood cells fall to the bottom of a test tube. Some people with rheumatic disease have an elevated ESR or sedimentation rate (cells fall quickly to the bottom of the test tube), showing that there is inflammation in the body. Not all children with active joint inflammation have an elevated ESR.

- **X-rays**—X-rays are needed if the doctor suspects injury to the bone or unusual bone development. Early in the disease, some x-rays can show cartilage damage. In general, x-rays are more useful later in the disease, when bones may be affected.

- **Other diseases**—Because there are many causes of joint pain and swelling, the doctor must rule out other conditions before diagnosing JRA. These include physical injury, bacterial or viral infection, Lyme disease, inflammatory bowel disease, lupus, dermatomyositis, and some forms of cancer. The doctor may use additional laboratory tests to help rule out these and other possible conditions.

Treatment

The special expertise of rheumatologists in caring for patients with JRA is extremely valuable. Pediatric rheumatologists are trained in both pediatrics and rheumatology and are best equipped to deal with the complex problems of children with arthritis and other rheumatic diseases. However, there are very few such specialists, and some areas of the country have none at all. In such circumstances, a team approach involving the child's pediatrician and a rheumatologist with experience in both adult and pediatric rheumatic disease provides optimal care for children with arthritis. Other important members of the team include physical therapists and occupational therapists.

The main goals of treatment are to preserve a high level of physical and social functioning and maintain a good quality of life. To achieve these goals, doctors recommend treatments to reduce swelling; maintain full movement in the affected joints; relieve pain; and identify, treat, and prevent complications. Most children with JRA need medication and physical therapy to reach these goals.

Several types of medication and therapy are available to treat JRA:

- **Nonsteroidal anti-inflammatory drugs (NSAIDs)**—Aspirin, ibuprofen (Motrin, Advil, Nuprin), and naproxen or naproxen sodium (Naprosyn, Aleve) are examples of NSAIDs. They often are the first type of medication used. Most doctors do not treat children with aspirin because of the possibility that it will cause bleeding problems, stomach upset, liver problems, or Reye syndrome. But for some children, aspirin in the correct dose (measured by blood test) can control JRA symptoms effectively with few serious side effects. If the doctor prefers not to use aspirin, other NSAIDs are available.

- **Disease-modifying anti-rheumatic drugs (DMARDs)**—If NSAIDs do not relieve symptoms of JRA, the doctor is likely to prescribe this type of medication. DMARDs slow the progression of JRA, but because they take weeks or months to relieve symptoms, they often are taken with a NSAID. Various types of DMARDs are available. Doctors are likely to use one type of DMARD, methotrexate, for children with JRA.

- **Corticosteroids**—In children with very severe JRA, stronger medicines may be needed to stop serious symptoms such as inflammation of the sac around the heart (pericarditis). Corticosteroids like prednisone may be added to the treatment plan to control severe symptoms. This medication can be given either intravenously (directly into the vein) or by mouth. Corticosteroids can interfere with a child's normal growth and can cause other side effects, such as a round face, weakened bones, and increased susceptibility to infections. Once the medication controls severe symptoms, the doctor may reduce the dose gradually and eventually stop it completely. Because it can be dangerous to stop taking corticosteroids suddenly, it is important that the patient carefully follow the doctor's instructions about how to take or reduce the dose.

- **Biologic agents**—Children with polyarticular JRA who have gotten little relief from other drugs may be given one of a new class of drug treatments called biologic agents. Etanercept (Enbrel), for example, is such an agent. It blocks the actions of tumor necrosis factor (TNF), a naturally occurring protein in the body that helps cause inflammation.

- **Physical therapy**—Exercise is an important part of a child's treatment plan. It can help to maintain muscle tone and preserve and recover the range of motion of the joints. A physiatrist (rehabilitation specialist) or a physical therapist can design an appropriate exercise program for a person with JRA. The specialist also may recommend using splints and other devices to help maintain normal bone and joint growth.

- **Complementary and alternative medicine**—Many adults seek alternative ways of treating arthritis, such as special diets or supplements. Although these methods may not be harmful in and of themselves, no research to date shows that they help. Some people have tried acupuncture, in which thin needles are inserted at specific points in the body. Others have tried glucosamine and chondroitin sulfate, two natural substances found in and around cartilage cells, for osteoarthritis of the knee. Some alternative or complementary approaches may help a child to cope with or reduce some of the stress of living with a chronic illness. If the doctor feels the approach has value and will not harm the child, it can be incorporated into the treatment plan. However, it is important not to neglect regular health care or treatment of serious symptoms.

Family Life

JRA affects the entire family who must cope with the special challenges of this disease. JRA can strain a child's participation in social and after-school activities and make school work more difficult. There are several things that family members can do to help the child do well physically and emotionally.

- Treat the child as normally as possible.

- Ensure that the child receives appropriate medical care and follows the doctor's instructions. Many treatment options are available, and because JRA is different in each child, what works for one may not work for another.

- Encourage exercise and physical therapy for the child.

- Work closely with the school to develop a suitable lesson plan for the child and to educate the teacher and the child's classmates about JRA.

- Explain to the child that getting JRA is nobody's fault. Some children believe that JRA is a punishment for something they did.

- Consider joining a support group. The American Juvenile Arthritis Organization runs support groups for people with JRA and their families. Support group meetings provide the chance to talk to other young people and parents of children with JRA and may help a child and the family cope with the condition.

- Work with therapists or social workers to adapt more easily to the lifestyle change JRA may bring.

Physical Activity

Although pain sometimes limits physical activity, exercise is important to reduce the symptoms of JRA and maintain function and range of motion of the joints. Most children with JRA can fully participate in physical activities and sports when their symptoms are under control. During a disease flare-up, the doctor may advise limiting certain activities depending on the joints involved. Once the flare-up is over, a child can start regular activities again. Swimming is particularly useful because it uses many joints and muscles without putting weight on the joints. A doctor or physical therapist can recommend exercises and activities.

Additional Information

American Juvenile Arthritis Organization (AJAO)
P.O. Box 7669
Atlanta, GA 30357-0669
Toll-Free: 800-568-4045
Phone: 404-965-7888
Website: http://www.arthritis.org
E-mail: help@arthritis.org

AJAO is part of the National Arthritis Foundation. This organization is the primary nonprofit group devoted to childhood rheumatic diseases. It has information about JRA, support groups, and pediatric rheumatology centers around the country.

Section 35.3

Rheumatoid Arthritis

Excerpted from "Handout on Health: Rheumatoid Arthritis," National Institute of Arthritis and Musculoskeletal and Skin Diseases (NIAMS), NIH Publication No. 04–4179, revised May 2004.

Features of Rheumatoid Arthritis

Rheumatoid arthritis is an inflammatory disease that causes pain, swelling, stiffness, and loss of function in the joints. It has several special features that make it different from other kinds of arthritis. For example, rheumatoid arthritis generally occurs in a symmetrical pattern, meaning that if one knee or hand is involved, the other one also is. The disease often affects the wrist joints and the finger joints closest to the hand. It can also affect other parts of the body besides the joints. In addition, people with rheumatoid arthritis may have fatigue, occasional fevers, and a general sense of not feeling well.

Rheumatoid arthritis affects people differently. For some people, it lasts only a few months or a year or two and goes away without causing any noticeable damage. Other people have mild or moderate forms of the disease, with periods of worsening symptoms called flares, and periods in which they feel better called remissions. Still others have a severe form of the disease that is active most of the time, lasts for many years or a lifetime, and leads to serious joint damage and disability.

Although rheumatoid arthritis can have serious effects on a person's life and well-being, current treatment strategies—including pain-relieving drugs and medications that slow joint damage, a balance between rest and exercise, and patient education and support programs—allow most people with the disease to lead active and productive lives. In recent years, research has led to a new understanding of rheumatoid arthritis and has increased the likelihood that, in time, researchers will find even better ways to treat the disease.

How Rheumatoid Arthritis Develops and Progresses

The Joints

A joint is a place where two bones meet. The ends of the bones are covered by cartilage, which allows for easy movement of the two bones.

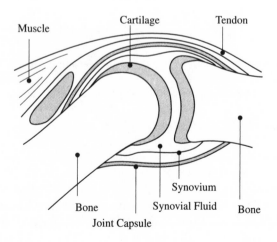

Figure 35.1. *Normal Joint*

The joint is surrounded by a capsule that protects and supports it. The joint capsule is lined with a type of tissue called synovium, which produces synovial fluid, a clear substance that lubricates and nourishes the cartilage and bones inside the joint capsule.

Like many other rheumatic diseases, rheumatoid arthritis is an autoimmune disease (auto means self), so-called because a person's immune system, which normally helps protect the body from infection and disease, attacks joint tissues for unknown reasons. White blood cells, the agents of the immune system, travel to the synovium and cause inflammation (synovitis), characterized by warmth, redness, swelling, and pain—typical symptoms of rheumatoid arthritis. During the inflammation process, the normally thin synovium becomes thick and makes the joint swollen and puffy to the touch.

As rheumatoid arthritis progresses, the inflamed synovium invades and destroys the cartilage and bone within the joint. The surrounding muscles, ligaments, and tendons that support and stabilize the joint become weak and unable to work normally. These effects lead to the pain and joint damage often seen in rheumatoid arthritis. Researchers studying rheumatoid arthritis now believe that it begins to damage bones during the first year or two that a person has the disease, one reason why early diagnosis and treatment are so important.

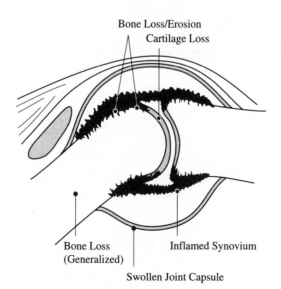

Figure 35.2. Joint Affected by Rheumatoid Arthritis

Other Parts of the Body

Some people with rheumatoid arthritis also have symptoms in places other than their joints. Many people with rheumatoid arthritis develop anemia, or a decrease in the production of red blood cells. Other effects that occur less often include neck pain and dry eyes and mouth. Very rarely, people may have inflammation of the blood vessels, the lining of the lungs, or the sac enclosing the heart.

Occurrence and Impact of Rheumatoid Arthritis

Scientists estimate that about 2.1 million people, or between 0.5 and 1 percent of the U.S. adult population, have rheumatoid arthritis. Interestingly, some recent studies have suggested that the overall number of new cases of rheumatoid arthritis actually may be going down. Scientists are investigating why this may be happening.

Rheumatoid arthritis occurs in all races and ethnic groups. Although the disease often begins in middle age and occurs with increased frequency in older people, children and young adults also develop it. Like some other forms of arthritis, rheumatoid arthritis occurs much more frequently in women than in men. About two to three times as many women as men have the disease.

By all measures, the financial and social impact of all types of arthritis, including rheumatoid arthritis, is substantial, both for the Nation and for individuals. From an economic standpoint, the medical and surgical treatment for rheumatoid arthritis and the wages lost because of disability caused by the disease add up to billions of dollars annually.

Daily joint pain is an inevitable consequence of the disease, and most patients also experience some degree of depression, anxiety, and feelings of helplessness. For some people, rheumatoid arthritis can interfere with normal daily activities, limit job opportunities, or disrupt the joys and responsibilities of family life. However, there are arthritis self-management programs that help people cope with the pain and other effects of the disease and help them lead independent and productive lives.

Searching for the Causes of Rheumatoid Arthritis

Scientists still do not know exactly what causes the immune system to turn against itself in rheumatoid arthritis, but research over the last few years has begun to piece together the factors involved.

Genetic (inherited) factors: Scientists have discovered that certain genes known to play a role in the immune system are associated with a tendency to develop rheumatoid arthritis. Some people with rheumatoid arthritis do not have these particular genes; still others have these genes, but never develop the disease. These somewhat contradictory data suggest that a person's genetic makeup plays an important role in determining if he or she will develop rheumatoid arthritis, but it is not the only factor. What is clear, however, is that more than one gene is involved in determining whether a person develops rheumatoid arthritis and how severe the disease will become.

Environmental factors: Many scientists think that something must occur to trigger the disease process in people whose genetic makeup makes them susceptible to rheumatoid arthritis. A viral or bacterial infection appears likely, but the exact agent is not yet known. This does not mean that rheumatoid arthritis is contagious: a person cannot catch it from someone else.

Other factors: Some scientists also think that a variety of hormonal factors may be involved. Women are more likely to develop rheumatoid arthritis than men, pregnancy may improve the disease, and the disease may flare after a pregnancy. Breast feeding may also aggravate the disease. Contraceptive use may alter a person's likelihood of developing rheumatoid arthritis. Scientists think that levels of the immune system molecules interleukin 12 (IL-12) and tumor necrosis factor-alpha (TNF-a) may change along with the changing hormone levels seen in pregnant women. This change may contribute to the swelling and tissue destruction seen in rheumatoid arthritis. These hormones, or possibly deficiencies or changes in certain hormones, may promote the development of rheumatoid arthritis in a genetically susceptible person who has been exposed to a triggering agent from the environment.

Even though all the answers are not known, one thing is certain: rheumatoid arthritis develops as a result of an interaction of many factors. Researchers are trying to understand these factors and how they work together.

Diagnosing and Treating Rheumatoid Arthritis

Diagnosing and treating rheumatoid arthritis requires a team effort involving the patient and several types of health care professionals. A person can go to his or her family doctor, internist, or to a rheumatologist. A rheumatologist is a doctor who specializes in arthritis and other diseases of the joints, bones, and muscles. As treatment progresses, other professionals often help. These may include nurses, physical or occupational therapists, orthopaedic surgeons, psychologists, and social workers.

Studies have shown that patients who are well informed and participate actively in their own care have less pain and make fewer visits to the doctor than do other patients with rheumatoid arthritis. Patient education and arthritis self-management programs, as well as support groups, help people to become better informed and to participate in their own care. Self-management programs teach about rheumatoid arthritis and its treatments, exercise and relaxation approaches, communication between patients and health care providers, and problem solving.

Diagnosis

Rheumatoid arthritis can be difficult to diagnose in its early stages for several reasons. First, there is no single test for the disease. In addition, symptoms differ from person to person and can be more severe in some people than in others. Also, symptoms can be similar to those of other types of arthritis and joint conditions, and it may take some time for other conditions to be ruled out. Finally, the full range of symptoms develops over time, and only a few symptoms may be present in the early stages. As a result, doctors use a variety of the following tools to diagnose the disease and to rule out other conditions:

Medical history: This is the patient's description of symptoms and when and how they began. Good communication between patient and doctor is especially important here. For example, the patient's description of pain, stiffness, and joint function, and how these change over time is critical to the doctor's initial assessment of the disease and how it changes over time.

Physical examination: This includes the doctor's examination of the joints, skin, reflexes, and muscle strength.

Laboratory tests: One common test is for rheumatoid factor, an antibody that is present eventually in the blood of most people with rheumatoid arthritis. (An antibody is a special protein made by the immune system that normally helps fight foreign substances in the body.) However, not all people with rheumatoid arthritis test positive for rheumatoid factor, especially early in the disease. Also, some people test positive for rheumatoid factor, yet never develop the disease. Other common laboratory tests include a white blood cell count, a blood test for anemia, and a test of the erythrocyte sedimentation rate (ESR), which measures inflammation in the body. C-reactive protein is another common test that measures disease activity.

X-rays: X-rays are used to determine the degree of joint destruction. They are not useful in the early stages of rheumatoid arthritis before bone damage is evident, but they can be used later to monitor the progression of the disease.

Treatment

Doctors use a variety of approaches to treat rheumatoid arthritis. These are used in different combinations and at different times during the course of the disease and are chosen according to the patient's individual situation. No matter what treatment the doctor and patient choose, the goals are the same: to relieve pain, reduce inflammation, slow down or stop joint damage, and improve the person's sense of well-being and ability to function.

Good communication between the patient and doctor is necessary for effective treatment. Talking to the doctor can help ensure that exercise and pain management programs are provided as needed, and that drugs are prescribed appropriately. Talking to the doctor can also help people who are making decisions about surgery.

Certain activities, medications, and surgery can help improve a person's ability to function independently and maintain a positive outlook. Rheumatoid arthritis treatments may include:

- **Rest and exercise:** People with rheumatoid arthritis need a good balance between rest and exercise, with more rest when the disease is active and more exercise when it is not. Rest helps to reduce active joint inflammation and pain and to fight fatigue. Exercise is important for maintaining healthy and strong muscles, preserving joint mobility, and maintaining flexibility. Exercise can also help people sleep well, reduce pain, maintain a positive attitude, and lose weight. Exercise programs should take into account the person's physical abilities, limitations, and changing needs.

- **Joint care:** Some people find using a splint for a short time around a painful joint reduces pain and swelling by supporting the joint and letting it rest. Other ways to reduce stress on joints include self-help devices (for example, zipper pullers, long-handled shoe horns); devices to help with getting on and off chairs, toilet seats, and beds; and changes in the ways that a person carries out daily activities.

- **Stress reduction:** People with rheumatoid arthritis face emotional challenges as well as physical ones. The emotions they feel because of the disease—fear, anger, and frustration—combined with any pain and physical limitations can increase their stress level. Although there is no evidence that stress plays a role in causing rheumatoid arthritis, it can make living with the disease difficult at times. Stress also may affect the amount of pain a person feels. There are a number of successful techniques for coping with stress. Regular rest periods can help, as can relaxation, distraction, or visualization exercises. Exercise programs, participation in support groups, and good communication with the health care team are other ways to reduce stress.

- **Healthful diet:** With the exception of several specific types of oils, there is no scientific evidence that any specific food or nutrient helps or harms people with rheumatoid arthritis. However, an overall nutritious diet with enough—but not an excess of—calories, protein, and calcium is important. Some people may need to be careful about drinking alcoholic beverages because of the medications they take for rheumatoid arthritis. Those taking methotrexate may need to avoid alcohol altogether because one of the most serious long-term side effects of methotrexate is liver damage.

- **Climate:** Some people notice that their arthritis gets worse when there is a sudden change in the weather. However, there is no evidence that a specific climate can prevent or reduce the effects of rheumatoid arthritis. Moving to a new place with a different climate usually does not make a long-term difference in a person's rheumatoid arthritis.

- **Medications:** Most people who have rheumatoid arthritis take medications. Some medications are used only for pain relief; others are used to reduce inflammation. Still others, often called disease-modifying antirheumatic drugs (DMARDs), are used to try to slow the course of the disease.

- **Surgery:** Several types of surgery are available to patients with severe joint damage. The primary purpose of these procedures is to reduce pain, improve the affected joint's function, and improve the patient's ability to perform daily activities. However, surgery is not for everyone, and the decision should be made only after careful consideration by patient and doctor. Together they should discuss the patient's overall health, the condition of the joint or tendon that will be operated on, and the reason for, as well as the risks and benefits of, the surgical procedure. Cost may be another factor. Commonly performed surgical procedures include joint replacement, tendon reconstruction, and synovectomy.

- *Joint replacement:* This is the most frequently performed surgery for rheumatoid arthritis, and it is done primarily to relieve pain and improve or preserve joint function. Artificial joints are not always permanent and may eventually have to be replaced. This may be an important consideration for young people.

- *Tendon reconstruction:* Rheumatoid arthritis can damage and even rupture tendons, the tissues that attach muscle to bone. This surgery, which is used most frequently on the hands, reconstructs the damaged tendon by attaching an intact tendon to it. This procedure can help to restore hand function, especially if the tendon is completely ruptured.

- *Synovectomy:* In this surgery, the doctor actually removes the inflamed synovial tissue. Synovectomy by itself is seldom performed now because not all of the tissue can be removed, and it eventually grows back. Synovectomy is done as part of reconstructive surgery, especially tendon reconstruction.

- **Routine monitoring and ongoing care:** Regular medical care is important to monitor the course of the disease, determine the effectiveness and any negative effects of medications, and change therapies as needed. Monitoring typically includes regular visits to the doctor. It also may include blood, urine, and other laboratory tests and x-rays. People with rheumatoid arthritis may want to discuss preventing osteoporosis with their doctors as part of their long-term, ongoing care. Osteoporosis is a condition in which bones become weakened and fragile. Having rheumatoid arthritis increases the risk of developing osteoporosis for both men and women, particularly if a person takes corticosteroids.

- **Alternative and complementary therapies:** Special diets, vitamin supplements, and other alternative approaches have been suggested for treating rheumatoid arthritis. Although many of these approaches may not be harmful in and of themselves, controlled scientific studies either have not been conducted on them or have found no definite benefit to these therapies. Some alternative or complementary approaches may help the patient cope or reduce some of the stress associated with living with a chronic illness. As with any therapy, patients should discuss the benefits and drawbacks with their doctors before beginning an alternative or new type of therapy. If the doctor feels the approach has value and will not be harmful, it can be incorporated into a patient's treatment plan.

Hope for the Future

Scientists are making rapid progress in understanding the complexities of rheumatoid arthritis: how and why it develops, why some people get it and others do not, why some people get it more severely than others. Results from research are having an impact today, enabling people with rheumatoid arthritis to remain active in life, family, and work far longer than was possible 20 years ago. There is also hope for tomorrow, as researchers begin to apply new technologies such as stem cell transplantation and novel imaging techniques. (Stem cells have the capacity to differentiate into specific cell types, which gives them the potential to change damaged tissue in which they are placed.) These and other advances will lead to an improved quality of life for people with rheumatoid arthritis.

Additional Information

National Institute of Arthritis and Musculoskeletal and Skin Diseases
Information Clearinghouse/NIH
1 AMS Circle
Bethesda, MD 20892-3675
Toll-Free: 877-22-NIAMS (64267)
Phone: 301-495-4484
TTY: 301-565-2966
Fast Facts: 301-881-2731 (to receive information by fax)
Website: http://www.nih.gov/niams/healthinfo
E-mail: niamsinfo@mail.nih.gov

American College of Rheumatology (ACR)
1800 Century Pl., Suite 250
Atlanta, GA 30345
Phone: 404-633-3777
Fax: 404-633-1870
Website: http://www.rheumatology.org
E-mail: acr@rheumatology.org

The College provides referrals to rheumatologists and physical and occupational therapists that have experience working with people who have rheumatoid arthritis. The organization also provides educational materials and guidelines.

Arthritis Foundation
P.O. Box 7660
Atlanta, GA 30357-0669
Toll-Free: 800-568-4045
Phone: 404-965-7888
Website: http://www.arthritis.org
E-mail: help@arthritis.org

The Arthritis Foundation is the major voluntary organization devoted to supporting arthritis research and providing educational and other services to individuals with arthritis. It also provides up-to-date information on research and treatment, nutrition, alternative therapies, and self-management strategies. Chapters nationwide offer exercise programs, classes, support groups, physician referral services, and free literature.

Chapter 36

Autoimmune Hepatitis

Autoimmune hepatitis is a disease in which the body's immune system attacks liver cells. This causes the liver to become inflamed (hepatitis). Researchers think a genetic factor may predispose some people to autoimmune diseases. About 70 percent of those with autoimmune hepatitis are women, most between the ages of 15 and 40. The disease is usually quite serious, and if not treated, gets worse over time. It is usually chronic, meaning it can last for years, and can lead to cirrhosis (scarring and hardening) of the liver and eventually liver failure.

Autoimmune hepatitis is classified as either type I or II. Type I is the most common form in North America. It occurs at any age and is more common among women than men. About half of those with type I have other autoimmune disorders, such as type 1 diabetes, proliferative glomerulonephritis, thyroiditis, Graves disease, Sjögren syndrome, autoimmune anemia, and ulcerative colitis. Type II autoimmune hepatitis is less common, typically affecting girls ages 2 to 14, although adults can have it too.

Symptoms

Fatigue is probably the most common symptom of autoimmune hepatitis. Other symptoms include the following:

"Autoimmune Hepatitis," National Institute of Diabetes and Digestive and Kidney Diseases (NIDDK), NIH Publication 04–4761, March 2004.

- enlarged liver
- jaundice
- itching
- skin rashes
- joint pain
- abdominal discomfort
- fatigue
- spider angiomas (abnormal blood vessels) on the skin
- nausea
- vomiting
- loss of appetite
- dark urine
- pale or gray colored stools

People in advanced stages of the disease are more likely to have symptoms such as fluid in the abdomen (ascites) or mental confusion. Women may stop having menstrual periods.

Symptoms of autoimmune hepatitis range from mild to severe. Because severe viral hepatitis or hepatitis caused by a drug—for example, certain antibiotics—has the same symptoms, tests may be needed for an exact diagnosis. Your doctor should also review and rule out all your medicines before diagnosing autoimmune hepatitis.

Diagnosis

Your doctor will make a diagnosis based on your symptoms, blood tests, and liver biopsy.

- **Blood tests.** A routine blood test for liver enzymes can help reveal a pattern typical of hepatitis, but further tests, especially for autoantibodies, are needed to diagnose autoimmune hepatitis. Antibodies are proteins made by the immune system to fight off bacteria and viruses. In autoimmune hepatitis, the immune system makes antinuclear antibodies (ANA), antibodies against smooth muscle cells (SMA), or liver and kidney microsomes (anti-LKM). The pattern and level of these antibodies help define the type of autoimmune hepatitis (type I or type II). Blood tests also help distinguish autoimmune hepatitis from viral hepatitis (such

288

as hepatitis B or C) or a metabolic disease (such as Wilson disease).

- **Liver biopsy.** A tiny sample of your liver tissue, examined under a microscope, can help your doctor accurately diagnose autoimmune hepatitis and tell how serious it is. You will go to a hospital or outpatient surgical facility for this procedure.

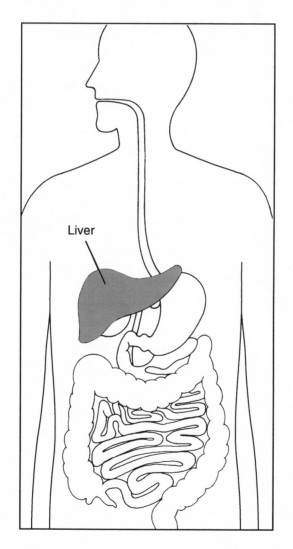

Figure 36.1. Autoimmune Hepatitis Affects the Liver.

Treatment

Treatment works best when autoimmune hepatitis is diagnosed early. With proper treatment, autoimmune hepatitis can usually be controlled. In fact, recent studies show that sustained response to treatment not only stops the disease from getting worse, but also may actually reverse some of the damage. The primary treatment is medicine to suppress (slow down) an overactive immune system.

Both types of autoimmune hepatitis are treated with daily doses of a corticosteroid called prednisone. Your doctor may start you on a high dose—20 to 60 milligrams (mg) per day—and lower the dose to 5 to 15 mg/day as the disease is controlled. The goal is to find the lowest possible dose that will control your disease.

Another medicine, azathioprine (Imuran) is also used to treat autoimmune hepatitis. Like prednisone, azathioprine suppresses the immune system, but in a different way. It helps lower the dose of prednisone needed, thereby reducing its side effects. Your doctor may prescribe azathioprine, in addition to prednisone, once your disease is under control.

Most people will need to take prednisone, with or without azathioprine, for years. Some people take it for life. Corticosteroids may slow down the disease, but everyone is different. In about one out of every three people, treatment can eventually be stopped. After stopping, it is important to carefully monitor your condition, and promptly report any new symptoms to your doctor because the disease may return and be even more severe, especially during the first few months after stopping treatment.

In about 7 out of 10 people, the disease goes into remission, with a lessening of severity of symptoms within 2 years of starting treatment. A portion of persons with a remission will see the disease return within 3 years, so treatment may be necessary on and off for years, if not for life.

Side Effects

Both prednisone and azathioprine have side effects. Because high doses of prednisone are needed to control autoimmune hepatitis, managing side effects is very important. However, most side effects appear only after a long period of time.

Some possible side effects of prednisone are:

- weight gain,
- anxiety and confusion,

- thinning of the bones (osteoporosis),
- thinning of the hair and skin,
- diabetes,
- high blood pressure,
- cataracts, and
- glaucoma.

Azathioprine can lower your white blood cell count and sometimes causes nausea and poor appetite. Rare side effects are allergic reaction, liver damage, and pancreatitis (inflammation of the pancreas gland with severe stomach pain).

Other Treatments

People who do not respond to standard immune therapy or who have severe side effects may benefit from other immunosuppressive agents like mycophenolate mofetil, cyclosporine, or tacrolimus. People who progress to end stage liver disease (liver failure) and/or cirrhosis may need a liver transplant. Transplantation has a 1-year survival rate of 90 percent and a 5-year survival rate of 70 to 80 percent.

Points to Remember

- Autoimmune hepatitis is a long-term disease in which your body's immune system attacks liver cells.

- The disease is diagnosed using various blood tests and a liver biopsy.

- With proper treatment, autoimmune hepatitis can usually be controlled. The main treatment is medicine that suppresses the body's overactive immune system.

Additional Information

American Liver Foundation
75 Maiden Lane, Suite 603
New York, NY 10038
Toll-Free: 800-465-4837
Phone: 212-668-1000
Fax: 212-483-8179
Website: http://www.liverfoundation.org
E-mail: info@liverfoundation.org

National Institute of Diabetes and Digestive and Kidney Diseases (NIDDK)

Information Clearinghouse
5 Information Way
Bethesda, MD 20892-3560
Toll-Free: 800-860-8747
Phone: 301-654-3810
Website: http://www.niddk.nih.gov

Chapter 37

Autoimmune Lymphoproliferative Syndrome (ALPS)

Doctors at the National Institutes of Health (NIH) saw a child who had immune system symptoms that did not fit any previously known disorders. They began to study these problems in 1990. Since then, dozens of other children and adults with similar problems have been identified and followed at NIH. In 1995, this newly identified condition was named autoimmune lymphoproliferative syndrome or ALPS. By August 1999, 58 individuals from 35 families had been diagnosed with ALPS. These families come from all over the country and are of many different racial backgrounds.

Clinical Features of ALPS

Some signs of ALPS are ones that people can feel or see, and some of them can be detected only by laboratory tests. Not all people with ALPS will have all of its possible symptoms. Some people have only a few. ALPS symptoms often include the following:

- An enlarged spleen
- Enlarged lymph nodes, especially in the neck and underarms
- An enlarged liver
- Skin rashes
- Frequent nose bleeds

Excerpted from "Learning about Autoimmune Lymphoproliferative Syndrome (ALPS)," National Human Genome Research Institute (NHGRI), updated April 2004.

- Anemia (low blood counts)
- An increase in certain types of white blood cells (including double-negative T cells)
- An increased life-span of some white blood cells that are no longer needed
- An alteration in a gene

What Is ALPS?

ALPS is a rare disease that affects both children and adults. ALPS stands for autoimmune lymphoproliferative (lim-fo-pro-lif'-er-a-tive) syndrome. Each of these three words helps describe the main features of this condition. The word autoimmune (self-immune) identifies ALPS as a disease of the immune system. The tools used to fight germs turn against our own cells and cause problems. The word lymphoproliferative describes the unusually large numbers of white blood cells (called lymphocytes (lim'-fo-sites)) stored in the lymph nodes and spleens of people with ALPS. The word syndrome refers to the many common symptoms shared by ALPS patients.

Doctors are still learning about ALPS. Based on experiences at the NIH, the following is believed to be true:

- ALPS is a disorder that develops in early childhood.
- ALPS is not cancer; it is not contagious; it is not AIDS.
- There is a wide spectrum of illness in ALPS. For some, it is very mild; for others, it is more severe.
- Once a person has ALPS, he or she does not become sicker and sicker over time. In fact, the problems seem to improve as children get to be teenagers and young adults.
- Most people with ALPS have episodes of autoimmune problems. These can happen at any age, but they appear worse in childhood.

Types of Autoimmune Problems

Common autoimmune problems in ALPS include:

- Very low red blood cell counts (hemolytic anemia) that can make one weak.
- Very low platelet counts (immune-mediated thrombocytopenia, or ITP) that cause bruises and nose bleeds, and may pose a risk

for hemorrhage (excessive bleeding). Little spots called petechiae (pet-eek'-ia) may also show up on the skin when platelets are low.

- Very low white blood cell counts (autoimmune neutropenia), creating a risk for bacterial infection.

- Less often, other autoimmune problems can occur in almost any organ—skin, liver, kidney, and nerves are examples.

What Happens in ALPS?

To better understand how ALPS works, imagine that you have a respiratory infection, perhaps the flu. The cells in the nose and throat send out a message to the immune system to start making more lymphocytes to fight the flu. New troops of lymphocytes come to the nose and throat to seek out and destroy the cells infected with the flu virus. Once the virus is conquered, the lymphocytes get a message that their job is done and they are no longer needed. At this point, it is normal for most of the fighter cells to disintegrate through a process called apoptosis (a-pop-TO-sis).

The immune systems of people with ALPS are efficient in fighting germs. The problem in ALPS happens after an infection is gone. In ALPS, apoptosis does not work as well as it should. In other words, the troops (lymphocytes) do not hear the message that the war is over. As a result, excess T and B cells gather in the lymph glands, liver, and spleen. We can detect the extra cells in people with ALPS by looking for high numbers of double-negative T cells. In general, these extra T cells do not cause a problem.

Sometimes in ALPS, the B cells make a mistake. Instead of making antibodies to be custom-designed against germs, the B cells make antibodies against platelets, red blood cells, or other cells. This causes autoimmune problems. The antibodies become stuck to the platelets and red blood cells, which then get stuck in the spleen. The spleen has to work extra hard to filter out the sticky cells. This is another reason why the spleen gets so big.

Management of ALPS

There is no cure for ALPS. However, most of its complications can be treated and prevented. Management of ALPS involves:

- **Diagnosis.** You probably know from experience that this may take months or years until you find a doctor who recognizes the features of ALPS.

- **Counseling and education.** The more you know about ALPS and how to recognize its symptoms and signs, the better you will be able to manage it.

- **Knowing what is treatable.** Unfortunately, ways have not been found which permanently make the swelling of lymph nodes go down or to fix the problem with apoptosis.

- **Therapies.** Complications of ALPS, including the many different autoimmune problems, can be treated successfully. ALPS can be managed through close communication with doctors as symptoms and signs arise.

Managing Enlarged Spleens in ALPS

Virtually all people with ALPS have an oversized spleen. Usually, it is not necessary to remove the spleen unless there are severe problems like anemia. However, removing a spleen carries both risks and benefits, which doctors and patients must carefully consider before deciding what to do.

Benefits of Splenectomy

- It will be easier to regulate and control blood counts.
- There is less discomfort.
- There is no longer a risk of spleen rupture, a very serious problem, should it occur.

Risks of Splenectomy

- After splenectomy, people with ALPS are missing an organ which helps protect against infection. The chances of getting certain bacterial infections increase, so people with ALPS must get some vaccines to avoid these infections.

- After the spleen is removed, people with ALPS may need to take antibiotics for many years to help prevent specific bacterial infections.

Managing Autoimmune Problems in ALPS

Steroids are the first line of treatment for autoimmune episodes, like hemolytic anemia and ITP. One common steroid is prednisone. It is often given for a short time, but sometimes it is needed for longer periods. When prednisone is not enough to treat the episode, other drugs, such as Imuran and cyclosporin, may also be prescribed. Steroids have saved lives and have dramatically reduced the complications in some people with ALPS. However, like all treatments, steroids have some disadvantages, so they should not be used too much or for too long.

Possible Long-Term Side Effects of Steroids

- Thinning of bones
- Poor wound healing
- Difficulty in fighting infection
- Diabetes
- Cataracts of the eyes
- Mood swings
- Weight gain

The body starts to rely on the steroids and the amount has to be slowly reduced.

Treatments

- **Blood transfusions** are useful to replace red blood cells when anemia is severe.

- **Vaccines** are important to help prevent infections. In addition to all the childhood vaccinations, it is important to get a yearly flu shot and boosters as needed. People with allergies to eggs should discuss this with their doctor prior to receiving a flu shot.

- **Gene therapy** is unfortunately not likely to work for ALPS.

Genetic Connection

Children can inherit ALPS from one of their parents. The process of apoptosis is controlled by several genes. Most people with ALPS have an altered gene that plays a major role in apoptosis. The altered gene may be passed from one generation to the next.

What is the Fas gene?

Genetic changes or mutations have been found that seem to be factors in the development of ALPS. In over 83 percent of the ALPS patients, an alteration has been found in a gene that encodes a cell component, or protein, called *Fas*. This alteration causes the gene to produce abnormal *Fas* protein. It is not completely understand how abnormal *Fas* protein leads to ALPS, but it clearly does. Identification of other genetic and non-genetic factors that contribute to the development of ALPS is still needed.

The *Fas* protein is one of several proteins that are important for apoptosis, the normal process through which cells die. *Fas* controls the life span of certain cells, particularly the lymphocytes. Like people, cells have a normal life span in which they grow, do their job, and then die. The mutated *Fas* protein does not work well, and cannot give the cells the message that it is time to die. Although most ALPS patients have one normal and one altered copy of the *Fas* gene, the altered protein is able to interfere with the function of the normal one.

However, *Fas* mutations do not explain all cases of ALPS. About 17 percent of people with ALPS do not have a *Fas* mutation. In some of them there are alterations in other proteins known as *Fas*-ligand and Caspase-10. In some ALPS patients a genetic alteration has not yet been found. Also, there are many relatives of ALPS patients who have a *Fas* mutation and do not have ALPS. It is believed that other genes and environmental factors also play a role determining which people get ALPS.

Are children at risk if a parent has a Fas gene mutation?

There are many people who have no signs of ALPS, yet have a *Fas* mutation. Individuals with a *Fas* mutation have a 50/50 chance of passing the *Fas* mutation on to their children. That means that each child has a 50 percent chance of inheriting the unaffected gene and a 50 percent chance of inheriting the altered gene. This chance is the same for each child. In other words, if you have 5 children and they have each inherited the *Fas* mutation, the sixth child still has the same 50/50 risk of inheriting the *Fas* mutation. Of the children who inherit the *Fas* mutation, approximately half of them will develop some features of ALPS. This figure is based on the 98 people studied so far at NIH who have a *Fas* gene mutation. Of these 98 people with the *Fas* gene mutation, 48 have enough symptoms to be diagnosed with ALPS and additional persons have some features of ALPS. Children who have inherited the unaltered *Fas* gene have almost no chance of developing ALPS.

Is ALPS contagious?

ALPS is not infectious.

Is it safe to play contact sports?

Sometimes doctors recommend that people with enlarged spleens not play contact sports. When the spleen is large, it is fragile and there is a risk of rupture. The NIH encourages people with large spleens to wear spleen guards. A spleen guard is a piece of fiberglass that is molded to a person's stomach. It is easily wrapped around your stomach and held in place under your shirt. In general, the spleen guard is worn whenever someone is involved in an activity at high risk for stomach injury, such as contact sports.

Additional Information

NIH Clinical Center
Patient Recruitment and Public Liaison Office
10 Cloister Ct., Building 61
Bethesda, MD 20892-4754
Toll-Free: 800-411-1222
Toll-Free TTY: 866-411-1010
TTY (local): 301-594-9774
Fax: 301-480-9793
Website: http://clinicalstudies.info.nih.gov/detail/A_1993-I-0063.html
E-mail: prpl@mail.cc.nih.gov

Physicians from around the country refer families suspected of having ALPS to be evaluated at the NIH Clinical Center. Their blood is studied for specific laboratory findings related to ALPS. After reviewing the medical records and lab results, the team invites those who may have ALPS to NIH for evaluation and follow-up. Many referrals have been received indicating that ALPS may be more common than once thought.

There is a genetic component to ALPS. However, the development of ALPS in families with mutations in apoptosis genes is not straightforward. Therefore, ALPS family members have been invited to join the NIH study by providing a small sample of their blood in order to help answer research questions.

Each person who is interested in participating in the ALPS study will have a chance to discuss study details with the investigators. Each person will be asked to read and sign a consent form. All of the tests, evaluations, and treatments at the NIH are free.

Chapter 38

Behçet Disease

What is Behçet disease?

The disease was first described in 1937 by Dr. Hulusi Behçet, a dermatologist in Turkey. Behçet disease is now recognized as a chronic condition that causes canker sores or ulcers in the mouth and on the genitals, and inflammation in parts of the eye. In some people, the disease also results in arthritis (swollen, painful, stiff joints), skin problems, and inflammation of the digestive tract, brain, and spinal cord.

Who gets Behçet disease?

Behçet disease is common in the Middle East, Asia, and Japan; it is rare in the United States. In Middle Eastern and Asian countries, the disease affects more men than women. In the United States, the opposite is true. Behçet disease tends to develop in people in their 20s or 30s, but people of all ages can develop this disease.

What causes Behçet disease?

The exact cause of Behçet disease is unknown. Most symptoms of the disease are caused by inflammation of the blood vessels. Inflammation is a characteristic reaction of the body to injury or disease and

Excerpted from "Questions and Answers about Behçet's Disease," National Institute of Arthritis and Musculoskeletal and Skin Diseases (NIAMS), NIH Publication No. 04–5026, April 2004.

is marked by four signs: swelling, redness, heat, and pain. Doctors think that an autoimmune reaction may cause the blood vessels to become inflamed, but they do not know what triggers this reaction. Under normal conditions, the immune system protects the body from diseases and infections by killing harmful foreign substances, such as germs, that enter the body. In an autoimmune reaction, the immune system mistakenly attacks and harms the body's own tissues.

Behçet disease is not contagious; it is not spread from one person to another. Researchers think that two factors are important for a person to get Behçet disease. First, it is believed that abnormalities of the immune system make some people susceptible to the disease. Scientists think that this susceptibility may be inherited; that is, it may be due to one or more specific genes. Second, something in the environment, possibly a bacterium or virus, might trigger or activate the disease in susceptible people.

What are the symptoms of Behçet disease?

Behçet disease affects each person differently. Some people have only mild symptoms, such as canker sores or ulcers in the mouth or on the genitals. Others have more severe signs, such as meningitis, which is an inflammation of the membranes that cover the brain and spinal cord. Meningitis can cause fever, a stiff neck, and headaches. More severe symptoms usually appear months or years after a person notices the first signs of Behçet disease. Symptoms can last for a long time or may come and go in a few weeks. Typically, symptoms appear, disappear, and then reappear. The times when a person is having symptoms are called flares. Different symptoms may occur with each flare; the problems of the disease often do not occur together. To help the doctor diagnose Behçet disease and monitor its course, patients may want to keep a record of which symptoms occur and when. Because many conditions mimic Behçet disease, physicians must observe the lesions (injuries) caused by the disorder in order to make an accurate diagnosis.

The five most common symptoms of Behçet disease are mouth sores, genital sores, other skin lesions, inflammation of parts of the eye, and arthritis.

- **Mouth sores** (known as oral aphthosis [af-THO-sis] and aphthous stomatitis) affect almost all patients with Behçet disease. Individual sores or ulcers are usually identical to canker sores, which are common in many people. They are often the first symptom that a person notices and may occur long before any other symptoms appear. The sores usually have a red border and several may appear at the same time. They may be painful and can make eating difficult. Mouth sores go away in 10 to 14 days, but often come back. Small sores usually heal without scarring, but larger sores may scar.

- **Genital sores** affect more than half of all people with Behçet disease and most commonly appear on the scrotum in men and vulva in women. The sores look similar to the mouth sores and may be painful. After several outbreaks, they may cause scarring.

- **Skin problems** are a common symptom of Behçet disease. Skin sores often look red or resemble pus-filled bumps or a bruise. The sores are red and raised, and typically appear on the legs and on the upper torso. In some people, sores or lesions may appear when the skin is scratched or pricked. When doctors suspect that a person has Behçet disease, they may perform a pathergy test in which they prick the skin with a small needle; 1 to 2 days after the test, people with Behçet disease may develop a red bump where the doctor pricked the skin. However, only half of the Behçet patients in Middle Eastern countries and Japan have this reaction. It is less commonly observed in patients from the United States, but if this reaction occurs, then Behçet disease is likely.

- **Uveitis** (yoo-vee-EYE-tis) involves inflammation of the middle or back part of the eye (the uvea) including the iris, and occurs in more than half of all people with Behçet disease. This symptom is more common among men than women and typically begins within 2 years of the first symptoms. Eye inflammation can cause blurred vision; rarely, it causes pain and redness. Because partial loss of vision or blindness can result if the eye frequently becomes inflamed, patients should report these symptoms to their doctor immediately.

- **Arthritis**, which is inflammation of the joints, occurs in more than half of all patients with Behçet disease. Arthritis causes pain, swelling, and stiffness in the joints, especially in the knees, ankles, wrists, and elbows. Arthritis that results from Behçet disease usually lasts a few weeks and does not cause permanent damage to the joints.

In addition to mouth and genital sores, other skin lesions, eye inflammation, and arthritis, Behçet disease may also cause blood clots and inflammation in the central nervous system and digestive organs.

Blood Clots: About 16 percent of patients with Behçet disease have blood clots resulting from inflammation in the veins (thrombophlebitis), usually in the legs. Symptoms include pain and tenderness in the affected area. The area may also be swollen and warm. Because thrombophlebitis can have severe complications, people should report symptoms to their doctor immediately. A few patients may experience artery problems such as aneurysms (balloon-like swelling of the artery wall).

Central Nervous System: Behçet disease affects the central nervous system in about 23 percent of all patients with the disease in the United States. The central nervous system includes the brain and spinal cord. Its function is to process information and coordinate thinking, behavior, sensation, and movement. Behçet disease can cause inflammation of the brain and the thin membrane that covers and protects the brain and spinal cord. This condition is called meningoencephalitis. People with meningoencephalitis may have fever, headache, stiff neck, and difficulty coordinating movement, and should report any of these symptoms to their doctor immediately. If this condition is left untreated, a stroke (blockage or rupture of blood vessels in the brain) can result.

Digestive Tract: Rarely, Behçet disease causes inflammation and ulceration (sores) throughout the digestive tract that are identical to the aphthous lesions in the mouth and genital area. This leads to abdominal pain, diarrhea, and/or bleeding. Because these symptoms are very similar to symptoms of other diseases of the digestive tract, such as ulcerative colitis and Crohn disease, careful evaluation is essential to rule out these other diseases.

How is Behçet disease diagnosed?

Diagnosing Behçet disease is very difficult because no specific test confirms it. Less than half of patients initially thought to have Behçet disease actually have it. When a patient reports symptoms, the doctor must examine the patient and rule out other conditions with similar symptoms. Because it may take several months or even years for all the common symptoms to appear, the diagnosis may not be made for a long time. A patient may even visit several different kinds of doctors before the diagnosis is made.

These symptoms are key to a diagnosis of Behçet disease:

• Mouth sores at least three times in 12 months.

- Any two of the following symptoms: recurring genital sores, eye inflammation with loss of vision, characteristic skin lesions, or positive pathergy (skin prick test).

Besides finding these signs, the doctor must rule out other conditions with similar symptoms, such as Crohn disease and reactive arthritis. The doctor also may recommend that the patient see an eye specialist to identify possible complications related to eye inflammation. A dermatologist may perform a biopsy of mouth, genital, or skin lesions to help distinguish Behçet from other disorders.

What kind of doctor treats a patient with Behçet disease?

Because the disease affects different parts of the body, a patient probably will see several different doctors. It may be helpful to both the doctors and the patient for one doctor to manage the complete treatment plan. This doctor can coordinate the treatments and monitor any side effects from the various medications that the patient takes.

A rheumatologist (a doctor specializing in arthritis and other inflammatory disorders) often manages a patient's treatment and treats joint disease. The following specialists also treat other symptoms that affect the different body systems:

- Gynecologist—treats genital sores in women
- Urologist—treats genital sores in men
- Dermatologist—treats genital sores in men and women, and skin and mucous membrane problems
- Ophthalmologist—treats eye inflammation
- Gastroenterologist—treats digestive tract symptoms
- Hematologist—treats disorders of the blood
- Neurologist—treats central nervous system symptoms

How is Behçet disease treated?

Although there is no cure for Behçet disease, people usually can control symptoms with proper medication, rest, exercise, and a healthy lifestyle. The goal of treatment is to reduce discomfort and prevent serious complications such as disability from arthritis or blindness. The type of medicine and the length of treatment depend on the person's symptoms and their severity. It is likely that a combination of treatments will be needed to relieve specific symptoms. Patients should tell each of their doctors about all of the medicines they are taking so that the doctors can coordinate treatment.

Topical Medicine: Topical medicine is applied directly on the sores to relieve pain and discomfort. For example, doctors prescribe rinses, gels, or ointments. Creams are used to treat skin and genital sores. The medicine usually contains corticosteroids (which reduce inflammation), other anti-inflammatory drugs, or an anesthetic, which relieves pain.

Oral Medicine: Doctors also prescribe medicines taken by mouth to reduce inflammation throughout the body, suppress the overactive immune system, and relieve symptoms. Doctors may prescribe one or more of the medicines described to treat the various symptoms of Behçet disease.

- *Corticosteroids*—Prednisone is a corticosteroid prescribed to reduce pain and inflammation throughout the body for people with severe joint pain, skin sores, eye disease, or central nervous system symptoms. Patients must carefully follow the doctor's instructions about when to take prednisone and how much to take. It also is important not to stop taking the medicine suddenly, because the medicine alters the body's production of the natural corticosteroid hormones. Long-term use of prednisone can have side effects such as osteoporosis (a disease that leads to bone fragility), weight gain, delayed wound healing, persistent heartburn, and elevated blood pressure. However, these side effects are rare when prednisone is taken at low doses for a short time. It is important that patients see their doctor regularly to monitor possible side effects. Corticosteroids are useful in early stages of disease and for acute severe flares. They are of limited use for long-term management of central nervous system and serious eye complications.

- *Immunosuppressive drugs*—These medicines (in addition to corticosteroids) help control an overactive immune system, which occurs in Behçet disease, reduce inflammation throughout the body, and can lessen the number of disease flares. Doctors may use immunosuppressive drugs when a person has eye disease or central nervous system involvement. These medicines are very strong and can have serious side effects. Patients must see their doctor regularly for blood tests to detect and monitor side effects.

Doctors may use one or more of the following immunosuppressive drugs depending on the person's specific symptoms.

- *Azathioprine*—Most commonly prescribed for people with organ transplants because it suppresses the immune system, azathioprine is now used for people with Behçet disease to treat uveitis and other uncontrolled disease manifestations. This medicine can upset the stomach and may reduce production of new blood cells by the bone marrow.

- *Chlorambucil or Cyclophosphamide*—Doctors may use these drugs to treat uveitis and meningoencephalitis. People taking either agent must see their doctor frequently because either can have serious side effects, such as permanent sterility and cancers of the blood. Patients have regular blood tests to monitor blood counts of white cells and platelets.

- *Cyclosporine*—Like azathioprine, doctors prescribe this medicine for people with organ transplants. When used by patients with Behçet disease, cyclosporine reduces uveitis and uncontrolled disease in other organs. To reduce the risk of side effects, such as kidney and liver disease, the doctor can adjust the dose. Patients must tell their doctor if they take any other medicines, because some medicines affect the way the body uses cyclosporine.

- *Colchicine*—Commonly used to treat gout, which is a form of arthritis, colchicine reduces inflammation throughout the body. The medicine sometimes is used to treat arthritis, mucous membrane, and skin symptoms in patients with Behçet disease. A research study in Turkey suggested that the medication works best for males with the disorder. Common side effects of colchicine include nausea, vomiting, and diarrhea. The doctor can decrease the dose to relieve these side effects.

- *Combination treatment*—Cyclosporine is sometimes used with azathioprine when one alone fails. Prednisone along with an immunosuppressive drug is a common combination.

If these medicines do not reduce the symptoms, doctors may use other drugs such as methotrexate. Methotrexate (Rheumatrex, Trexall), which is also used to treat various kinds of cancer as well as rheumatoid arthritis, can relieve Behçet symptoms because it suppresses the immune system and reduces inflammation throughout the body.

Rest and Exercise: Although rest is important during flares, doctors usually recommend moderate exercise, such as swimming or walking, when the symptoms have improved or disappeared. Exercise can help people with Behçet disease keep their joints strong and flexible.

What is the prognosis for a person with Behçet disease?

Most people with Behçet disease can lead productive lives and control symptoms with proper medicine, rest, and exercise. Doctors can use many medicines to relieve pain, treat symptoms, and prevent complications. When treatment is effective, flares usually become less frequent. Many patients eventually enter a period of remission (a disappearance of symptoms). In some people, treatment does not relieve symptoms, and gradually more serious symptoms such as eye disease may occur. Serious symptoms may appear months or years after the first signs of Behçet disease.

What are researchers trying to learn about Behçet disease?

Researchers are exploring possible genetic, bacterial, and viral causes of Behçet disease as well as improved drug treatment. For example, genetic studies show strong association of the gene HLA-B51 with the disease, but the exact role of this gene in the development of Behçet is uncertain. Researchers hope to identify genes that increase a person's risk for developing Behçet disease. Studies of these genes and how they work may provide new understanding of the disease and possibly new treatments.

Researchers are also investigating factors in the environment, such as bacteria or viruses that may trigger Behçet disease. They are particularly interested in whether *Streptococcus*, the bacterium that causes strep throat, is associated with Behçet disease. Many people with Behçet disease have had several strep infections. In addition, researchers suspect that herpesvirus type 1, a virus that causes cold sores, may be associated with Behçet disease.

Finally, researchers are identifying other medicines to better treat Behçet disease. Tumor necrosis factor (TNF) inhibitors are a class of

Behçet Disease

drugs that reduce joint inflammation. Although serious side effects have been reported for TNF inhibitors, they have shown some promise in treating Behçet disease. Examples of TNF inhibitors include etanercept and infliximab. Also, interferon alpha, a protein that helps fight infection, has shown promise in treating Behçet disease. Thalidomide, which is believed to be a TNF inhibitor, appears effective in treating severe mouth sores, but its use is experimental and side effects are a concern. Thalidomide is not used to treat women of childbearing age because it causes severe birth defects.

Additional Information

American Academy of Dermatology (AAD)
P.O. Box 4014
Schaumberg, IL 60168-4014
Toll-Free: 888-462-3376
Phone: 847-330-0230
Fax: 847-330-0050
Website: http://www.aad.org

American Behçet's Disease Association
P.O. Box 19952
Amarillo, TX 79114
Toll-Free: 800-723-4238
Website: http://www.behcets.com

American College of Rheumatology (ACR)
1800 Century Pl., Suite 250
Atlanta, GA 30345
Phone: 404-633-3777
Fax: 404-633-1870
Website: http://www.rheumatology.org
E-mail: acr@rheumatology.org

American Skin Association (ASA)
346 Park Ave. S., 4th Floor
New York, NY 10010
Toll-Free: 800-499-SKIN (7546)
Phone: 212-889-4858
Fax: 212-889-4959
Website: http://www.americanskin.org
E-mail: info@americanskin.org

Arthritis Foundation
P.O. Box 7660
Atlanta, GA 30357-0669
Toll-Free: 800-568-4045
Phone: 404-965-7888
Website: http://www.arthritis.org
E-mail: help@arthritis.org

National Eye Institute
31 Center Dr., MSC 2510
Bethesda, MD 20892-2510
Phone: 301-496-5248
Website: http://www.nei.nih.gov

National Institute of Arthritis and Musculoskeletal and Skin Diseases
Information Clearinghouse/NIH
1 AMS Circle
Bethesda, MD 20892-3675
Toll-Free: 877-22-NIAMS (64267)
Phone: 301-495-4484
TTY: 301-565-2966
Fast Facts: 301-881-2731 (to receive information by fax)
Website: http://www.nih.gov/niams/healthinfo
E-mail: niamsinfo@mail.nih.gov

National Institute of Neurological Disorders and Stroke
P.O. Box 5801
Bethesda, MD 20824
Toll-Free: 800-352-9424
Phone: 301-496-5751
TTY: 301-468-5981
Website: http://www.ninds.nih.gov

Chapter 39

Celiac Disease

Celiac disease is a digestive disease that damages the small intestine and interferes with absorption of nutrients from food. People who have celiac disease cannot tolerate a protein called gluten, which is found in wheat, rye, and barley. When people with celiac disease eat foods containing gluten, their immune system responds by damaging the small intestine. Specifically, tiny finger-like protrusions, called villi, on the lining of the small intestine are lost. Nutrients from food are absorbed into the bloodstream through these villi. Without villi, a person becomes malnourished—regardless of the quantity of food eaten.

Because the body's own immune system causes the damage, celiac disease is considered an autoimmune disorder. However, it is also classified as a disease of malabsorption because nutrients are not absorbed. Celiac disease is also known as celiac sprue, nontropical sprue, and gluten-sensitive enteropathy.

Celiac disease is a genetic disease, meaning that it runs in families. Sometimes the disease is triggered—or becomes active for the first time—after surgery, pregnancy, childbirth, viral infection, or severe emotional stress.

Symptoms

Celiac disease affects people differently. Some people develop symptoms as children, others as adults. One factor thought to play a role

Excerpted from "Celiac Disease," National Institute of Diabetes and Digestive and Kidney Diseases (NIDDK), NIH Publication No. 04–4269, February 2004.

in when and how celiac appears is whether and how long a person was breast fed—the longer one was breast fed, the later symptoms of celiac disease appear and the more atypical the symptoms. Other factors include the age at which one began eating foods containing gluten and how much gluten is eaten.

Symptoms may or may not occur in the digestive system. For example, one person might have diarrhea and abdominal pain, while another person has irritability or depression. In fact, irritability is one of the most common symptoms in children.

Symptoms of celiac disease may include one or more of the following:

- recurring abdominal bloating and pain
- chronic diarrhea
- weight loss
- pale, foul-smelling stool
- unexplained anemia (low count of red blood cells)
- gas
- bone pain
- behavior changes
- muscle cramps
- fatigue
- delayed growth
- failure to thrive in infants
- pain in the joints
- seizures
- tingling numbness in the legs (from nerve damage)
- pale sores inside the mouth, called aphthous ulcers
- painful skin rash, called dermatitis herpetiformis
- tooth discoloration or loss of enamel
- missed menstrual periods (often because of excessive weight loss)

Anemia, delayed growth, and weight loss are signs of malnutrition—not getting enough nutrients. Malnutrition is a serious problem for anyone, but particularly for children because they need adequate nutrition to develop properly.

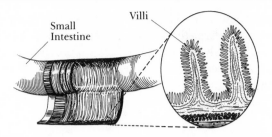

Figure 39.1. Villi on the lining of the small intestine help absorb nutrients.

Some people with celiac disease may not have symptoms. The undamaged part of their small intestine is able to absorb enough nutrients to prevent symptoms. However, people without symptoms are still at risk for the complications of celiac disease.

Diagnosing Celiac Disease

Diagnosing celiac disease can be difficult because some of its symptoms are similar to those of other diseases, including irritable bowel syndrome, Crohn disease, ulcerative colitis, diverticulosis, intestinal infections, chronic fatigue syndrome, and depression. Recently, researchers discovered that people with celiac disease have higher than normal levels of certain antibodies in their blood. Antibodies are produced by the immune system in response to substances that the body perceives to be threatening. To diagnose celiac disease, physicians test blood to measure levels of antibodies to endomysium and tissue transglutaminase.

If the tests and symptoms suggest celiac disease, the physician may remove a tiny piece of tissue from the small intestine to check for damage to the villi. This is done in a procedure called a biopsy: the physician eases a long, thin tube called an endoscope through the mouth and stomach into the small intestine, and then takes a sample of tissue using instruments passed through the endoscope. Biopsy of the small intestine is the best way to diagnose celiac disease.

Screening

Screening for celiac disease involves testing asymptomatic people for the antibodies. Americans are not routinely screened for celiac disease. However, because celiac disease is hereditary, family members—particularly first-degree relatives—of people who have been

313

diagnosed may need to be tested for the disease. About 10 percent of an affected person's first-degree relatives (parents, siblings, or children) will also have the disease. The longer a person goes undiagnosed and untreated, the greater the chance of developing malnutrition and other complications.

Treatment

The only treatment for celiac disease is to follow a gluten-free diet—that is, to avoid all foods that contain gluten. For most people, following this diet will stop symptoms, heal existing intestinal damage, and prevent further damage. Improvements begin within days of starting the diet, and the small intestine is usually completely healed—meaning the villi are intact and working—in 3 to 6 months. (It may take up to 2 years for older adults.)

The gluten-free diet is a lifetime requirement. Eating any gluten, no matter how small an amount, can damage the intestine. This is true for anyone with the disease, including people who do not have noticeable symptoms. Depending on a person's age at diagnosis, some problems, such as delayed growth and tooth discoloration, may not improve.

A small percentage of people with celiac disease do not improve on the gluten-free diet. These people often have severely damaged intestines that cannot heal even after they eliminate gluten from their diet. Because their intestines are not absorbing enough nutrients, they may need to receive intravenous nutrition supplements. Drug treatments are being evaluated for unresponsive celiac disease. These patients may need to be evaluated for complications of the disease.

Gluten-Free Diet

A gluten-free diet means avoiding all foods that contain wheat (including spelt, triticale, and kamut), rye, and barley—in other words, most grain, pasta, cereal, and many processed foods. Despite these restrictions, people with celiac disease can eat a well-balanced diet with a variety of foods, including bread and pasta. For example, instead of wheat flour, people can use potato, rice, soy, or bean flour. Or, they can buy gluten-free bread, pasta, and other products from special food companies.

Whether people with celiac disease should avoid oats is controversial because some people have been able to eat oats without having a reaction. Scientists are doing studies to find out whether people with celiac disease can tolerate oats. Until the studies are complete, people with celiac disease should follow their physician or dietitian's advice about eating oats. A dietitian is a health care professional who specializes in food and nutrition. Plain meat, fish, rice, fruits, and vegetables do not contain gluten, so people with celiac disease can eat as much of these foods as they like.

The gluten-free diet is complicated. It requires a completely new approach to eating that affects a person's entire life. People with celiac disease have to be extremely careful about what they buy for lunch at school or work, eat at cocktail parties, or grab from the refrigerator for a midnight snack. Eating out can be a challenge as the person with celiac disease learns to scrutinize the menu for foods with gluten and question the waiter or chef about possible hidden sources of gluten. Hidden sources of gluten include additives, preservatives, and stabilizers found in processed food, medicines, and mouthwash. If ingredients are not itemized, you may want to check with the manufacturer of the product. With practice, screening for gluten becomes second nature.

A dietitian can help people learn about their new diet. Also, support groups are particularly helpful for newly diagnosed people and their families as they learn to adjust to a new way of life.

Complications of Celiac Disease

Damage to the small intestine and the resulting problems with nutrient absorption put a person with celiac disease at risk for several diseases and health problems.

- Lymphoma and adenocarcinoma are types of cancer that can develop in the intestine.

- Osteoporosis is a condition in which the bones become weak, brittle, and prone to breaking. Poor calcium absorption is a contributing factor to osteoporosis.

- Miscarriage and congenital malformation of the baby, such as neural tube defects, are risks for untreated pregnant women with celiac disease because of malabsorption of nutrients.

- Short stature results when childhood celiac disease prevents nutrient absorption during the years when nutrition is critical to a child's normal growth and development. Children who are diagnosed and treated before their growth stops may have a catch-up period.

- Seizures, or convulsions, result from inadequate absorption of folic acid. Lack of folic acid causes calcium deposits, called calcifications, to form in the brain, which in turn cause seizures.

Incidence of Celiac Disease

Celiac disease is the most common genetic disease in Europe. In Italy about 1 in 250 people and in Ireland about 1 in 300 people have celiac disease. Recent studies have shown that it may be more common in Africa, South America, and Asia than previously believed.

Until recently, celiac disease was thought to be uncommon in the United States. However, studies have shown that celiac disease occurs in an estimated 1 in 133 Americans. Among people who have a first-degree relative diagnosed with celiac, as many as 1 in 22 people may have the disease. A recent study in which random blood samples from the Red Cross were tested for celiac disease suggests that as many as 1 in every 250 Americans may have it. Celiac disease could be under-diagnosed in the United States for a number of reasons:

- Celiac symptoms can be attributed to other problems.

- Many doctors are not knowledgeable about the disease.

- Only a handful of U.S. laboratories are experienced and skilled in testing for celiac disease.

More research is needed to find out the true prevalence of celiac disease among Americans.

Diseases Linked to Celiac Disease

People with celiac disease tend to have other autoimmune diseases as well, including the following:

- dermatitis herpetiformis
- thyroid disease
- systemic lupus erythematosus
- type 1 diabetes
- liver disease
- collagen vascular disease
- rheumatoid arthritis
- Sjögren syndrome

The connection between celiac and these diseases may be genetic.

Dermatitis Herpetiformis

Dermatitis herpetiformis (DH) is a severe itchy, blistering skin disease caused by gluten intolerance. DH is related to celiac disease because both are autoimmune disorders caused by gluten intolerance, but they are separate diseases. The rash usually occurs on the elbows, knees, and buttocks. Although people with DH do not usually have digestive symptoms, they often have the same intestinal damage as people with celiac disease.

DH is diagnosed by a skin biopsy, which involves removing a tiny piece of skin near the rash and testing it for the IgA antibody. DH is treated with a gluten-free diet and medication to control the rash, such as dapsone or sulfapyridine. Drug treatment may last several years.

Points to Remember

- People with celiac disease cannot tolerate gluten, a protein in wheat, rye, barley, and possibly oats.

- Celiac disease damages the small intestine and interferes with nutrient absorption.

- Treatment is important because people with celiac disease could develop complications like cancer, osteoporosis, anemia, and seizures.

- A person with celiac disease may or may not have symptoms.

- Diagnosis involves blood tests and biopsy.

- Because celiac disease is hereditary, family members of a person with celiac disease may need to be tested.

- Celiac disease is treated by eliminating all gluten from the diet. The gluten-free diet is a lifetime requirement.

Additional Information

American Celiac Society
P.O. Box 23455
New Orleans, LA 70183-0455
Phone: 504-737-3293
E-mail: amerceliacsoc@onebox.com

American Dietetic Association
120 S. Riverside Plaza, Suite 2000
Chicago, IL 60606-6995
Toll-Free: 800-877-1600
Website: http://www.eatright.org/Public
E-mail: hotline@eatright.org

Celiac Disease Foundation
13251 Ventura Blvd., #1
Studio City, CA 91604
Phone: 818-990-2354
Fax: 818-990-2379
Website: http://www.celiac.org
E-mail: cdf@celiac.org

Celiac Sprue Association/USA Inc.
P.O. Box 31700
Omaha, NE 68131-0700
Toll-Free: 877-CSA-4CSA (272-4272)
Phone: 402-558-0600
Fax: 402-558-1347
Website: http://www.csaceliacs.org
E-mail: celiacs@csaceliacs.org

Gluten Intolerance Group (GIG) of North America
15110 10th Ave. S.W., Suite A
Seattle, WA 98166
Phone: 206-246-6652
Fax: 206-246-6531
Website: http://www.gluten.net
E-mail: info@gluten.net

National Institute of Diabetes and Digestive and Kidney Diseases (NIDDK)
Information Clearinghouse
5 Information Way
Bethesda, MD 20892-3560
Toll-Free: 800-860-8747
Phone: 301-654-3810
Website: http://www.niddk.nih.gov

Chapter 40

Devic Syndrome

Devic syndrome is a rare autoimmune central nervous system disorder characterized by transverse myelitis (in which the fatty, protective covering of the spinal cord breaks down) and optic neuritis (in which inflammation of the optic nerve causes loss of vision and eye pain). It is considered a special form of multiple sclerosis (MS) with a severe and rapid course. The disorder affects the optic nerve and the nerves in the spinal cord. In Devic syndrome, the fatty sheath that protects these nerves is lost. Individuals may experience vision impairment and various degrees of paralysis, as well as incontinence. The disorder is closely linked with MS and lupus, but usually appears before any symptoms of MS are noted. If an isolated disease episode affecting the spinal cord and optic nerve occurs after an infection or common cold, it is considered a post-infectious acute demyelinated encephalomyelitis (ADE) rather than Devic syndrome.

Is there any treatment?

There is currently no standard treatment for Devic syndrome. Generally, treatment is symptomatic and supportive. Corticosteroids may be prescribed. Treatment for ADE may include corticosteroids, intravenous immunoglobulin, and intravenous methylprednisolone

---

"Devic's Syndrome Information Page," National Institute of Neurological Disorders and Stroke (NINDS), updated February 9, 2005.

What is the prognosis?

Devic syndrome is fatal in many patients. Some ADE patients achieve complete or nearly complete recovery while others may have residual deficits. Some severe cases of ADE may be fatal.

What research is being done?

The National Institute of Neurological Disorders and Stroke (NINDS) supports an extensive research program of basic studies to increase understanding of how the nervous system works. A major goal of this research is to develop methods for repairing damaged nerves and restoring full use and strength to injured areas.

Additional Information

Multiple Sclerosis Foundation
6350 N. Andrews Ave.
Ft. Lauderdale, FL 33309-2130
Toll-Free: 888-MSFOCUS (673-6287)
Phone: 954-776-6805
Fax: 954-351-0630
Website: http://www.msfocus.org
E-mail: support@msfocus.org

National Eye Institute (NEI)
31 Center Drive MSC 2510
Bethesda, MD 20892-2510
Phone: 301-496-5248
Website: http://www.nei.nih.gov

Chapter 41

Type 1 Diabetes: Insulin-Dependent

"We thought he had the flu."

"She was thirsty, and she kept running to the bathroom. The school nurse suspected a bladder infection."

"He felt tired and was losing weight. We blamed it on exams."

Diabetes is a great pretender, and its first symptoms are often mistaken for those of more common childhood problems—it may be the last illness that parents suspect when they bring their child to see a doctor. Yet 210,000 people under the age of 20 already have the condition.

The parents of a child who is diagnosed with diabetes have a big adjustment ahead: They must understand the condition and help their child control it and cope with it. But with care, encouragement, and some good practical knowledge about diabetes, parents can become their child's most important allies in learning to live with the condition.

What is diabetes?

Diabetes is a condition that affects how the body handles glucose, a simple sugar that is the major energy source for the body and is

This information was provided by KidsHealth, one of the largest resources online for medically reviewed health information written for parents, kids, and teens. For more articles like this one, visit www.KidsHealth.org, or www.Teens Health.org. © 2004 The Nemours Center for Children's Health Media, a division of The Nemours Foundation.

derived from the foods we eat. Blood levels of glucose are controlled primarily by a hormone called insulin—a chemical produced by beta cells in the pancreas (a gland located near the stomach).

Normally, soon after we eat, beta cells in the pancreas secrete insulin into the bloodstream to help our bodies handle glucose absorbed into the blood from digested food. Insulin allows glucose to enter individual body cells for use as fuel. It also directs the way glucose is stored in fat cells (as fat) and in the liver (as glycogen).

When children develop diabetes, it's usually because the pancreas stops producing enough insulin. From the beginning of their illness, they must depend on insulin injections to control their blood glucose levels (currently, insulin can't be taken by mouth because it's destroyed by the body's digestive juices). This type of diabetes is known as insulin-dependent diabetes mellitus (IDDM), but it can also be called type 1 diabetes or juvenile diabetes.

When insulin-dependent diabetes mellitus affects a child, the child's own immune system attacks and destroys the beta cells in the pancreas that produce insulin. Although children with insulin-dependent diabetes mellitus probably inherit a genetic tendency for developing this type of diabetes, their immune systems still need some sort of trigger to set off beta cell destruction. Although exact trigger or triggers aren't known for certain, researchers suspect that viruses may be involved in some cases.

Insulin-dependent diabetes mellitus is different from non-insulin-dependent diabetes mellitus (NIDDM) (also called adult-onset or type 2 diabetes), the most common form of the disease when all age groups are considered. Although type 2 diabetes is more common in adults, the disorder is being seen more often in children and teens in recent years. Higher rates of children who are overweight or obese are probably contributing to this trend.

This form of diabetes doesn't result from destruction of the cells that make insulin (as in type 1 diabetes)—instead, it stems from the body's "resistance" to the effects of insulin, often associated with obesity. Adults and children with non-insulin-dependent diabetes mellitus may control their diabetes with diet, exercise, and sometimes medicines taken by mouth. But in some cases of non-insulin-dependent diabetes mellitus, these treatments alone may not control the condition adequately and the patient must use insulin.

How does diabetes affect the body?

Once insulin-producing beta cells are destroyed, the child's pancreas can't replace them. As beta cells die, insulin levels in the blood drop, and glucose can no longer enter the body's cells to be used as an energy source. Without insulin, body cells are starved for glucose fuel, even as glucose levels rise higher and higher in the blood. The body interprets messages from these "hungry" cells and the low blood insulin levels as signals that the child is starving from lack of food, so the brain's appetite centers push the child to eat more (in other words, his or her appetite increases). The body also activates other anti-starvation hormone systems to begin breaking down muscle and stored fat to produce more glucose and alternative fuels (so the child loses weight).

As the kidneys flush out excess glucose from the blood via urine, the child needs to urinate more frequently and in larger volumes (a symptom called polyuria). In response to this large loss of body water through increased urination, the child becomes very thirsty. He or she drinks unusually large amounts of water or other liquids (polydipsia) in an attempt to keep the levels of body water normal.

As the child's body breaks down fats, by-products called fatty acids and ketones build up in the blood. Rising levels of ketones can trigger episodes of rapid, deep breathing (called Kussmaul respirations) and give the child's breath a fruity smell. As the child's blood fills with abnormally high levels of acid and other body chemicals, abdominal pain, nausea, and vomiting occur. High levels of acid in the body also affect the brain, which causes the child to become very sleepy or even lose consciousness. This condition is known as diabetic ketoacidosis.

In addition to short-term problems, diabetes can also cause long-term complications. Heart disease and stroke are two to four times more common in people with diabetes than in those without it. Diabetes is also the leading cause of blindness in people over age 20, and it's the leading cause of end-stage renal disease, the most severe cause of kidney damage.

People with diabetes are also at higher risk for high blood pressure; periodontal disease (severe gum disease that can lead to tooth loss); nerve problems that can cause numbness or pain in the extremities, particularly the feet; and disease of the blood vessels that supply the legs and feet that can result in gangrene and lead to amputations. However, research has shown that better control of diabetes can significantly reduce a person's risk of developing these problems.

What are the first symptoms?

Parents of a child with classic symptoms of diabetes may notice that their son or daughter is abnormally thirsty, needs to urinate frequently, and has been losing weight in spite of a good appetite. But this is only one possible set of symptoms. Sometimes, the first sign of diabetes is bedwetting in a child who has always been dry at night. Other times, in girls, it's a vaginal yeast infection (also called a *Candida* infection).

About 25% of children have already progressed to diabetic ketoacidosis by the time they first see the doctor. Because these children may vomit and complain of abdominal pain, their symptoms can be mistaken for the flu or appendicitis. If the condition isn't recognized and treatment isn't started, the other symptoms of diabetic ketoacidosis develop: rapid and deep breathing, fruity breath odor, and possible loss of consciousness.

Doctors diagnose diabetes by testing for glucose and ketones in the urine and by measuring glucose levels in the blood.

What's it like for kids with insulin-dependent diabetes?

Children with diabetes grow up with the task of monitoring and controlling their body's glucose levels, which involves:

- following a balanced diet to control their intake of carbohydrates (sugars and starches in food that release glucose into the blood).

- getting regular exercise to help control their blood glucose levels and reduce their risk of long-term complications of diabetes (such as heart and blood vessel disease).

- checking their blood glucose levels several times each day by testing a small blood sample with a glucose meter.

- giving themselves insulin injections (based on their blood glucose levels) according to a plan that's been worked out with their doctor beforehand.

Living with diabetes is a challenge, no matter what a child's age, but young children and teens often have special issues to deal with. Young children may not understand why the blood samples and insulin injections are necessary and may be angry and uncooperative.

Teens may feel different from their peers and may struggle through times when they want to live a more spontaneous lifestyle than their diabetes regime allows. Even when they faithfully follow their treatment schedule, teens with diabetes may feel frustrated when the natural adolescent body changes and the surge of growth hormone—a hormone that tends to raise blood glucose—may make their diabetes somewhat harder to control.

Are there advances in the treatment of diabetes?

Fortunately, new products and equipment are being developed every day to help children cope with the special problems of growing up with diabetes. Devices that may make blood sugar testing and insulin injections easier and more effective are being continuously developed. Some, such as the insulin pump, are already in use.

Researchers are also working on techniques to deliver insulin through nasal sprays, inhalers, patches, and pills. The genetically engineered human insulin now used has replaced older forms of insulin that were more likely to cause skin problems and allergic reactions. Scientists also are perfecting revolutionary new glucose monitors that would make traditional blood sampling obsolete.

The development of devices that can continuously and accurately measure a person's blood sugar are the key to producing an "artificial pancreas." With such a system, the blood sugar readings from a sensing device are fed into a computerized insulin pump, which can then dispense the precise amount of insulin the person needs. This kind of reliable and practically wearable or implantable system could enable a person with diabetes to achieve excellent blood sugar nearly effortlessly.

A potential "cure" for diabetes involving transplantation of insulin-producing pancreatic cells is now possible, too, but not perfected. Scientists are making progress in finding safe ways to protect the transplanted cells from being attacked and destroyed by the body's immune defenses.

Researchers are also testing ways to stop diabetes before it starts. Currently, the U.S. government's National Institute of Diabetes and Digestive and Kidney Diseases (NIDDK) is studying nondiabetic relatives of people with insulin-dependent diabetes mellitus to see if they can prevent diabetes in those who may have inherited an increased risk for the disease.

Until scientists have perfected ways to better treat and possibly even prevent diabetes, you can help your child lead a happier, healthier life by giving constant encouragement, arming yourself with diabetes information, and making sure your child eats right, exercises, and stays on top of glucose levels every day.

Chapter 42

Glomerulonephritis

Definition: Glomerulonephritis is a type of kidney disease caused by inflammation of the internal kidney structures (glomeruli).

Causes, Incidence, and Risk Factors

Glomerulonephritis (GN) may be a temporary and reversible condition, or it may be progressive. Progressive glomerulonephritis may result in destruction of the kidney glomeruli, chronic renal failure, and end stage renal disease. The disease may be caused by specific problems with the body's immune system, but the precise cause of most cases is unknown.

Damage to the glomeruli with subsequent impaired filtering causes blood and protein to be lost in the urine. Because symptoms develop gradually, the disorder may be discovered when there is an abnormal urinalysis during routine physical or examination for unrelated disorders. Glomerulonephritis can cause hypertension and may only be discovered as a cause of hypertension that is difficult to control.

It may develop after survival of the acute phase of rapidly progressive glomerulonephritis. In about one-fourth of people with chronic glomerulonephritis, there is no prior history of kidney disease, and the disorder first appears as chronic renal failure.

Specific disorders that are associated with glomerulonephritis include:

- Focal segmental glomerulosclerosis (FSG)
- Goodpasture syndrome
- IgA (immunoglobulin A) nephropathy
- IgM mesangial proliferative glomerulonephritis
- Lupus nephritis
- Membranoproliferative GN I
- Membranoproliferative GN II
- Post-streptococcal GN
- Rapidly progressive (crescentic) glomerulonephritis
- Rapidly progressive glomerulonephritis (RPGN).

Symptoms

- Blood in the urine (dark, rust-colored, or brown urine)
- Foamy urine

Chronic renal failure symptoms that gradually develop may include:

- Unintentional weight loss
- Nausea, vomiting
- General ill feeling (malaise)
- Fatigue
- Headache
- Frequent hiccups
- Generalized itching
- Decreased urine output
- Need to urinate at night
- Easy bruising or bleeding
- Decreased alertness
  - Drowsiness, somnolence, lethargy
  - Confusion, delirium
  - Coma
- Muscle twitching
- Muscle cramps
- Seizures

- Increased skin pigmentation (hyperpigmentation)—skin may appear yellow or brown
- Decreased sensation in the hands, feet, or other areas.

Additional symptoms that may be associated with this disease:

- Excessive urination
- Nosebleed
- High blood pressure
- Blood in the vomit or in stools

Signs and Tests

High blood pressure may be present along with abnormal urinalysis. Laboratory tests may reveal anemia or indicate reduced kidney functioning, including azotemia (accumulation of nitrogenous wastes such as creatinine and urea). Later, signs of chronic renal failure may be apparent, including edema, polyneuropathy, and signs of fluid overload including abnormal heart and lung sounds.

- A urinalysis may show blood, casts, protein, or some other abnormality.
- Findings on kidney or abdominal ultrasound, kidney or abdominal CT scan, or IVP are non-specific.
- A chest x-ray may show fluid overload.
- A kidney biopsy may show one of the forms of chronic glomerulonephritis or non-specific scarring of the glomeruli.

This disease may also alter the results of the following tests:

- Urine specific gravity
- Urine concentration test
- Uric acid, urine
- Total protein
- Urine red blood count (RBC)
- Urine protein
- Creatinine clearance
- Urine creatinine
- Complement component 3

- Complement
- Blood urea nitrogen (BUN)
- Anti-glomerular basement membrane
- Albumin

Treatment

Treatment varies depending on the cause of the disorder, and the type and severity of symptoms. The primary treatment goal is control of symptoms. Hypertension may be difficult to control, and it is generally the most important aspect of treatment.

Various antihypertensive medications may be used to attempt to control high blood pressure. Corticosteroids, immunosuppressives, or other medications may be used to treat some of the causes of chronic glomerulonephritis.

Dietary restrictions on salt, fluids, protein, and other substances may be recommended to aid control of hypertension or renal failure.

Dialysis or kidney transplantation may be necessary to control symptoms of renal failure and to sustain life.

Support Groups

The stress of illness can often be helped by joining support groups where members share common experiences and problems.

Expectations (Prognosis)

The outcome varies depending on the cause. Some types of glomerulonephritis may have spontaneous remission.

If nephrotic syndrome is present and can be controlled, other symptoms may be controlled. If nephrotic syndrome is present and cannot be controlled, end-stage renal disease may result.

The disorder generally progresses at widely variable rates.

Complications

- Nephrotic syndrome
- Acute nephritic syndrome
- Chronic renal failure
- End-stage renal disease
- Hypertension

- Malignant hypertension
- Fluid overload—congestive heart failure, pulmonary edema
- Chronic or recurrent urinary tract infection
- Increased susceptibility to other infections

Calling Your Health Care Provider

Call your health care provider if disorders associated with increased risk of glomerulonephritis are present, or if symptoms indicating glomerulonephritis develop.

Prevention

There is no specific prevention for most cases of glomerulonephritis. Some cases may be prevented by avoiding or limiting exposure to organic solvents, mercury, and nonsteroidal anti-inflammatory analgesics.

Chapter 43

Goodpasture Syndrome

Goodpasture syndrome is a rare disease that can affect the lungs and kidneys. It is an autoimmune disease, a condition in which the body's own defense system reacts against some part of the body itself. When the immune system is working normally, it creates antibodies to fight off germs. In Goodpasture syndrome, the immune system makes antibodies that attack the lungs and kidneys. Why this happens is uncertain. A combination of factors has been implicated, among them the presence of an inherited component and exposure to certain chemicals.

Goodpasture syndrome can cause people to cough up blood or feel a burning sensation when urinating. But its first signs may be vague, like fatigue, nausea, dyspnea (difficulty breathing), or pallor. These signs are followed by kidney involvement, represented first by small amounts of blood in the urine, protein in the urine, and other clinical and laboratory findings.

To diagnose Goodpasture syndrome, doctors use a blood test, but a kidney biopsy (or a lung biopsy) may be necessary to check for the presence of the harmful antibody.

Goodpasture syndrome is treated with oral immunosuppressive drugs (cyclophosphamide and corticosteroids) to keep the immune system from making antibodies. Corticosteroid drugs may be given intravenously to control bleeding in the lungs. A process called plasmapheresis

---

"Goodpasture's Syndrome," National Institute of Diabetes and Digestive and Kidney Diseases (NIDDK), NIH Publication No. 03–4558, June 2003.

(PLAZ-ma-fer-REE-sis) may be helpful and necessary to remove the harmful antibodies from the blood; this is usually done in combination with the immunosuppressive drug treatment.

Goodpasture syndrome may last only a few weeks or as long as 2 years. Bleeding in the lungs can be very serious in some cases. But Goodpasture syndrome does not usually lead to permanent lung damage. Damage to the kidneys, however, may be long-lasting. If the kidneys fail, dialysis to remove waste products and extra fluid from the blood or kidney transplantation may become necessary.

Additional Information

National Kidney Foundation
30 East 33rd St.
New York, NY 10016
Toll-Free: 800-622-9010
Phone: 212-889-2210
Website: http://www.kidney.org
E-mail: info@kidney.org

National Kidney and Urologic Diseases Information Clearinghouse
3 Information Way
Bethesda, MD 20892-3580
Toll-Free: 800-891-5390
Phone: 301-654-4415
Fax: 703-738-4929
Website: http://kidney.niddk.nih.gov
E-mail: nkudic@info.niddk.nih.gov

Chapter 44

Guillain-Barré Syndrome

Guillain-Barré (ghee-yan bah-ray) syndrome is a disorder in which the body's immune system attacks part of the peripheral nervous system. The first symptoms of this disorder include varying degrees of weakness or tingling sensations in the legs. In many instances the weakness and abnormal sensations spread to the arms and upper body. These symptoms can increase in intensity until certain muscles cannot be used at all; and, when severe, the patient is almost totally paralyzed. In these cases the disorder is life-threatening—potentially interfering with breathing, and at times, with blood pressure or heart rate. It is considered a medical emergency. Such a patient is often put on a respirator to assist with breathing, and is watched closely for problems such as an abnormal heart beat, infections, blood clots, and high or low blood pressure. Most patients, however, recover from even the most severe cases of Guillain-Barré syndrome, although some continue to have a certain degree of weakness.

Guillain-Barré syndrome can affect anybody. It can strike at any age, and both sexes are equally prone to the disorder. The syndrome is rare, however, afflicting only about one person in 100,000. Usually Guillain-Barré occurs a few days or weeks after the patient has had symptoms of a respiratory or gastrointestinal viral infection. Occasionally surgery or vaccinations will trigger the syndrome.

"Guillain-Barré Syndrome Fact Sheet," National Institute of Neurological Disorders and Stroke (NINDS), NIH Publication No. 01–2902, updated February 9, 2005.

After the first clinical manifestations of the disease, the symptoms can progress over the course of hours, days, or weeks. Most people reach the stage of greatest weakness within the first 2 weeks after symptoms appear, and by the third week of the illness 90 percent of all patients are at their weakest.

Cause of Guillain-Barré

No one yet knows why Guillain-Barré strikes some people and not others. Nor does anyone know exactly what sets the disease in motion.

What scientists do know is that the body's immune system begins to attack the body itself, causing what is known as an autoimmune disease. Usually the cells of the immune system attack only foreign material and invading organisms. In Guillain-Barré syndrome, however, the immune system starts to destroy the myelin sheath that surrounds the axons of many peripheral nerves, or even the axons themselves (axons are long, thin extensions of the nerve cells; they carry nerve signals). The myelin sheath surrounding the axon speeds up the transmission of nerve signals and allows the transmission of signals over long distances.

In diseases in which the peripheral nerves' myelin sheaths are injured or degraded, the nerves cannot transmit signals efficiently. That is why the muscles begin to lose their ability to respond to the brain's commands, commands that must be carried through the nerve network. The brain also receives fewer sensory signals from the rest of the body, resulting in an inability to feel textures, heat, pain, and other sensations. Alternately, the brain may receive inappropriate signals that result in tingling, crawling-skin, or painful sensations. Because the signals to and from the arms and legs must travel the longest distances they are most vulnerable to interruption. Therefore, muscle weakness and tingling sensations usually first appear in the hands and feet and progress upwards.

When Guillain-Barré is preceded by a viral or bacterial infection, it is possible that the virus has changed the nature of cells in the nervous system so that the immune system treats them as foreign cells. It is also possible that the virus makes the immune system less discriminating about what cells it recognizes as its own, allowing some of the immune cells, such as certain kinds of lymphocytes and macrophages, to attack the myelin. Sensitized T lymphocytes cooperate with B lymphocytes to produce antibodies against components of the myelin sheath and may contribute to destruction of the myelin. Scientists are investigating these and other possibilities to find why the immune system goes awry in Guillain-Barré syndrome and other autoimmune diseases. The cause and course of Guillain-Barré syndrome is an active area of neurological investigation, incorporating the cooperative efforts of neurological scientists, immunologists, and virologists.

Diagnosis

Guillain-Barré is called a syndrome rather than a disease because it is not clear that a specific disease-causing agent is involved. A syndrome is a medical condition characterized by a collection of symptoms (what the patient feels) and signs (what a doctor can observe or measure). The signs and symptoms of the syndrome can be quite varied, so doctors may, on rare occasions, find it difficult to diagnose Guillain-Barré in its earliest stages.

Several disorders have symptoms similar to those found in Guillain-Barré, so doctors examine and question patients carefully before making a diagnosis. Collectively, the signs and symptoms form a certain pattern that helps doctors differentiate Guillain-Barré from other disorders. For example, physicians will note whether the symptoms appear on both sides of the body (most common in Guillain-Barré), and the quickness with which the symptoms appear (in other disorders, muscle weakness may progress over months rather than days or weeks). In Guillain-Barré, reflexes such as knee jerks are usually lost. Because the signals traveling along the nerve are slower, a nerve conduction velocity (NCV) test may aid in the diagnosis. In Guillain-Barré patients, the cerebrospinal fluid that bathes the spinal cord and brain contains more protein than usual. Therefore, a physician may decide to perform a spinal tap, a procedure in which the doctor inserts a needle into the patient's lower back to draw cerebrospinal fluid from the spinal column.

Treatment

There is no known cure for Guillain-Barré syndrome. However, there are therapies that lessen the severity of the illness and accelerate the recovery in most patients. There are also a number of ways to treat the complications of the disease.

Currently, plasmapheresis and high-dose immunoglobulin therapy are used. Both are equally effective, but immunoglobulin is easier to administer. Plasmapheresis is a method by which whole blood is removed from the body and processed so that the red and white blood cells are separated from the plasma, or liquid portion of the blood. The blood cells are then returned to the patient without the plasma, which the body quickly replaces. Scientists still do not know exactly why plasmapheresis works, but the technique seems to reduce the severity and duration of the Guillain-Barré episode. This may be because the plasma portion of the blood contains elements of the immune system that may be toxic to the myelin.

In high-dose immunoglobulin therapy, doctors give intravenous injections of the proteins that the immune system uses naturally to attack invading organisms. Investigators have found that giving high doses of these immunoglobulins, derived from a pool of thousands of normal donors, to Guillain-Barré patients can lessen the immune attack on the nervous system. Investigators do not know why or how this works, although several hypotheses have been proposed.

The use of steroid hormones has also been tried as a way to reduce the severity of Guillain-Barré, but controlled clinical trials have demonstrated that this treatment not only is ineffective, but may even have a deleterious effect on the disease.

The most critical part of the treatment for this syndrome consists of keeping the patient's body functioning during recovery of the nervous system. This sometimes requires placing the patient on a respirator, a heart monitor, or other machines that assist body functions. The need for this sophisticated machinery is one reason why Guillain-Barré syndrome patients are usually treated in hospitals, often in an intensive care ward. In the hospital, doctors can also look for and treat the many problems that can afflict any paralyzed patient—complications such as pneumonia or bed sores.

Often, even before recovery begins, caregivers may be instructed to manually move the patient's limbs to help keep the muscles flexible and strong. Later, as the patient begins to recover limb control, physical therapy begins. Carefully planned clinical trials of new and experimental therapies are the key to improving the treatment of patients with Guillain-Barré syndrome. Such clinical trials begin with the research of basic and clinical scientists who, working with clinicians, identify new approaches to treating patients with the disease.

Prognosis

Guillain-Barré syndrome can be a devastating disorder because of its sudden and unexpected onset. In addition, recovery is not necessarily quick. As noted, patients usually reach the point of greatest weakness or paralysis days or weeks after the first symptoms occur. Symptoms then stabilize at this level for a period of days, weeks, or months. The recovery period may take as little as a few weeks, or as long as a few years. About 30 percent of those with Guillain-Barré still have a residual weakness after 3 years. About 3 percent may suffer a relapse of muscle weakness and tingling sensations many years after the initial attack.

Guillain-Barré syndrome patients face not only physical difficulties, but emotionally painful periods as well. It is often extremely difficult for patients to adjust to sudden paralysis and dependence on others for help with routine daily activities. Patients sometimes need psychological counseling to help them adapt.

Research

Scientists are concentrating on finding new treatments and refining existing ones. Scientists are also looking at the workings of the immune system to find which cells are responsible for beginning and carrying out the attack on the nervous system. The fact that so many cases of Guillain-Barré begin after a viral or bacterial infection suggests that certain characteristics of some viruses and bacteria may activate the immune system inappropriately. Investigators are searching for those characteristics. Certain proteins or peptides in viruses and bacteria may be the same as those found in myelin, and the generation of antibodies to neutralize the invading viruses or bacteria could trigger the attack on the myelin sheath.

Additional Information

Guillain-Barré Syndrome Foundation International
P.O. Box 262
Wynnewood, PA 19096
Phone: 610-667-0131
Fax: 610-667-7036
Website: http://www.guillain-barre.com
E-mail: info@gbsfi.com

National Institute of Neurological Disorders and Stroke
P.O. Box 5801
Bethesda, MD 20824
Toll-Free: 800-352-9424
Phone: 301-496-5751
TTY: 301-468-5981
Website: http://www.ninds.nih.gov

Chapter 45

Idiopathic Thrombocytopenic Purpura

What is idiopathic thrombocytopenic purpura (ITP)?

ITP stands for idiopathic thrombocytopenic purpura. *Idiopathic* means that the cause is unknown. *Thrombocytopenic* means the blood does not have enough platelets. *Purpura* means a person has excessive bruising. You may also hear ITP called immune thrombocytopenic purpura.

In people with ITP, all of the blood cells are normal except for the blood platelets. Platelets are the tiny cells that seal minor cuts and wounds and form blood clots. A person with too few platelets bruises easily and bleeds for a long time after being injured. Tiny red dots on the skin, called petechiae (pe-TEEK-ee-ay) might also appear. When the platelet count is very low, the person with ITP might have nosebleeds that are hard to stop, or might have bleeding in the intestines.

What causes ITP?

The cause of ITP is not known. People with ITP form antibodies that destroy their blood platelets. Normally, antibodies are a healthy response to bacteria or viruses. In people with ITP, however, the antibodies attack the body's own blood platelets.

Who gets ITP?

There are 2 types of ITP. One type affects children, and the other type affects adults. In children, the usual age for getting ITP is 2 to 4 years of age. Most adults with ITP are young women, but it can occur in anyone. ITP does not run in families.

How does ITP affect children?

ITP is different in children than in adults. Most children with ITP have a very low platelet count that causes sudden bleeding. The usual symptoms are bruises and the tiny red dots on the skin. Nosebleeds and bleeding gums are also common.

How is ITP diagnosed?

Your doctor can diagnose ITP by asking questions about your health and doing a physical exam. Your doctor may take a blood sample and look at it under a microscope.

How is ITP treated in children?

Because most children recover with no treatment, many doctors recommend just watching them carefully and taking care of the bleeding symptoms. Children do not have to go to the hospital if good care is available at home. However, some doctors recommend a short treatment with prednisone pills or intravenous infusions (given in a vein) of gamma globulin to increase the platelet count more quickly. Both medicines have some side effects.

How does ITP affect adults?

In most adults, ITP lasts much longer than it does in children. At the time of diagnosis, most adults have noticed increased bleeding and easy bruising for several weeks, or even months. In women, increased menstrual blood flow is a major sign.

Many adults have only mild thrombocytopenia. In fact, quite a few people have no bleeding symptoms. They are only diagnosed with ITP when their blood is checked for another reason and a low blood platelet count is found.

How is ITP treated in adults?

Treatment of ITP in adults is aimed at increasing the blood platelet count. This is not the same as curing the disease. Patients may take prednisone for several weeks, even a month or longer. However, when the medicine is stopped, the platelet counts may get low again.

If prednisone does not help enough, the spleen can be removed. The spleen makes most of the antibodies that destroy the blood platelets. It also destroys old or damaged blood cells. In an otherwise healthy young person, removal of the spleen is not a serious operation.

What about ITP in pregnant women?

Diagnosing ITP during pregnancy can be difficult, because platelet counts may be low for other reasons. About 5% of women have mildly low platelet counts at the end of a normal pregnancy. The cause of this is unknown. The platelet count goes back to normal right after delivery.

A baby born to a mother with ITP may have a low blood platelet count a few days to a few weeks after birth. These babies are usually kept in the hospital for several days for observation (watching to make sure they are okay) before they go can home.

Additional Information

Platelet Disorder Support Association
P.O. Box 61533
Potomac, MD 20859
Toll-Free: 87-PLATELET (877-528-3538)
Phone: 301-770-6636
Fax: 301-770-6638
Website: http://www.itppeople.com
E-mail: pdsa@pdsa.org

Chapter 46

Inflammatory Bowel Disease

Chapter Contents

Section 46.1

Crohn Disease

"Crohn's Disease," National Institute of Diabetes and Digestive and Kidney Diseases (NIDDK), NIH Publication No. 03-3410, January 2003.

Crohn disease causes inflammation in the small intestine. Crohn disease usually occurs in the lower part of the small intestine, called the ileum, but it can affect any part of the digestive tract, from the mouth to the anus. The inflammation extends deep into the lining of the affected organ. The inflammation can cause pain and can make the intestines empty frequently, resulting in diarrhea. Crohn disease is an inflammatory bowel disease (IBD), the general name for diseases that cause inflammation in the intestines. Crohn disease can be difficult to diagnose because its symptoms are similar to other intestinal disorders such as irritable bowel syndrome and to another type

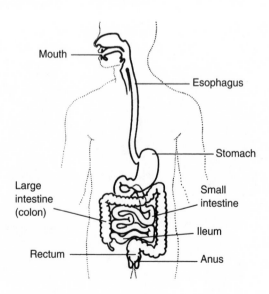

***Figure 46.1.** The Digestive System*

of IBD called ulcerative colitis. Ulcerative colitis causes inflammation and ulcers in the top layer of the lining of the large intestine.

Crohn disease affects men and women equally and seems to run in some families. About 20 percent of people with Crohn disease have a blood relative with some form of IBD, most often a brother or sister, sometimes a parent or child. Crohn disease may also be called ileitis, enteritis, regional enteritis, chronic cicatrizing enteritis, granulomatous enteritis, or distal ileitis.

What Causes Crohn Disease?

Theories about what causes Crohn disease abound, but none has been proven. The most popular theory is that the body's immune system reacts to a virus or a bacterium by causing ongoing inflammation in the intestine. People with Crohn disease tend to have abnormalities of the immune system, but doctors do not know whether these abnormalities are a cause or result of the disease. Crohn disease is not caused by emotional distress.

Symptoms

The most common symptoms of Crohn disease are abdominal pain, often in the lower right area, and diarrhea. Rectal bleeding, weight loss, and fever may also occur. Bleeding may be serious and persistent, leading to anemia. Children with Crohn disease may suffer delayed development and stunted growth.

Diagnosis

A thorough physical exam and a series of tests may be required to diagnose Crohn disease. Blood tests may be done to check for anemia, which could indicate bleeding in the intestines. Blood tests may also uncover a high white blood cell count, which is a sign of inflammation somewhere in the body. By testing a stool sample, the doctor can tell if there is bleeding or infection in the intestines.

The doctor may do an upper gastrointestinal (GI) series to look at the small intestine. For this test, the patient drinks barium, a chalky solution that coats the lining of the small intestine, before x-rays are taken. The barium shows up white on x-ray film, revealing inflammation or other abnormalities in the intestine. The doctor may also do a colonoscopy. For this test, the doctor inserts an endoscope—a long, flexible, lighted tube linked to a computer and TV monitor—into the anus to see the inside of the large intestine. The doctor will be able to see any inflammation or bleeding. During the exam, the doctor may do a biopsy, which involves taking a sample of tissue from the lining of the intestine to view with a microscope. If these tests show Crohn disease, more x-rays of both the upper and lower digestive tract may be necessary to see how much is affected by the disease.

Complications

The most common complication is blockage of the intestine. Blockage occurs because the disease tends to thicken the intestinal wall with swelling and scar tissue, narrowing the passage. Crohn disease may also cause sores, or ulcers, that tunnel through the affected area into surrounding tissues such as the bladder, vagina, or skin. The areas around the anus and rectum are often involved. The tunnels, called fistulas, are a common complication and often become infected. Sometimes fistulas can be treated with medicine, but in some cases they may require surgery.

Nutritional complications are common in Crohn disease. Deficiencies of proteins, calories, and vitamins are well documented in Crohn disease. These deficiencies may be caused by inadequate dietary intake, intestinal loss of protein, or poor absorption (malabsorption).

Other complications associated with Crohn disease include arthritis, skin problems, inflammation in the eyes or mouth, kidney stones, gallstones, or other diseases of the liver and biliary system. Some of these problems resolve during treatment for disease in the digestive system, but some must be treated separately.

Treatment

Treatment for Crohn disease depends on the location and severity of disease, complications, and response to previous treatment. The goals of treatment are to control inflammation, correct nutritional deficiencies, and relieve symptoms like abdominal pain, diarrhea, and rectal bleeding. Treatment may include drugs, nutrition supplements, surgery, or a combination of these options. At this time, treatment can help control the disease, but there is no cure.

Some people have long periods of remission, sometimes years, when they are free of symptoms. However, the disease usually recurs at various times over a person's lifetime. This changing pattern of the disease means one cannot always tell when a treatment has helped. Predicting when a remission may occur or when symptoms will return is not possible. Someone with Crohn disease may need medical care for a long time, with regular doctor visits to monitor the condition.

Drug Therapy

Most people are first treated with drugs containing mesalamine, a substance that helps control inflammation. Sulfasalazine is the most commonly used of these drugs. Patients who do not benefit from it or who cannot tolerate it may be put on other mesalamine-containing drugs, generally known as 5-ASA agents, such as Asacol, Dipentum, or Pentasa. Possible side effects of mesalamine preparations include nausea, vomiting, heartburn, diarrhea, and headache.

Some patients take corticosteroids to control inflammation. These drugs are the most effective for active Crohn disease, but they can cause serious side effects, including greater susceptibility to infection.

Drugs that suppress the immune system are also used to treat Crohn disease. Most commonly prescribed are 6-mercaptopurine and a related drug, azathioprine. Immunosuppressive agents work by blocking the immune reaction that contributes to inflammation. These drugs may cause side effects like nausea, vomiting, and diarrhea, and may lower a person's resistance to infection. When patients are treated with a combination of corticosteroids and immunosuppressive drugs, the dose of corticosteroids can eventually be lowered. Some studies suggest that immunosuppressive drugs may enhance the effectiveness of corticosteroids.

The U.S. Food and Drug Administration has approved the drug infliximab (brand name, Remicade) for the treatment of moderate to severe Crohn disease that does not respond to standard therapies (mesalamine substances, corticosteroids, immunosuppressive agents), and for the treatment of open, draining fistulas. Infliximab, the first treatment approved specifically for Crohn disease, is an anti-tumor necrosis factor (TNF) substance. TNF is a protein produced by the immune system that may cause the inflammation associated with Crohn disease. Anti-TNF removes TNF from the bloodstream before it reaches the intestines, thereby preventing inflammation. Investigators will continue to study patients taking infliximab to determine its long-term safety and efficacy.

Antibiotics are used to treat bacterial overgrowth in the small intestine caused by stricture, fistulas, or prior surgery. For this common problem, the doctor may prescribe one or more of the following antibiotics: ampicillin, sulfonamide, cephalosporin, tetracycline, or metronidazole.

Diarrhea and crampy abdominal pain are often relieved when the inflammation subsides, but additional medication may also be necessary. Several antidiarrheal agents could be used, including diphenoxylate,

loperamide, and codeine. Patients who are dehydrated because of diarrhea will be treated with fluids and electrolytes.

Nutrition Supplementation

The doctor may recommend nutritional supplements, especially for
children whose growth has been slowed. Special high-calorie liquid
formulas are sometimes used for this purpose. A small number of
patients may need periods of feeding by vein. This can help patients
who need extra nutrition temporarily, those whose intestines need to
rest, or those whose intestines cannot absorb enough nutrition from
food.

Surgery

Surgery to remove part of the intestine can help Crohn disease,
but cannot cure it. The inflammation tends to return next to the area
of intestine that has been removed. Many Crohn disease patients require surgery, either to relieve symptoms that do not respond to medical therapy, or to correct complications such as blockage, perforation,
abscess, or bleeding in the intestine.

Some people who have Crohn disease in the large intestine need
to have their entire colon removed in an operation called colectomy.
A small opening is made in the front of the abdominal wall, and the
tip of the ileum is brought to the skin's surface. This opening, called
a stoma, is where waste exits the body. The stoma is about the size of
a quarter and is usually located in the right lower part of the abdomen near the belt-line. A pouch is worn over the opening to collect
waste, and the patient empties the pouch as needed. The majority of
colectomy patients go on to live normal, active lives. Sometimes only
the diseased section of intestine is removed and no stoma is needed.
In this operation, the intestine is cut above and below the diseased
area and reconnected.

Because Crohn disease often recurs after surgery, people considering it should carefully weigh its benefits and risks compared with
other treatments. Surgery may not be appropriate for everyone. People
faced with this decision should get as much information as possible
from doctors, nurses who work with colon surgery patients (enterostomal therapists), and other patients. Patient advocacy organizations
can suggest support groups and other information resources.

People with Crohn disease may feel well and be free of symptoms
for substantial spans of time when their disease is not active. Despite

the need to take medication for long periods of time and occasional hospitalizations, most people with Crohn disease are able to hold jobs, raise families, and function successfully at home and in society.

Can diet control Crohn disease?

No special diet has been proven effective for preventing or treating this disease. Some people find their symptoms are made worse by milk, alcohol, hot spices, or fiber. People are encouraged to follow a nutritious diet and avoid any foods that seem to worsen symptoms. But there are no consistent rules. People should take vitamin supplements only on their doctor's advice.

Is pregnancy safe for women with Crohn disease?

Research has shown that the course of pregnancy and delivery is usually not impaired in women with Crohn disease. Even so, women with Crohn disease should discuss the matter with their doctors before pregnancy. Most children born to women with Crohn disease are unaffected. Children who do get the disease are sometimes more severely affected than adults, with slowed growth and delayed sexual development in some cases.

Hope Through Research

Researchers continue to look for more effective treatments. Examples of investigational treatments include:

- **Anti-TNF.** Research has shown that cells affected by Crohn disease contain a cytokine, a protein produced by the immune system, called tumor necrosis factor (TNF). TNF may be responsible for the inflammation of Crohn disease. Anti-TNF is a substance that finds TNF in the bloodstream, binds to it, and removes it before it can reach the intestines and cause inflammation. In studies, anti-TNF seems particularly helpful in closing fistulas.

- **Interleukin 10.** Interleukin 10 (IL-10) is a cytokine that suppresses inflammation. Researchers are now studying the effectiveness of synthetic IL-10 in treating Crohn disease.

- **Antibiotics.** Antibiotics are now used to treat the bacterial infections that often accompany Crohn disease, but some research suggests that they might also be useful as a primary treatment for active Crohn disease.

- **Budesonide.** Researchers recently identified a new corticosteroid called budesonide that appears to be as effective as other corticosteroids, but causes fewer side effects.

- **Methotrexate and cyclosporine.** These are immunosuppressive drugs that may be useful in treating Crohn disease. One potential benefit of methotrexate and cyclosporine is that they appear to work faster than traditional immunosuppressive drugs.

- **Natalizumab.** Natalizumab is an experimental drug that reduces symptoms and improves the quality of life when tested in people with Crohn disease. The drug decreases inflammation by binding to immune cells and preventing them from leaving the bloodstream and reaching the areas of inflammation.

- **Zinc.** Free radicals—molecules produced during fat metabolism, stress, and infection, among other things—may contribute to inflammation in Crohn disease. Free radicals sometimes cause cell damage when they interact with other molecules in the body. The mineral zinc removes free radicals from the bloodstream. Studies are underway to determine whether zinc supplementation might reduce inflammation.

Section 46.2

Ulcerative Colitis

"Ulcerative Colitis," National Institute of Diabetes and Digestive and
Kidney Diseases (NIDDK), NIH Publication No. 03–1597, April 2003.

Ulcerative colitis is a disease that causes inflammation and sores,
called ulcers, in the lining of the large intestine. The inflammation
usually occurs in the rectum and lower part of the colon, but it may
affect the entire colon. Ulcerative colitis rarely affects the small intestine except for the end section, called the terminal ileum. Ulcerative colitis may also be called colitis or proctitis.

The inflammation makes the colon empty frequently, causing diarrhea. Ulcers form in places where the inflammation has killed the
cells lining the colon; the ulcers bleed and produce pus.

Ulcerative colitis is an inflammatory bowel disease (IBD), the general name for diseases that cause inflammation in the small intestine and colon. Ulcerative colitis can be difficult to diagnose because
its symptoms are similar to other intestinal disorders and to another
type of IBD called Crohn disease. Crohn disease differs from ulcerative colitis because it causes inflammation deeper within the intestinal wall. Also, Crohn disease usually occurs in the small intestine,
although it can also occur in the mouth, esophagus, stomach, duode-
num, large intestine, appendix, and anus.

Ulcerative colitis may occur in people of any age, but most often it
starts between ages 15 and 30, or less frequently between ages 50 and
70. Children and adolescents sometimes develop the disease. Ulcerative colitis affects men and women equally and appears to run in
some families.

Cause of Ulcerative Colitis

Theories about what causes ulcerative colitis abound, but none
have been proven. The most popular theory is that the body's immune
system reacts to a virus or a bacterium by causing ongoing inflammation in the intestinal wall. People with ulcerative colitis have abnormalities of the immune system, but doctors do not know whether

these abnormalities are a cause or a result of the disease. Ulcerative colitis is not caused by emotional distress or sensitivity to certain foods or food products, but these factors may trigger symptoms in some people.

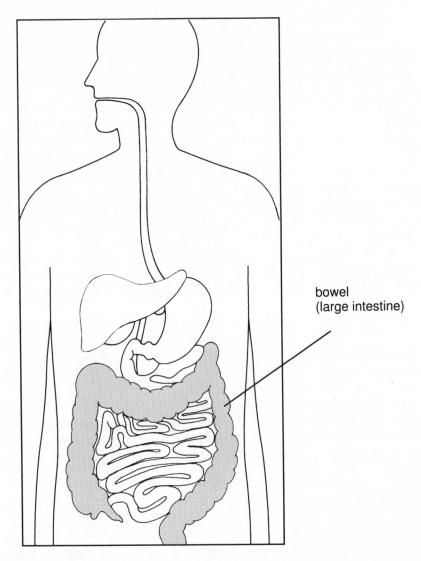

bowel
(large intestine)

Figure 46.2. The Large Intestine (Source: "What I Need to Know about Irritable Bowel Syndrome," National Institute of Diabetes and Digestive and Kidney Diseases (NIDDK), NIH Publication No. 03–4686, April 2003.)

Symptoms

The most common symptoms of ulcerative colitis are abdominal pain and bloody diarrhea. Patients also may experience the following:

- fatigue
- weight loss
- loss of appetite
- rectal bleeding
- loss of body fluids and nutrients

About half of patients have mild symptoms. Others suffer frequent fever, bloody diarrhea, nausea, and severe abdominal cramps. Ulcerative colitis may also cause problems such as arthritis, inflammation of the eye, liver disease (hepatitis, cirrhosis, and primary sclerosing cholangitis), osteoporosis, skin rashes, and anemia. No one knows for sure why problems occur outside the colon. Scientists think these complications may occur when the immune system triggers inflammation in other parts of the body. Some of these problems go away when the colitis is treated.

Diagnosis

A thorough physical exam and a series of tests may be required to diagnose ulcerative colitis. Blood tests may be done to check for anemia, which could indicate bleeding in the colon or rectum. Blood tests may also uncover a high white blood cell count, which is a sign of inflammation somewhere in the body. By testing a stool sample, the doctor can detect bleeding or infection in the colon or rectum.

The doctor may do a colonoscopy or sigmoidoscopy. For either test, the doctor inserts an endoscope—a long, flexible, lighted tube connected to a computer and TV monitor—into the anus to see the inside of the colon and rectum. The doctor will be able to see any inflammation, bleeding, or ulcers on the colon wall. During the exam, the doctor may do a biopsy, which involves taking a sample of tissue from the lining of the colon to view with a microscope. A barium enema x-ray of the colon may also be required. This procedure involves filling the colon with barium, a chalky white solution. The barium shows up white on x-ray film, allowing the doctor a clear view of the colon, including any ulcers or other abnormalities that might be there.

Treatment for Ulcerative Colitis

Treatment for ulcerative colitis depends on the seriousness of the disease. Most people are treated with medication. In severe cases, a patient may need surgery to remove the diseased colon. Surgery is the only cure for ulcerative colitis.

Some people whose symptoms are triggered by certain foods are able to control the symptoms by avoiding foods that upset their intestines, like highly seasoned foods, raw fruits and vegetables, or milk sugar (lactose). Each person may experience ulcerative colitis differently, so treatment is adjusted for each individual. Emotional and psychological support is important.

Some people have remissions—periods when the symptoms go away—that last for months or even years. However, most patients' symptoms eventually return. This changing pattern of the disease means one cannot always tell when a treatment has helped. Some people with ulcerative colitis may need medical care for some time, with regular doctor visits to monitor the condition.

Drug Therapy

The goal of therapy is to induce and maintain remission, and to improve the quality of life for people with ulcerative colitis. Several types of drugs are available.

- **Aminosalicylates,** drugs that contain 5-aminosalicylic acid (5-ASA), help control inflammation. Sulfasalazine is a combination of sulfapyridine and 5-ASA and is used to induce and maintain remission. The sulfapyridine component carries the anti-inflammatory 5-ASA to the intestine. However, sulfapyridine may lead to side effects such as nausea, vomiting, heartburn, diarrhea, and headache. Other 5-ASA agents such as olsalazine, mesalamine, and balsalazide, have a different carrier, offer fewer side effects, and may be used by people who cannot take sulfasalazine. 5-ASAs are given orally, through an enema, or in a suppository, depending on the location of the inflammation in the colon. Most people with mild or moderate ulcerative colitis are treated with this group of drugs first.

- **Corticosteroids,** such as prednisone and hydrocortisone, also reduce inflammation. They may be used by people who have moderate to severe ulcerative colitis or who do not respond to 5-ASA drugs. Corticosteroids, also known as steroids, can be given orally, intravenously, through an enema, or in a suppository depending on the location of the inflammation. These drugs can cause side effects such as weight gain, acne, facial hair, hypertension, mood swings, and an increased risk of infection. For this reason, they are not recommended for long-term use.

- **Immunomodulatory drugs,** such as azathioprine and 6-mercapto-purine (6-MP), reduce inflammation by affecting the immune system. They are used for patients who have not responded to 5-ASAs or corticosteroids or who are dependent on corticosteroids. However, immunomodulatory drugs are slow-acting and may take up to 6 months before the full benefit is seen. Patients taking these drugs are monitored for complications including pancreatitis and hepatitis, a reduced white blood cell count, and an increased risk of infection. Cyclosporine-A may be used with 6-MP or azathioprine to treat active, severe ulcerative colitis in people who do not respond to intravenous corticosteroids.

Other drugs may be given to relax the patient or to relieve pain, diarrhea, or infection.

Hospitalization

Occasionally, symptoms are severe enough that the person must be hospitalized. For example, a person may have severe bleeding or severe diarrhea that causes dehydration. In such cases the doctor will try to stop diarrhea and loss of blood, fluids, and mineral salts. The patient may need a special diet, feeding through a vein, medications, or sometimes surgery.

Surgery

About 25 percent to 40 percent of ulcerative colitis patients must eventually have their colons removed because of massive bleeding, severe illness, rupture of the colon, or risk of cancer. Sometimes the doctor will recommend removing the colon if medical treatment fails or if the side effects of corticosteroids or other drugs threaten the patient's health. Surgery to remove the colon and rectum, known as proctocolectomy, is followed by one of the following:

- **Ileostomy,** in which the surgeon creates a small opening in the abdomen, called a stoma, and attaches the end of the small intestine, called the ileum, to it. Waste will travel through the small intestine and exit the body through the stoma. The stoma is about the size of a quarter and is usually located in the lower right part of the abdomen near the belt line. A pouch is worn over the opening to collect waste, and the patient empties the pouch as needed.

- **Ileoanal anastomosis**, or pull-through operation, which allows the patient to have normal bowel movements because it preserves part of the anus. In this operation, the surgeon removes the diseased part of the colon and the inside of the rectum, leaving the outer muscles of the rectum. The surgeon then attaches the ileum to the inside of the rectum and the anus, creating a pouch. Waste is stored in the pouch and passed through the anus in the usual manner. Bowel movements may be more frequent and watery than before the procedure. Inflammation of the pouch (pouchitis) is a possible complication.

Not every operation is appropriate for every person. Which surgery to have depends on the severity of the disease and the patient's needs, expectations, and lifestyle. People faced with this decision should get as much information as possible by talking to their doctors, to nurses who work with colon surgery patients (enterostomal therapists), and to other colon surgery patients. Patient advocacy organizations can direct people to support groups and other information resources.

Most people with ulcerative colitis will never need to have surgery. If surgery does become necessary, however, some people find comfort in knowing that after the surgery, the colitis is cured and most people go on to live normal, active lives.

Research

Researchers are always looking for new treatments for ulcerative colitis. Therapies that are being tested for usefulness in treating the disease include:

- **Biologic agents.** These include monoclonal antibodies, interferons, and other molecules made by living organisms. Researchers modify these drugs to act specifically, but with decreased side effects, and are studying their effects in people with ulcerative colitis.

- **Budesonide.** This corticosteroid may be nearly as effective as prednisone in treating mild ulcerative colitis, and it has fewer side effects.

- **Heparin.** Researchers are examining whether the anticoagulant heparin can help control colitis.

- **Nicotine.** In an early study, symptoms improved in some patients who were given nicotine through a patch or an enema. (This use of nicotine is still experimental—the findings do not mean that people should go out and buy nicotine patches or start smoking.)

- **Omega-3 fatty acids.** These compounds, naturally found in fish oils, may benefit people with ulcerative colitis by interfering with the inflammatory process.

Is colon cancer a concern?

About 5 percent of people with ulcerative colitis develop colon cancer. The risk of cancer increases with the duration and the extent of involvement of the colon. For example, if only the lower colon and rectum are involved, the risk of cancer is no higher than normal. However, if the entire colon is involved, the risk of cancer may be as much as 32 times the normal rate.

Sometimes precancerous changes occur in the cells lining the colon. These changes are called dysplasia. People who have dysplasia are more likely to develop cancer than those who do not. Doctors look for signs of dysplasia when doing a colonoscopy or sigmoidoscopy and when examining tissue removed during the test.

According to the 2002 updated guidelines for colon cancer screening, people who have had IBD throughout their colon for at least 8 years, and those who have had IBD in only the left colon for 12 to 15 years should have a colonoscopy with biopsies every 1 to 2 years to check for dysplasia. Such screening has not been proven to reduce the risk of colon cancer, but it may help identify cancer early should it develop. These guidelines were produced by an independent expert panel and endorsed by numerous organizations, including the American Cancer Society, the American College of Gastroenterology, the American Society of Colon and Rectal Surgeons, and the Crohn's and Colitis Foundation of America Inc., among others.

Additional Information

Crohn's and Colitis Foundation of America
386 Park Ave. S., 17th Floor
New York, NY 10016-8804
Toll-Free: 800-932-2423
Crohn's and Colitis Foundation of America (continued on next page)

Website: http://www.ccfa.org
E-mail: info@ccfa.org

International Foundation for Functional Gastrointestinal Disorders (IFFGD) Inc.
P.O. Box 170864
Milwaukee, WI 53217-8076
Toll-Free: 888-964-2001
Phone: 414-964-1799
Fax: 414-964-7176
Website: http://www.iffgd.org
E-mail: iffgd@iffgd.org

National Institute of Diabetes and Digestive and Kidney Diseases (NIDDK)
Information Clearinghouse
5 Information Way
Bethesda, MD 20892-3560
Toll-Free: 800-860-8747
Phone: 301-654-3810
Website: http://www.niddk.nih.gov

Reach Out for Youth with Ileitis and Colitis, Inc.
84 Northgate Circle
Melville, NY 11747
Phone: 631-293-3102
Fax: 631-293-3103
Website: http://www.reachoutforyouth.org
E-mail: reachoutforyouth@reachoutforyouth.org

United Ostomy Association, Inc.
19772 MacArthur Blvd., #200
Irvine, CA 92612-2405
Toll-Free: 800-826-0826
Phone: 949-660-8624
Fax: 949-660-9262
Website: http://www.uoa.org
E-mail: uoa@deltanet.com

Chapter 47

Inflammatory Myopathies

Chapter Contents

Section 47.1

What Is Myositis?

What is myositis? (my oe SIE tis)

Myositis is the general term used to describe swelling of the muscles. Injury, infection, and even exercise can cause muscle swelling. The swelling will go away once the injury or infection is treated, or once you rest your muscles from exercise. Certain medicines can also cause some muscle swelling that goes away once you stop taking the medicine.

Often people who have temporary myositis from one of these causes become concerned when they read about the serious, chronic form of myositis. This chapter is referring to inflammatory myopathies.

What are inflammatory myopathies?

Myositis is used in the medical terms of dermatomyositis (DM), polymyositis (PM), inclusion-body myositis (IBM), and juvenile forms of myositis (JM or JPM). These are all considered inflammatory myopathies. Inflammatory myopathies are diseases of the muscle where there is swelling and loss of muscle.

Inflammatory myopathies are thought to be autoimmune diseases, meaning the body's immune system, which normally fights infections and viruses, does not stop fighting once the infection or virus is gone. The immune system then attacks the body's own normal, healthy tissue through inflammation or swelling. All of these diseases can cause muscle weakness, but each type is different.

Some early signs of myositis include:

- Trouble rising from a chair, climbing stairs, or lifting arms.
- Tired feeling after standing or walking.
- Trouble swallowing or breathing.

Testing for myositis: Your doctor may run some tests, including a physical examination, blood tests, electromyogram (EMG), and a muscle biopsy. A myositis diagnosis is often confirmed by the muscle biopsy. If you think you or someone you know may have DM, PM, IBM, JM or JPM, talk to your doctor right away. It is important to start treatment as soon as possible.

Section 47.2

Dermatomyositis

What is dermatomyositis? What are the signs and symptoms?

Dermatomyositis (DM) affects people of any age or sex, but is found in more women than men. DM is thought to be an autoimmune disease, meaning the body's immune system, which normally fights infections and viruses, does not stop fighting once the infection or virus is gone. The immune system then attacks the body's own normal, healthy tissue through inflammation or swelling.

DM is the easiest type of myositis to diagnose because of the skin rash. The DM rash looks patchy, dusky, and red or purple. It is found on the eyelids, cheeks, nose, back, upper chest, elbows, knees, and knuckles. Some people also have hardened bumps under the skin, called calcinosis. The rash is often seen before muscle weakness is felt. The skin rash and weak muscles are caused by inflammation, or swelling in the blood vessels under the skin and in the muscles—vasculitis.

Muscle weakness usually happens over a period of days, weeks, or months. Patients who have the skin rash, but feel no muscle weakness, have amyopathic DM, or DM sine myositis. The weakness begins with muscles that are closest to and within the trunk of the body. Neck, hip, back, and shoulder muscles are examples. Some DM patients have muscle pain and difficulty swallowing, or dysphagia.

363

What tests will the doctor run to decide if I have dermatomyositis?

Your doctor may first ask you questions about your health in general, including your health history. The doctor will want to know when you first saw signs of the skin rash or muscle weakness. He or she will then look at your skin and muscles for signs of DM.

Finally, the doctor may ask the hospital's lab to run one or more of the following tests:

- Blood tests for muscle enzymes (including creatine phosphokinase (CPK) and aldolase tests)
- Muscle biopsy
- Magnetic resonance imaging (MRI)
- Electromyogram (EMG)

There may be other tests to rule out another type of disease or condition. If you have questions about any test, be sure to talk with your doctor or lab technician.

How is dermatomyositis treated?

Many patients do well with oral prednisone. This is a steroid medicine that stops your body from attacking the muscle by slowing down your immune system. If prednisone does not work for you, there are other treatments, including methotrexate; hydroxychloroquine, also known as Plaquenil; and cyclosporine. Some DM patients respond to intravenous immunoglobulin, a medicine given through a needle for a few hours each time.

Your doctor might also want you to do special exercises or a rehabilitation program. Someone will show you how to do the exercises and help you, to make sure that you are doing them right.

Talk with your doctor about DM. If you have DM, it is important to start treatment as soon as possible. Patients that are diagnosed and treated quickly have better results.

Section 47.3

Polymyositis

What is polymyositis? What are the signs and symptoms?

Polymyositis (PM) is found mostly in people over the age of 20.
More women than men have PM. PM is thought to be an autoimmune
disease, meaning the body's immune system, which normally fights
infections and viruses, does not stop fighting once the infection or virus is gone. The immune system then attacks the body's own normal,
healthy tissue through inflammation or swelling.

PM does not cause a rash. Muscle weakness usually happens over
days, weeks, or months. The weakness begins with muscles closest to
and within the trunk of the body. Neck, hip, back, and shoulder muscles are examples. Some patients also have weakness in muscles far-
ther from the trunk, like hands and fingers. Many PM patients have
trouble swallowing, or dysphagia. Some patients have trouble breathing and muscle pain.

What tests will the doctor run to see if I have polymyositis?

Your doctor may first ask you questions about your health in general, including your health history. He or she will want to know when
you first saw signs of muscle weakness or pain. The doctor may test
your muscles to see how strong they are.

Finally, the doctor may ask the hospital's lab to run one or more of
the following tests:

- Blood tests for muscle enzymes (including creatine phosphokinase (CPK) and aldolase tests)

- Muscle biopsy

- Magnetic resonance imaging (MRI)

- Electromyogram (EMG)

The doctor may ask for more tests to rule out another disease or condition. If you have any questions about any tests, be sure to talk to your doctor.

How is polymyositis treated?

There are treatments for PM. Many patients do well with oral prednisone. This is a steroid medicine that stops your body from attacking the muscle by slowing down your immune system. If prednisone does not work for you, there are other treatments.

Your doctor might also want you to do special exercises or a rehabilitation program. Someone will show you how to do the exercises to make sure that you are doing them right.

Talk with your doctor about polymyositis (PM). If you have PM, it is important to start treatment as soon as possible. Patients that are diagnosed and treated quickly have better results. If you do not respond to treatment, you may need to be tested again to make sure that you do not have inclusion-body myositis (IBM).

Section 47.4

Inclusion-Body Myositis

What is inclusion-body myositis? What are the signs and symptoms?

Inclusion-body myositis, or IBM for short, is found in more men than women. Signs of IBM usually start after age 50. A small number of IBM cases may be hereditary, or passed through your parents. IBM is thought to be an autoimmune disease, meaning the body's immune system, which normally fights infections and viruses, does not stop fighting once the infection or virus is gone. The immune system then attacks the body's own normal, healthy tissue through inflammation or swelling.

IBM is slower than the other types of myositis. Muscle weakness happens over months or years. Most muscles are affected including neck, hip, back, shoulder, wrist, and finger muscles. Many IBM patients notice shrinking, or atrophy, in the arms and thighs as the muscles become weaker. Trouble swallowing—dysphagia—is a common problem for IBM patients. Weakness of face muscles is sometimes seen.

How will the doctor test for IBM?

Your doctor may ask you questions about your health in general, including when you first saw signs of muscle weakness. He or she may also test your muscles to see how strong they are, then ask the hospital's lab to run a number of tests. These tests may include the following:

- Blood tests for muscle enzymes (including creatine phosphokinase (CPK) and aldolase tests)
- Muscle biopsy
- Magnetic resonance imaging (MRI)
- Electromyogram (EMG)

The doctor may ask for more tests to rule out another disease or condition. If you have any questions about any tests, be sure to talk to your doctor.

How is inclusion-body myositis treated?

There is no sure treatment for IBM, but you have choices. A few IBM patients have responded to certain treatments including prednisone and intravenous immunoglobulin (IVIG). Special exercises, or physical therapy, might help you stay active. Someone will show you how to do the exercises to make sure that you are doing them right. Talk with your doctor about IBM. If you have IBM, it is important to be diagnosed as soon as possible.

Section 47.5

Juvenile Dermatomyositis

What is juvenile dermatomyositis? What are the signs and symptoms?

Juvenile dermatomyositis, or JM for short, is a disease found in children under the age of 18. JM affects 3,000 to 5,000 children in the United States. JM is thought to be an autoimmune disease. In an autoimmune disease, the body's immune system, which normally fights infections and diseases, fights the body's own tissues and cells. The immune system fights infections or injuries through inflammation or swelling. The other forms of myositis (polymyositis and inclusion-body myositis) are not as common in children as in adults.

The first sign of JM is usually a skin rash. The rash may be red and patchy, like dry skin; a red or purple color on the eyelids or cheeks that may look more like allergies; or both. JM patients can have weak muscles at the same time they see the skin rash, or the weak muscles may come after the rash over days, weeks, or months. The weaker muscles are usually closer to the body (for example, neck, shoulders, back, and stomach), and you may notice your child having trouble climbing or standing from a seated position. The skin rash and weak muscles are caused by inflammation, or swelling in the blood vessels under the skin and in the muscles called vasculitis.

Other signs may include falling, weaker voice (dysphonia), or problems swallowing (dysphagia). About half of the children with JM have pain in their muscles.

Some children may have calcinosis or contractures. Contractures happen when the muscle shortens and causes the joint to stay bent. Exercising the muscles can keep contractures from happening.

How will the doctor know my child has JM?

Your doctor may first ask you and your child questions about your child's health in general, including when you saw the first signs of weakness or rash. The doctor will also look at your child's skin and muscles, looking for signs of JM. Finally, the doctor may ask the hospital's lab to run one or more of the following tests:

- Blood tests for muscle enzymes (including creatine phosphokinase (CPK) and aldolase tests)
- Muscle biopsy
- Magnetic resonance imaging (MRI)
- Electromyogram (EMG)

How can juvenile dermatomyositis be treated?

Most doctors first treat JM with prednisone, which is also called a steroid, corticosteroid, or prednisolone. Prednisone will slow the body's immune system since the immune system is attacking normal, healthy tissue. Side effects of prednisone include weight gain, mood changes, rounder face, and slowed growth. Prednisone also affects children's bones, so doctors may have them take a calcium supplement to help keep their bones healthy and strong. Other possible medicines include methotrexate; hydroxychloroquine, also known as Plaquenil; and cyclosporine.

Doctors often work with physical therapists to find an exercise program that is right for each JM patient. Exercise helps the muscles and joints stay strong and flexible. A balanced and healthy diet is also important for the JM patient.

Talk with your doctor about JM. If your child has JM, it is important to start treatment as soon as possible. Patients who are diagnosed and treated quickly have better results in general.

Additional Information

Myositis Association
1233 20th Street, N.W., Suite 402
Washington, DC 20036
Phone: 202-887-0088
Fax: 202-466-8940
Website: http://www.myositis.org
E-mail: tma@myositis.org

The Myositis Association has a quarterly newsletter especially for JM families, with information for parents and special pages for children. It is sent to every member affected by JM.

Chapter 48

Lambert-Eaton Myasthenic Syndrome (LEMS)

What is Lambert-Eaton myasthenic syndrome?

Lambert-Eaton myasthenic syndrome (LEMS) is a disorder of the neuromuscular junction—the site where nerve cells meet muscle cells and help activate the muscles. It is caused by a disruption of electrical impulses between these nerve and muscle cells. LEMS is an autoimmune condition; in such disorders the immune system, which normally protects the body from foreign organisms, mistakenly attacks the body's own tissues. The disruption of electrical impulses is associated with antibodies produced as a consequence of this autoimmunity. Symptoms include muscle weakness, a tingling sensation in the affected areas, fatigue, and dry mouth. LEMS is closely associated with cancer, in particular small cell lung cancer. More than half the individuals diagnosed with LEMS also develop small cell lung cancer. LEMS may appear up to 3 years before cancer is diagnosed.

Is there any treatment?

There is no cure for LEMS. Treatment is directed at decreasing the autoimmune response (through the use of steroids, plasmapheresis, or high-dose intravenous immunoglobulin) or improving the transmission of the disrupted electrical impulses by giving drugs such as diamino pyridine or pyridostigmine bromide (Mestinon). For patients

"Lambert-Eaton Myasthenic Syndrome Information Page," National Institute of Neurological Disorders and Stroke (NINDS), updated February 09, 2005.

with small cell lung cancer, treatment of the cancer is the first priority.

What is the prognosis?

The prognosis for individuals with LEMS varies. Those with LEMS not associated with malignancy have a benign overall prognosis. Generally the presence of cancer determines the prognosis.

What research is being done?

The NINDS supports research on neuromuscular disorders such as LEMS with the ultimate goal of finding ways to treat, prevent, and cure them.

Additional Information

American Autoimmune-Related Diseases Association, Inc. (AARDA)
22100 Gratiot Ave.
East Detroit, MI 48021
Toll-Free: 800-598-4668 (for literature requests)
Phone: 586-776-3900
Fax: 586-776-3903
Website: http://www.aarda.org
E-mail: aarda@aarda.org

Muscular Dystrophy Association
3300 E. Sunrise Drive
Tucson, AZ 85718
Toll-Free: 800-572-1717
Website: http://www.mdausa.org
E-mail: mda@mdausa.org

National Institute of Neurological Disorders and Stroke
P.O. Box 5801
Bethesda, MD 20824
Toll-Free: 800-352-9424
Phone: 301-496-5751
TTY: 301-468-5981
Website: http://www.ninds.nih.gov

National Organization for Rare Disorders (NORD)
55 Kansas Ave.
P.O. Box 1968
Danbury, CT 06813-1968
Toll-Free: 800-999-6673
Phone: 203-744-0100
TDD: 203-797-9590
Website: http://www.rarediseases.org
E-mail: orphan@rarediseases.org

Chapter 49

Lupus

Lupus, also called systemic lupus erythematosus (SLE), is a disease that affects the immune system. Normally, the immune system fights infections caused by germs. In lupus, instead of protecting the body, the immune system makes the mistake of attacking healthy cells. Lupus can affect almost any part of the body, including joints, skin, kidneys, heart, lungs, blood vessels, and brain. There is no way to know what part of the body will be affected. For most people though, lupus is a mild disease affecting only a few parts of the body, and some patients do not get inner organ problems (like in the heart and lungs), but do have skin and joint problems. Normally, lupus develops slowly, with symptoms that come and go. For some, it can cause serious and even life-threatening problems. Even for patients with diseases that hurt their organs, with good care and management and a strong partnership between a patient and her health care provider, the prognosis is good.

Incidence

Lupus affects up to 1.4 million people in the United States. About 9 out of 10 people who have lupus are women. Lupus is 3 times more common in black women than in white women. It is also more common in women of Hispanic/Latina, Asian, and American Indian descent. Black and Hispanic/Latina women tend to develop symptoms at an earlier age than other women. African Americans have more severe organ problems, especially with their kidneys.

"Lupus," National Women's Health Information Center (NWHIC), September 2003.

373

Types of Lupus

Systemic Lupus Erythematosus (SLE)

SLE is the most common type of lupus. SLE can affect many parts of the body including joints, skin, kidneys, lungs, heart, blood vessels, nervous system, blood, and brain. Although SLE usually develops in people between the ages of 15 and 44 years, it can occur in childhood or later in life. The signs of SLE vary, and there are usually periods of both illness and wellness (also called remission). Some people have just a few signs of the disease while others have more. Its symptoms can include the following:

- butterfly rash across the nose and cheeks
- skin rashes on parts of the body exposed to the sun
- sores in the mouth or nose
- painful or swollen joints
- fever
- weight loss
- hair loss
- fatigue
- chest pain when taking deep breaths
- purple or pale fingers or toes from cold or stress
- abdominal pain
- kidney inflammation
- headaches
- paranoia schizophrenia
- hallucinations
- depression
- trouble thinking
- memory problems
- seizures
- strokes
- blood clots

Discoid Lupus Erythematosus (DLE)

DLE just affects the skin. It does not affect other organs, like SLE. Its symptoms can include:

- A red, raised rash on the face, scalp, or other parts of the body. The rash may become thick and scaly and may last for days or years.

- Sores in the mouth or nose.

A small group of people with DLE later develop SLE. There is no way to know if someone with DLE will get SLE. A skin biopsy (removing a piece of skin to look at under a microscope) of the rash is taken to diagnose this type of lupus.

Drug-Induced Lupus

This type of lupus is a reaction to some prescription medicines. The symptoms of this type of lupus are similar to SLE, except it does not cause problems with the kidneys or central nervous system. It can take months to years of taking the medicine before symptoms appear. After the drug is discontinued, it could take days, weeks, or months for symptoms to go away.

Neonatal Lupus

While rare, some newborn babies of women with SLE or other immune system disorders get lupus. Babies with neonatal lupus may have a serious heart defect. About one-half of babies with neonatal lupus are born with a heart condition. This condition is permanent, but it can be treated with a pacemaker (a device that helps the heart set a rhythm). Other affected babies may have a skin rash or liver problems. Some babies have both heart and skin problems.

Causes

The cause of lupus is not known. It is likely that there is no single cause, but a combination of genetic, environmental, and possibly hormonal factors that work together to cause the disease. Lupus is not contagious—you cannot catch it from someone. No specific lupus gene has been found, but it does run in families.

Diagnosis

SLE may be hard to diagnose and is often mistaken for other diseases. For this reason, lupus has often been called the great imitator. No single test can tell if a person has lupus. There are many ways to diagnose SLE:

1. **Medical history.** Give your health care provider a complete, accurate medical history. This information, along with a physical exam and special tests, helps your doctor rule out other diseases that can be confused with lupus.

2. **Symptoms.** Having 4 (or more) of the 11 symptoms of lupus, as defined by the American College of Rheumatology.

3. **Lab tests.** The antinuclear antibody (ANA) test is a commonly used test. An antibody is a chemical the body makes to fight off infections. The test looks for the strength of your antibodies. Most people with lupus test positive for ANA. However, other health problems, like malaria (a disease from a mosquito bite), can also give you a positive test. That is why other tests may be needed.

Lupus Flares

When symptoms appear, it is called a flare. These may come and go. You may have swelling and rashes one week and no symptoms at all the next. You may find that your symptoms flare after you have been out in the sun or after a hard day at work. Even if you take medicine for lupus, you may find that there are times when the symptoms become worse. Learning to recognize that a flare is coming can help you take steps to cope with it. Many people feel very tired or have pain, a rash, a fever, stomach discomfort, headache, or dizziness just before a flare.

Take steps to prevent flares:

* Learn to recognize that a flare is coming.
* Try to set realistic goals and priorities.
* Limit the time you spend in the sun.
* Maintain a healthy diet.
* Develop coping skills to help limit stress.
* Get enough rest.
* Exercise moderately when possible.
* Develop a support system of family, friends, and health care providers.

Treatment

There is no known cure for lupus, but there are effective treatments. Most of the symptoms of lupus are from inflammation (swelling), so treatment focuses on reducing the swelling. Treatment may include taking these medicines:

- **Nonsteroidal anti-inflammatory drugs (NSAIDs).** NSAIDs are often used to reduce joint and muscle pain and inflammation in people who have mild SLE (mild pain or organs are not affected). There are many different types of NSAIDs, both prescription drugs and over-the-counter drugs. These include aspirin, ibuprofen, naproxen, and other medicines. Common side effects of NSAIDs can include stomach upset, heartburn, drowsiness, headache, and fluid retention. If you have any side effects, talk to your health care provider. NSAIDs can also cause problems in your blood, liver, and kidneys.

- **Antimalarial drugs.** Medicines used to prevent or treat malaria are used to treat joint pain, skin rashes, and ulcers. Two common antimalarials are hydroxychloroquine (Plaquenil) and chloroquine (Aralen). Side effects of antimalarials can include stomach upset, nausea, vomiting, diarrhea, headache, dizziness, blurred vision, insomnia, and itching.

- **Corticosteroid hormones.** These are powerful drugs that reduce inflammation in various tissues of the body. They can be taken by mouth, in creams applied to the skin, or by injection. Prednisone is a corticosteroid that is often used to treat lupus. Corticosteroids can have various side effects, so doctors try to use the lowest dose possible. Short-term side effects include swelling, increased appetite, weight gain, and emotional ups and downs. These side effects generally stop when the drug is stopped. Long-term side effects of corticosteroids can include stretch marks on the skin, excessive hair growth, weakened or damaged bones, high blood pressure, damage to the arteries, high blood sugar, infections, and cataracts. People with lupus who are using corticosteroids should talk to their health care provider about taking calcium supplements, vitamin D, or other drugs to reduce the risk of osteoporosis (weakened, fragile bones).

- **Immunosuppressive agents/chemotherapy.** These agents are used in serious cases of lupus, when major organs are losing their ability to function. These drugs suppress the immune system to limit the damage to the organ. Examples are azathioprine (Imuran) and cyclophosphamide (Cytoxan). These drugs can cause serious side effects including nausea, vomiting, hair loss, bladder problems, decreased fertility, and increased risk of cancer and infection.

Work closely with your health care provider to ensure that your treatment plan is as successful as possible. Because some treatments may cause harmful side effects, promptly report any new symptoms. It is also important not to stop or change treatments without talking to your health care provider first.

Is it safe for me to become pregnant?

Today, most women with lupus can safely become pregnant. With proper medical care, you can lower the risks of pregnancy and deliver a normal, healthy baby. However, you must carefully plan your pregnancy. Your disease should be under control or in remission for 12 months before you get pregnant. Find an obstetrician who is experienced in managing high-risk pregnancies, and who can work closely with your primary health care provider. Plan your delivery at a hospital that can manage high-risk patients and provide the specialized care you and your baby may need. Talk to your doctor about which medicines are safe to take while pregnant.

Women with lupus may face certain problems during the pregnancy. While flares are not caused by pregnancy, flares that do develop often occur during the first or second trimester or during the first few months following delivery. Most flares are mild and easily treated with small doses of corticosteroids. Another complication is pre-eclampsia. Pre-eclampsia causes a sudden increase in blood pressure, protein in the urine, or both. This is a serious condition that requires immediate treatment, and you might have to deliver your infant early.

Babies born to women with lupus have no greater chance of birth defects or mental retardation than do babies born to women without lupus. As your pregnancy progresses, your obstetrician will regularly check the baby's heartbeat and growth with sonograms (a machine that creates pictures of your baby's organs). Although giving birth to your baby early (prematurity) presents a danger to the baby, most problems can be successfully treated in a hospital that specializes in caring for premature newborns. About 3% of babies born to mothers with lupus will have neonatal lupus.

Breast feeding your baby is safe for mothers with lupus. If you are on medications and breast feeding, talk with your provider about how the medicine might affect your baby.

How can I tell the difference between symptoms of lupus and symptoms of pregnancy?

It may be hard to tell the difference. You may have symptoms from being pregnant that you mistake for lupus symptoms. Here are just some problems that may cause confusion:

- **Skin.** While pregnant, you may have red palms and a rash. Lupus can also cause a rash.

- **Joints.** Lupus can cause arthritis. Pregnancy can cause aching in your joints.

- **Lungs.** It may be hard for you to breathe if you have lupus. Pregnancy can also cause a shortness of breath and hyperventilation.

Talk to your health care provider about how to tell the difference between the physical changes you will have during your pregnancy and symptoms of lupus.

How can I cope with the stress of having lupus?

Staying healthy takes extra effort and care for women with lupus. Sometimes, women with lupus may feel tired, and you may need extra rest because of your treatments. If you feel tired, make a point to allow yourself extra time in your schedule for rest. Some approaches that may help you to cope with lupus include the following:

- exercising
- relaxing, using techniques like meditation
- setting priorities for spending time and energy
- educating yourself about the disease
- having a good support system

A support system may include family, friends, health care providers, community organizations, and organized support groups. Participating in a support group can provide emotional help, boost self-esteem and morale, and help develop or improve coping skills. Also, talk to your family about how they can support your efforts to take care of yourself.

What research is being done on lupus?

There are many promising areas of research on lupus. Studies are looking at the safety of estrogen use (hormone therapy and birth control pills) by women with lupus; causes or risk factors for lupus (including behavior, genetics, environment, and culture); and lupus in minority women.

Additional Information

American Autoimmune-Related Diseases Association, Inc. (AARDA)
22100 Gratiot Ave.
East Detroit, MI 48021
Toll-Free: 800-598-4668 (for literature requests)
Phone: 586-776-3900
Fax: 586-776-3903
Website: http://www.aarda.org
E-mail: aarda@aarda.org

American College of Rheumatology (ACR)
1800 Century Pl., Suite 250
Atlanta, GA 30345
Phone: 404-633-3777
Fax: 404-633-1870
Website: http://www.rheumatology.org
E-mail: acr@rheumatology.org

Arthritis Foundation
P.O. Box 7660
Atlanta, GA 30357-0669
Toll-Free: 800-568-4045
Phone: 404-965-7888
Website: http://www.arthritis.org
E-mail: help@arthritis.org

Lupus Foundation of America, Inc.
2000 L Street, N.W., Suite 710
Washington, DC 20036
Toll-Free: 800-558-0121
Phone: 202-349-1155
Fax: 202-349-1156
Website: http://www.lupus.org
E-mail: lupusinfo@lupus.org

SLE Lupus Foundation, Inc.
149 Madison Ave., Suite 205
New York, NY 10016
Toll-Free: 800-74-LUPUS (58787)
Phone: 212-685-4118
Fax: 212-545-1843
Website: http://www.lupusny.org
E-mail: lupus@lupusny.org

Chapter 50

Multiple Sclerosis

Although multiple sclerosis (MS) was first diagnosed in 1849, the earliest known description of a person with possible MS dates from fourteenth century Holland. An unpredictable disease of the central nervous system, MS can range from relatively benign, to somewhat disabling, to devastating as communication between the brain and other parts of the body is disrupted.

The vast majority of patients are mildly affected, but in the worst cases MS can render a person unable to write, speak, or walk. A physician can diagnose MS in some patients soon after the onset of the illness. In others, however, physicians may not be able to readily identify the cause of the symptoms, leading to years of uncertainty and multiple diagnoses punctuated by baffling symptoms that mysteriously wax and wane.

What is multiple sclerosis?

During an MS attack, inflammation occurs in areas of the white matter of the central nervous system in random patches called plaques. This process is followed by destruction of myelin, the fatty covering that insulates nerve cell fibers in the brain and spinal cord. Myelin facilitates the smooth, high-speed transmission of electrochemical messages between the brain, the spinal cord, and the rest of the body; when it is damaged, neurological transmission of messages

Excerpted from "Multiple Sclerosis: Hope Through Research," National Institute of Neurological Disorders and Stroke (NINDS), updated March 4, 2005.

may be slowed or blocked completely, leading to diminished or lost function. The name multiple sclerosis signifies both the number (multiple) and condition (sclerosis, from the Greek term for scarring or hardening) of the demyelinated areas in the central nervous system.

How many people have MS?

No one knows exactly how many people have MS. It is believed that, currently, there are approximately 250,000 to 350,000 people in the United States with MS diagnosed by a physician. This estimate suggests that approximately 200 new cases are diagnosed each week.

Who gets MS?

Most people experience their first symptoms of MS between the ages of 20 and 40, but a diagnosis is often delayed. This is due to both the transitory nature of the disease and the lack of a specific diagnostic test—specific symptoms and changes in the brain must develop before the diagnosis is confirmed.

Although scientists have documented cases of MS in young children and elderly adults, symptoms rarely begin before age 15 or after age 60. Whites are more than twice as likely as other races to develop MS. In general, women are affected at almost twice the rate of men; however, among patients who develop the symptoms of MS at a later age, the gender ratio is more balanced.

MS is five times more prevalent in temperate climates—such as those found in the northern United States, Canada, and Europe—than in tropical regions. Furthermore, the age of 15 seems to be significant in terms of risk for developing the disease: some studies indicate that a person moving from a high-risk (temperate) to a low-risk (tropical) area before the age of 15 tends to adopt the risk (in this case, low) of the new area and vice versa. Other studies suggest that people moving after age 15 maintain the risk of the area where they grew up.

These findings indicate a strong role for an environmental factor in the cause of MS. It is possible that, at the time of or immediately following puberty, patients acquire an infection with a long latency period. Or, conversely, people in some areas may come in contact with an unknown protective agent during the time before puberty. Other studies suggest that the unknown geographic or climatic element may actually be simply a matter of genetic predilection and reflect racial and ethnic susceptibility factors.

Periodically, scientists receive reports of MS clusters. The most famous of these MS epidemics took place in the Faeroe Islands north of Scotland in the years following the arrival of British troops during World War II. Despite intense study of this and other clusters, no direct environmental factor has been identified. Nor has any definitive evidence been found to link daily stress to MS attacks, although there is evidence that the risk of worsening is greater after acute viral illnesses.

What causes MS?

Scientists have learned a great deal about MS in recent years; still, its cause remains elusive. Many investigators believe MS to be an autoimmune disease—one in which the body, through its immune system, launches a defensive attack against its own tissues. In the case of MS, it is the nerve-insulating myelin that comes under assault. Such assaults may be linked to an unknown environmental trigger, perhaps a virus.

Is MS inherited?

Increasing scientific evidence suggests that genetics may play a role in determining a person's susceptibility to MS. Some populations, such as Gypsies, Eskimos, and Bantus, never get MS. Native Indians of North and South America, the Japanese, and other Asian peoples have very low incidence rates. It is unclear whether this is due mostly to genetic or environmental factors.

In the population at large, the chance of developing MS is less than a tenth of one percent. However, if one person in a family has MS, that person's first-degree relatives—parents, children, and siblings—have a one to three percent chance of getting the disease.

Further indications that more than one gene is involved in MS susceptibility comes from studies of families in which more than one member has MS. Several research teams found that people with MS inherit certain regions on individual genes more frequently than people without MS. Of particular interest is the human leukocyte antigen (HLA) or major histocompatibility complex region on chromosome 6. HLAs are genetically determined proteins that influence the immune system. The HLA patterns of MS patients tend to be different from those of people without the disease.

Studies strengthen the theory that MS is the result of a number of factors rather than a single gene or other agent. Development of MS is likely to be influenced by the interactions of a number of genes, each of which (individually) has only a modest effect. Additional studies are needed to specifically pinpoint which genes are involved, determine their function, and learn how each gene's interactions with other genes and with the environment make an individual susceptible to MS. In addition to leading to better ways to diagnose MS, such studies should yield clues to the underlying causes of MS and, eventually, to better treatments or a way to prevent the disease.

What is the course of MS?

Each case of MS displays one of several patterns of presentation and subsequent course. Most commonly, MS first manifests itself as a series of attacks followed by complete or partial remissions as symptoms mysteriously lessen, only to return later after a period of stability. This is called relapsing-remitting (RR) MS. Primary-progressive (PP) MS is characterized by a gradual clinical decline with no distinct remissions, although there may be temporary plateaus or minor relief from symptoms. Secondary-progressive (SP) MS begins with a relapsing-remitting course followed by a later primary-progressive course. Rarely, patients may have a progressive-relapsing (PR) course in which the disease takes a progressive path punctuated by acute attacks. PP, SP, and PR are sometimes lumped together and called chronic progressive MS.

In addition, twenty percent of the MS population has a benign form of the disease in which symptoms show little or no progression after the initial attack; these patients remain fully functional. A few patients experience malignant MS, defined as a swift and relentless decline resulting in significant disability or even death shortly after disease onset. However, MS is very rarely fatal, and most people with MS have a fairly normal life expectancy.

Can life events affect the course of MS?

While there is no good evidence that daily stress or trauma affects the course of MS, there is data on the influence of pregnancy. Since MS generally strikes during childbearing years, a common concern among women with the disease is whether or not to have a baby. Studies on the subject have shown that MS has no adverse effects on the course of pregnancy, labor, or delivery; in fact symptoms often stabilize or remit during pregnancy. This temporary improvement is thought to relate to changes in a woman's immune system that allow her body to carry a baby: because every fetus has genetic material from the father as well as the mother, the mother's body should identify the growing fetus as foreign tissue and try to reject it in much the same way the body seeks to reject a transplanted organ. To prevent this from happening, a natural process takes place to suppress the mother's immune system in the uterus during pregnancy.

However, women with MS who are considering pregnancy need to be aware that certain drugs used to treat MS should be avoided during pregnancy and while breast feeding. These drugs can cause birth defects and can be passed to the fetus via blood and to an infant via breast milk. Among them are prednisone, corticotropin, azathioprine, cyclophosphamide, diazepam, phenytoin, carbamazepine, and baclofen.

Unfortunately, between 20 and 40 percent of women with MS do have a relapse in the three months following delivery. However, there is no evidence that pregnancy and childbirth affect the overall course of the disease one way or the other. Also, while MS is not in itself a reason to avoid pregnancy and poses no significant risks to the fetus, physical limitations can make childcare more difficult. Therefore, it is important that MS patients planning families discuss these issues with both their partner and physician.

What are the symptoms of MS?

Symptoms of MS may be mild or severe, of long duration or short, and may appear in various combinations, depending on the area of the nervous system affected. Complete or partial remission of symptoms, especially in the early stages of the disease, occurs in approximately 70 percent of MS patients.

The initial symptom of MS is often blurred or double vision, red-green color distortion, or even blindness in one eye. Inexplicably, visual problems tend to clear up in the later stages of MS. Inflammatory problems of the optic nerve may be diagnosed as retrobulbar or optic neuritis. Fifty-five percent of MS patients will have an attack of optic neuritis at some time or other and it will be the first symptom of MS in approximately 15 percent. This has led to general recognition of optic neuritis as an early sign of MS, especially if tests also reveal abnormalities in the patient's spinal fluid.

Most MS patients experience muscle weakness in their extremities and difficulty with coordination and balance at some time during the course of the disease. These symptoms may be severe enough to impair walking or even standing. In the worst cases, MS can produce partial or complete paralysis. Spasticity—the involuntary increased tone of muscles leading to stiffness and spasms—is common, as is fatigue. Fatigue may be triggered by physical exertion and improve with rest, or it may take the form of a constant and persistent tiredness.

Most people with MS also exhibit paresthesias, transitory abnormal sensory feelings such as numbness, prickling, or pins and needles sensations; uncommonly, some may also experience pain. Loss of sensation sometimes occurs. Speech impediments, tremors, and dizziness are other frequent complaints. Occasionally, people with MS have hearing loss.

Approximately half of all people with MS experience cognitive impairments such as difficulties with concentration, attention, memory, and poor judgment, but such symptoms are usually mild and are frequently overlooked. In fact, they are often detectable only through comprehensive testing. Patients themselves may be unaware of their cognitive loss; it is often a family member or friend who first notices a deficit. Such impairments are usually mild, rarely disabling, and intellectual and language abilities are generally spared.

Cognitive symptoms occur when lesions develop in brain areas responsible for information processing. These deficits tend to become more apparent as the information to be processed becomes more complex. Fatigue may also add to processing difficulties. Scientists do not yet know whether altered cognition in MS reflects problems with information acquisition, retrieval, or a combination of both. Types of memory problems may differ depending on the individual's disease course (relapsing-remitting, primary-progressive, etc.), but there does not appear to be any direct correlation between duration of illness and severity of cognitive dysfunction.

Depression, which is unrelated to cognitive problems, is another common feature of MS. In addition, about 10 percent of patients suffer from more severe psychotic disorders such as manic-depression and paranoia. Five percent may experience episodes of inappropriate euphoria and despair—unrelated to the patient's actual emotional state—known as laughing/weeping syndrome. This syndrome is thought to be due to demyelination in the brainstem, the area of the brain that controls facial expression and emotions, and is usually seen only in severe cases.

As the disease progresses, sexual dysfunction may become a problem. Bowel and bladder control may also be lost.

In about 60 percent of MS patients, heat—whether generated by temperatures outside the body or by exercise—may cause temporary worsening of many MS symptoms. In these cases, eradicating the heat eliminates the problem. Some temperature-sensitive patients find that a cold bath may temporarily relieve their symptoms. For the same reason, swimming is often a good exercise choice for people with MS.

The erratic symptoms of MS can affect the entire family as patients may become unable to work at the same time they are facing high medical bills and additional expenses for housekeeping assistance and modifications to homes and vehicles. The emotional drain on both patient and family is immeasurable. Support groups and counseling may help MS patients, their families, and friends find ways to cope with the many problems the disease can cause.

Possible Symptoms of Multiple Sclerosis

- Muscle weakness
- Spasticity
- Impairment of senses of pain, temperature, and touch
- Pain (moderate to severe)
- Ataxia
- Tremor
- Speech disturbances
- Vision disturbances
- Vertigo
- Bladder dysfunction
- Bowel dysfunction
- Sexual dysfunction
- Depression
- Euphoria
- Cognitive abnormalities
- Fatigue

How is MS diagnosed?

There is no single test that unequivocally detects MS. When faced with a patient whose symptoms, neurological exam results, and medical history suggest MS, physicians use a variety of tools to rule out other possible disorders and perform a series of laboratory tests which, if positive, confirm the diagnosis.

Imaging technologies such as magnetic resonance imaging (MRI) can help locate central nervous system lesions resulting from myelin loss. MRI is painless, noninvasive, and does not expose the body to radiation. It is often used in conjunction with the contrast agent gadolinium, which helps distinguish new plaques from old. However, since these lesions can also occur in several other neurological disorders, they are not absolute evidence of MS.

Several new MRI techniques may help quantify and characterize MS lesions that are too subtle to be detected using conventional MRI scans. While standard MRI provides an anatomical picture of lesions, magnetic resonance spectroscopy (MRS) yields information about the brain's biochemistry; specifically, it can measure the brain chemical N-acetyl aspartate. Decreased levels of this chemical can indicate nerve damage.

Magnetization transfer imaging (MTI) is able to detect white matter abnormalities before lesions can be seen on standard MRI scans by calculating the amount of free water in tissues. Demyelinated tissues and damaged nerves show increased levels of free (versus bound) water particles.

Diffusion-tensor magnetic resonance imaging (DT-MRI or DTI) measures the random motion of water molecules. Individual water molecules are constantly in motion, colliding with each other at extremely high speeds. This causes them to spread out, or diffuse. DT-MRI maps this diffusion to produce intricate, three-dimensional images indicating the size and location of demyelinated areas of the brain. Changes in this process can then be measured and correlated with disease progression.

Functional MRI (fMRI) uses radio waves and a strong magnetic field to measure the correlation between physical changes in the brain (such as blood flow) and mental functioning during the performance of cognitive tasks.

In addition to helping scientists and physicians better understand how MS develops—an important first step in devising new treatments—these approaches offer earlier diagnosis and enhance efforts to monitor disease progression and the effects of treatment.

Other tests that may be used to diagnosis MS include visual evoked potential (VEP) tests and studies of cerebrospinal fluid (the colorless liquid that circulates through the brain and spinal cord). VEP tests measure the speed of the brain's response to visual stimuli. VEP can sometimes detect lesions that the scanners miss, and is particularly useful when abnormalities seen on MRI do not meet the specific criteria for MS. Auditory and sensory evoked potentials have also been used in the past, but are no longer believed to contribute significantly to the diagnosis of MS. Like imaging technologies, VEP is helpful, but not conclusive because it cannot identify the cause of lesions.

Examination of cerebrospinal fluid can show cellular and chemical abnormalities often associated with MS. These abnormalities include increased numbers of white blood cells and higher-than-average amounts of protein, especially myelin basic protein and an antibody called immunoglobulin G. Physicians can use several different laboratory techniques to separate and graph the various proteins in MS patients' cerebrospinal fluid. This process often identifies the presence of a characteristic pattern called oligoclonal bands.

While it can still be difficult for the physician to differentiate between an MS attack and symptoms that can follow a viral infection or even an immunization, our growing understanding of disease mechanisms and the expanded use of MRI is enabling physicians to diagnose MS with far more confidence than ever before. Today, most patients who undergo a diagnostic evaluation for MS will be classified as either having MS or not having MS, although there are still cases where a person may have the clinical symptoms of MS, but not meet all the criteria to confirm a diagnosis of MS. In these cases, a diagnosis of possible MS is used.

A number of other diseases may produce symptoms similar to those seen in MS. Other conditions with an intermittent course and MS-like lesions of the brain's white matter include polyarteritis, lupus erythematosus, syringomyelia, tropical spastic paraparesis, some cancers, and certain tumors that compress the brainstem or spinal cord. Progressive multifocal leukoencephalopathy can mimic the acute stage of an MS attack. Physicians will also need to rule out stroke, neurosyphilis, spinocerebellar ataxias, pernicious anemia, diabetes, Sjögren disease, and vitamin B_{12} deficiency. Acute transverse myelitis may signal the first attack of MS, or it may indicate other problems such as infection with the Epstein-Barr or herpes simplex B viruses. Recent reports suggest that the neurological problems associated with Lyme disease may present a clinical picture much like MS.

Investigators are continuing their search for a definitive test for MS. Until one is developed, however, evidence of both multiple attacks and central nervous system lesions must be found before a diagnosis of MS is given.

Can MS be treated?

There is as yet no cure for MS. Many patients do well with no therapy at all, especially since many medications have serious side effects and some carry significant risks. Naturally occurring or spontaneous remissions make it difficult to determine therapeutic effects of experimental treatments; however, the emerging evidence that MRIs can chart the development of lesions is already helping scientists evaluate new therapies.

In the past, the principal medications physicians used to treat MS were steroids possessing anti-inflammatory properties. Studies suggest that intravenous methylprednisolone may be superior to the more traditional intravenous ACTH for patients experiencing acute relapses; no strong evidence exists to support the use of these drugs to treat progressive forms of MS. Also, there is some indication that steroids may be more appropriate for people with movement, rather than sensory, symptoms.

While steroids do not affect the course of MS over time, they can reduce the duration and severity of attacks in some patients. Because steroids can produce numerous adverse side effects (acne, weight gain, seizures, psychosis), they are not recommended for long-term use.

One of the most promising MS research areas involves naturally occurring antiviral proteins known as interferons. Three forms of beta interferon (Avonex, Betaseron, and Rebif) have now been approved by the Food and Drug Administration for treatment of relapsing-remitting MS. Beta interferon has been shown to reduce the number of exacerbations and may slow the progression of physical disability. When attacks do occur, they tend to be shorter and less severe. In addition, MRI scans suggest that beta interferon can decrease myelin destruction.

Investigators speculate that the effects of beta interferon may be due to the drug's ability to correct an MS-related deficiency of certain white blood cells that suppress the immune system and/or its ability to inhibit gamma interferon, a substance believed to be involved in MS attacks. Alpha interferon is also being studied as a possible treatment for MS. Common side effects of interferons include fever, chills, sweating, muscle aches, fatigue, depression, and injection site reactions.

Scientists continue their extensive efforts to create new and better therapies for MS. Goals of therapy are threefold: to improve recovery from attacks, to prevent or lessen the number of relapses, and to halt disease progression. Some therapies currently under investigation include:

- **Immunotherapy:** As evidence of immune system involvement in the development of MS has grown, trials of various new treatments to alter or suppress immune response are being conducted. Most of these therapies are, at this time, still considered experimental.

- **Nerve impulse conduction therapy:** Because the transmission of electrochemical messages between the brain and body is disrupted in MS, medications to improve the conduction of nerve impulses are being investigated.

- **Antigen therapy:** Trials of a synthetic form of myelin basic protein, called copolymer I (Copaxone), were successful, leading the FDA to approve the agent for the treatment of relapsing-remitting MS.

- **Cytokines:** Cytokines, the powerful chemicals produced by T cells, may be used to manipulate the immune system. Scientists are studying a variety of substances that may block harmful cytokines, such as those involved in inflammation, or that encourage the production of protective cytokines.

- **Remyelination:** Some studies focus on strategies to reverse the damage to myelin and oligodendrocytes (the cells that make and maintain myelin in the central nervous system), both of which are destroyed during MS attacks.

- **Diet:** Over the years, many people have tried to implicate diet as a cause of or treatment for MS. To date, clinical studies have not been able to confirm benefits from dietary changes.

- **Unproven Therapies:** MS is a disease with a natural tendency to remit spontaneously, and for which there is no universally effective treatment and no known cause. These factors open the door for an array of unsubstantiated claims of cures. At one time or another, many ineffective and even potentially dangerous therapies have been promoted as treatments for MS. None of these treatments is an effective therapy for MS or any of its symptoms.

Are any MS symptoms treatable?

While some scientists look for therapies that will affect the overall course of the disease, others are searching for new and better medications to control the symptoms of MS without triggering intolerable side effects. Symptoms which can be addressed through medical treatment include the following:

- Spasticity
- Weakness and ataxia (incoordination)
- Fatigue
- Bladder malfunctions
- Urinary problems and constipation
- Sexual dysfunction

- Depression
- Tremors

What recent advances have been made in MS research?

Many advances, on several fronts, have been made in the war against MS. Each advance interacts with the others, adding greater depth and meaning to each new discovery. Scientists are now able to visualize and follow the development of MS lesions in the brain and spinal cord using MRI; this ability is a tremendous aid in the assessment of new therapies and can speed the process of evaluating new treatments.

Other tools have been developed that make the painstaking work of teasing out the disease's genetic secrets possible. Such studies have strengthened scientists' conviction that MS is a disease with many genetic components, none of which is dominant. Immune system-related genetic factors that predispose an individual to the development of MS have been identified, and may lead to new ways to treat or prevent the disease. In fact, a treatment that may actually slow the course of the disease has been found and a growing number of therapies are now available that effectively treat some MS symptoms. In addition, there are a number of treatments under investigation that may curtail attacks or improve function of demyelinated nerve fibers. Over a dozen clinical trials testing potential therapies are underway, and additional new treatments are being devised and tested in animal models.

Additional Information

American Autoimmune-Related Diseases Association, Inc. (AARDA)
22100 Gratiot Ave.
East Detroit, MI 48021
Toll-Free: 800-598-4668 (for literature requests)
Phone: 586-776-3900
Fax: 586-776-3903
Website: http://www.aarda.org
E-mail: aarda@aarda.org

International Essential Tremor Foundation
P.O. Box 14005
Lenexa, KS 66285-4005
Toll-Free: 888-387-3667
Phone: 913-341-3880

Fax: 913-341-1296
Website: http://www.essentialtremor.org
E-mail: staff@essentialtremor.org

Multiple Sclerosis Foundation
6350 N. Andrews Ave.
Ft. Lauderdale, FL 33309-2130
Toll-Free: 888-MSFOCUS (673-6287)
Phone: 954-776-6805
Fax: 954-351-0630
Website: http://www.msfocus.org
E-mail: support@msfocus.org

National Institute of Neurological Disorders and Stroke
P.O. Box 5801
Bethesda, MD 20824
Toll-Free: 800-352-9424
Phone: 301-496-5751
TTY: 301-468-5981
Website: http://www.ninds.nih.gov

National Multiple Sclerosis Society
733 Third Ave., 6th Floor
New York, NY 10017-3288
Toll-Free: 800-344-4867
Phone: 212-986-3240
Fax: 212-986-7981
Website: http://www.nmss.org
E-mail: info@nmss.org

Well Spouse Foundation
63 W. Main St., Suite H
Freehold, NJ 07728
Toll-Free: 800-838-0879
Phone: 732-577-8899
Fax: 732-577-8644
Website: http://www.wellspouse.org
E-mail: info@wellspouse.org

Chapter 51

Myasthenia Gravis

Myasthenia gravis is a chronic autoimmune neuromuscular disease characterized by varying degrees of weakness of the skeletal (voluntary) muscles of the body. The name myasthenia gravis, which is Latin and Greek in origin, literally means grave muscle weakness. With current therapies, however, most cases of myasthenia gravis are not as grave as the name implies. In fact, for the majority of individuals with myasthenia gravis, life expectancy is not lessened by the disorder.

The hallmark of myasthenia gravis is muscle weakness that increases during periods of activity and improves after periods of rest. Certain muscles such as those that control eye and eyelid movement, facial expression, chewing, talking, and swallowing are often, but not always, involved in the disorder. The muscles that control breathing and neck and limb movements may also be affected.

Causes of Myasthenia Gravis

Myasthenia gravis is caused by a defect in the transmission of nerve impulses to muscles. It occurs when normal communication between the nerve and muscle is interrupted at the neuromuscular junction—the place where nerve cells connect with the muscles they control. Normally when impulses travel down the nerve, the nerve endings release a neurotransmitter substance called acetylcholine.

"Myasthenia Gravis Fact Sheet," National Institute of Neurological Disorders and Stroke (NINDS), NIH Publication No. 99–768, updated February 9, 2005.

Acetylcholine travels through the neuromuscular junction and binds to acetylcholine receptors which are activated and generate a muscle contraction. In myasthenia gravis, antibodies block, alter, or destroy the receptors for acetylcholine at the neuromuscular junction which prevents the muscle contraction from occurring. These antibodies are produced by the body's own immune system. Thus, myasthenia gravis is an autoimmune disease because the immune system—which normally protects the body from foreign organisms—mistakenly attacks itself.

The Thymus Gland in Myasthenia Gravis

The thymus gland, which lies in the upper chest area beneath the breastbone, plays an important role in the development of the immune system in early life. Its cells form a part of the body's normal immune system. The gland is somewhat large in infants, grows gradually until puberty, and then gets smaller and is replaced by fat with age. In adults with myasthenia gravis, the thymus gland is abnormal. It contains certain clusters of immune cells indicative of lymphoid hyperplasia—a condition usually found only in the spleen and lymph nodes during an active immune response. Some individuals with myasthenia gravis develop thymomas or tumors of the thymus gland. Generally thymomas are benign, but they can become malignant.

The relationship between the thymus gland and myasthenia gravis is not yet fully understood. Scientists believe the thymus gland may give incorrect instructions to developing immune cells, ultimately resulting in autoimmunity and the production of the acetylcholine receptor antibodies, thereby setting the stage for the attack on neuromuscular transmission.

Symptoms

Although myasthenia gravis may affect any voluntary muscle, muscles that control eye and eyelid movement, facial expression, and swallowing are most frequently affected. The onset of the disorder may be sudden. Symptoms often are not immediately recognized as myasthenia gravis.

In most cases, the first noticeable symptom is weakness of the eye muscles. In others, difficulty in swallowing and slurred speech may be the first signs. The degree of muscle weakness involved in myasthenia gravis varies greatly among patients, ranging from a localized form, limited to eye muscles (ocular myasthenia), to a severe or generalized form in which many muscles—sometimes including those that control breathing—are affected. Symptoms, which vary in type and severity, may include a drooping of one or both eyelids (ptosis); blurred or double vision (diplopia) due to weakness of the muscles that control eye movements; unstable or waddling gait; weakness in arms, hands, fingers, legs, and neck; a change in facial expression; difficulty in swallowing; shortness of breath; and impaired speech (dysarthria).

Incidence

Myasthenia gravis occurs in all ethnic groups and both genders. It most commonly affects young adult women (under 40) and older men (over 60), but it can occur at any age.

In neonatal myasthenia, the fetus may acquire immune proteins (antibodies) from a mother affected with myasthenia gravis. Generally, cases of neonatal myasthenia gravis are transient (temporary), and the child's symptoms usually disappear within 2–3 months after birth. Other children develop myasthenia gravis indistinguishable from adults. Myasthenia gravis in juveniles is common.

Myasthenia gravis is not directly inherited nor is it contagious. Occasionally, the disease may occur in more than one member of the same family.

Rarely, children may show signs of congenital myasthenia or congenital myasthenic syndrome. These are not autoimmune disorders, but are caused by defective genes that produce proteins in the acetylcholine receptor or in acetylcholinesterase.

Diagnosis

Unfortunately, a delay in diagnosis of one or two years is not unusual in cases of myasthenia gravis. Because weakness is a common symptom of many other disorders, the diagnosis is often missed in people who experience mild weakness or in those individuals whose weakness is restricted to only a few muscles.

The first steps of diagnosing myasthenia gravis include a review of the individual's medical history, and physical and neurological examinations. The signs a physician must look for are impairment of eye movements or muscle weakness without any changes in the individual's ability to feel things. If the doctor suspects myasthenia gravis, several tests are available to confirm the diagnosis.

A special blood test can detect the presence of immune molecules or acetylcholine receptor antibodies. Most patients with myasthenia gravis have abnormally elevated levels of these antibodies. However, antibodies may not be detected in patients with only ocular forms of the disease.

Another test is called the edrophonium test. This approach requires the intravenous administration of edrophonium chloride or Tensilon®, a drug that blocks the degradation (breakdown) of acetylcholine and temporarily increases the levels of acetylcholine at the neuromuscular junction. In people with myasthenia gravis involving the eye muscles, edrophonium chloride will briefly relieve weakness. Other methods to confirm the diagnosis include a version of nerve conduction study which tests for specific muscle fatigue by repetitive nerve stimulation. This test records weakening muscle responses when the nerves are repetitively stimulated. Repetitive stimulation of a nerve during a nerve conduction study may demonstrate decrements of the muscle action potential due to impaired nerve-to-muscle transmission.

A different test called single fiber electromyography (EMG), in which single muscle fibers are stimulated by electrical impulses, can also detect impaired nerve-to-muscle transmission. EMG measures the electrical potential of muscle cells. Muscle fibers in myasthenia gravis, as well as other neuromuscular disorders, do not respond as well to repeated electrical stimulation compared to muscles from normal individuals. Computed tomography (CT) may be used to identify an abnormal thymus gland or the presence of a thymoma.

A special examination called pulmonary function testing—which measures breathing strength—helps to predict whether respiration may fail and lead to a myasthenic crisis.

Treatment

Today, myasthenia gravis can be controlled. There are several therapies available to help reduce and improve muscle weakness. Medications used to treat the disorder include anticholinesterase agents such as neostigmine and pyridostigmine, which help improve neuromuscular transmission and increase muscle strength. Immunosuppressive drugs such as prednisone, cyclosporine, and azathioprine may also be used. These medications improve muscle strength by suppressing the production of abnormal antibodies. They must be used with careful medical follow-up because they may cause major side effects.

Thymectomy, the surgical removal of the thymus gland (which is abnormal in myasthenia gravis patients), reduces symptoms in more than 70 percent of patients without thymoma and may cure some individuals, possibly by re-balancing the immune system. Other therapies used to treat myasthenia gravis include plasmapheresis, a procedure in which abnormal antibodies are removed from the blood, and high-dose intravenous immune globulin which temporarily modifies the immune system and provides the body with normal antibodies from donated blood. These therapies may be used to help individuals during especially difficult periods of weakness. A neurologist will determine which treatment option is best for each individual depending on the severity of the weakness, which muscles are affected, and the individual's age and other associated medical problems.

Myasthenic Crisis

A myasthenic crisis occurs when the muscles that control breathing weaken to the point that ventilation is inadequate, creating a medical emergency and requiring a respirator for assisted ventilation. In patients whose respiratory muscles are weak, crises—which generally call for immediate medical attention—may be triggered by infection, fever, an adverse reaction to medication, or emotional stress.

Prognosis

With treatment, the outlook for most patients with myasthenia gravis is bright: they will have significant improvement of their muscle weakness, and they can expect to lead normal or nearly normal lives. Some cases of myasthenia gravis may go into remission temporarily and muscle weakness may disappear completely so that medications can be discontinued. Stable, long-lasting complete remissions are the goal of thymectomy. In a few cases, the severe weakness of myasthenia gravis may cause a crisis (respiratory failure), which requires immediate emergency medical care.

Additional Information

Myasthenia Gravis Foundation of America
1821 University Ave. W., Suite S256
St. Paul, MN 55104
Toll-Free: 800-541-5454
Phone: 651-917-6256
Fax: 651-917-1835
Website: http://www.myasthenia.org
E-mail: mgfa@myasthenia.org

Muscular Dystrophy Association
3300 E. Sunrise Drive
Tucson, AZ 85718
Toll-Free: 800-572-1717
Website: http://www.mdausa.org
E-mail: mda@mdausa.org

Chapter 52

Myocarditis

Definition: Myocarditis is an inflammation of the heart muscle.

Causes, Incidence, and Risk Factors

Myocarditis is an uncommon disorder caused by viral infections such as coxsackie virus, adenovirus, and echovirus. It may also occur during or after various viral, bacterial, or parasitic infections (such as polio, influenza, or rubella).

The condition may be caused by exposure to chemicals or allergic reactions to certain medications and it can be associated with autoimmune diseases.

The heart muscle becomes inflamed and weakened, causing symptoms of heart failure, which may mimic a heart attack.

Symptoms

- History of preceding viral illness
- Fever
- Chest pain that may resemble a heart attack
- Joint pain/swelling
- Abnormal heart beats
- Fatigue

"Myocarditis," © 2005 A.D.A.M., Inc. Reprinted with permission.

- Shortness of breath
- Leg edema
- Inability to lie flat

Total absence of symptoms is common.
Additional symptoms that may be associated with this disease:

- Syncope (fainting), often related to arrhythmias
- Decreased urine output
- Other symptoms consistent with a viral infection—headache, muscle aches, diarrhea, sore throat, rashes.

Signs and Tests

A physical examination may detect a rapid heartbeat (tachycardia) or abnormal heart beats, abnormal heart sounds (murmurs, extra heart sounds), fluid in the lungs, and fluid in the skin of the legs. In addition, other signs suggestive of an infection may be present: fever, rashes, red throat, itchy eyes, and swollen joints.

Tests used in the diagnosis of myocarditis include:

- Electrocardiogram (ECG)
- Chest x-ray
- Ultrasound of the heart (echocardiogram)—may show weak heart muscle, an enlarged heart, or fluid surrounding the heart
- White blood cell count
- Red blood cell count
- Blood cultures for infection
- Blood tests for antibodies against the heart muscle and the body itself
- Heart muscle biopsy—rarely performed.

Treatment

Treatment includes evaluation and treatment of underlying cause. This may require use of antibiotics, reduced level of activity, and low-salt diet. Steroids and other medications may be used to reduce inflammation. Diuretics (medicine to promote removal of body water via the urine) are also given.

If the heart muscle is very weak, standard medicines to treat heart failure are also used. Abnormal heart rhythm may require the use of additional medications, a pacemaker, or even a defibrillator. If a blood clot is present in the heart chamber, blood thinning medicine is given as well.

Expectations (Prognosis)

Myocarditis is very variable and the prognosis depends on the cause and the individual patient. Some may recover completely, while others may have permanent heart failure.

Complications

* Heart failure
* Pericarditis
* Cardiomyopathy

Calling Your Health Care Provider

Call your health care provider if symptoms of myocarditis occur, especially after a recent infection.

If you have myocarditis, call your health care provider (or get to the emergency room if symptoms are severe) if you experience increased swelling, chest pain, difficulty breathing, or other new symptoms.

Prevention

Prompt treatment of causative disorders may reduce the risk of myocarditis.

Chapter 53

Paraneoplastic Syndromes

Paraneoplastic syndromes are a group of rare degenerative disorders that are triggered by a person's immune system response to a neoplasm, or cancerous tumor. Neurologic paraneoplastic syndromes are believed to occur when cancer-fighting antibodies or white blood cells known as T cells mistakenly attack normal cells in the nervous system. These disorders typically affect middle-aged to older persons and are most common in persons with lung, ovarian, lymphatic, or breast cancer. Neurologic symptoms generally develop over a period of days to weeks and usually occur prior to tumor detection, which can complicate diagnosis. These symptoms may include difficulty in walking and/or swallowing, loss of muscle tone, loss of fine motor coordination, slurred speech, memory loss, vision problems, sleep disturbances, dementia, seizures, sensory loss in the limbs, and vertigo. Neurologic paraneoplastic syndromes include Lambert-Eaton myasthenic syndrome, stiff-person syndrome, encephalomyelitis (inflammation of the brain and spinal cord), myasthenia gravis, cerebellar degeneration, limbic and/or brainstem encephalitis, neuromyotonia, opsoclonus (involving eye movement), and sensory neuropathy.

Treatment

The cancer is treated first, followed by efforts to decrease the autoimmune response—either through steroids such as cortisone or prednisone, high-dose intravenous immunoglobulin, or irradiation.

"Paraneoplastic Syndromes Information Page," National Institute of Neurological Disorders and Stroke (NINDS), February 9, 2005.

Plasmapheresis, a process that cleanses antibodies from the blood, may ease symptoms in patients with paraneoplastic disorders that affect the peripheral nervous system. Speech and physical therapy may help patients regain some functions.

Prognosis

There are no cures for paraneoplastic syndromes and resulting progressive neurological damage. Generally the presence of cancer determines the diagnosis.

Research

Research on neurologic paraneoplastic syndromes is aimed at enhancing scientific understanding of them and evaluating new therapeutic interventions. Researchers are seeking to learn what causes the autoimmune response in these disorders. Studies are directed toward developing assays that detect different types of antibodies. Scientists also hope to develop animal models for these diseases, which may be used to determine effective treatment strategies.

Additional Information

American Autoimmune-Related Diseases Association, Inc. (AARDA)
22100 Gratiot Ave.
East Detroit, MI 48021
Toll-Free: 800-598-4668 (for literature requests)
Phone: 586-776-3900
Fax: 586-776-3903
Website: http://www.aarda.org
E-mail: aarda@aarda.org

National Cancer Institute(NCI)
Suite 3036A, MSC 8322
6116 Executive Blvd.
Bethesda, MD 20892-8322
Toll-Free: 800-4-CANCER (422-6237)

National Cancer Institute (NCI) continued
Toll-Free TTY: 800-332-8615
Website: http://www.cancer.gov
E-mail:
cancergovstaff@mail.nih.gov

National Organization for Rare Disorders (NORD)
55 Kansas Ave.
P.O. Box 1968
Danbury, CT 06813-1968
Toll-Free: 800-999-6673
Phone: 203-744-0100
TDD: 203-797-9590
Website: http://www.rarediseases.org
E-mail: orphan@rarediseases.org

Chapter 54

Pediatric Autoimmune Neuropsychiatric Disorders (PANDAS)

Is there a test for pediatric autoimmune neuropsychiatric disorders (PANDAS)?

No. The diagnosis of PANDAS is a clinical diagnosis, which means that there are no lab tests that can diagnose PANDAS. Instead clinicians use 5 diagnostic criteria for the diagnosis of PANDAS. At the present time the clinical features of the illness are the only means of determining whether or not a child might have PANDAS.

The diagnostic criteria for PANDAS are:

1. Presence of obsessive-compulsive disorder (OCD) and/or a tic disorder.

2. Pediatric onset of symptoms (age 3 years to puberty).

3. Episodic course of symptom severity.

4. Association with group A Beta-hemolytic streptococcal infection (a positive throat culture for strep or history of scarlet fever).

5. Association with neurological abnormalities (motoric hyperactivity, or adventitious movements, such as choreiform movements).

"PANDAS Frequently Asked Questions," National Institute of Mental Health (NIMH), August 2004.

What is an episodic course of symptoms?

Children with PANDAS seem to have dramatic ups and downs in their OCD and/or tic severity. Tics or OCD which are almost always present at a relatively consistent level do not represent an episodic course. Many kids with OCD or tics have good days and bad days, or even good weeks and bad weeks. However, patients with PANDAS have a very sudden onset or worsening of their symptoms followed by a slow, gradual improvement. If they get another strep infection, their symptoms suddenly worsen again. The increased symptom severity usually persists for at least several weeks, but may last for several months or longer. The tics or OCD then seem to gradually fade away, and the children often enjoy a few weeks or several months without problems. When they have another strep throat infection, the tics or OCD return just as suddenly and dramatically as they did previously.

My child has had strep throat before, and he has tics and/ or OCD. Does that mean he has PANDAS?

No. Many children have OCD and/or tics, and almost all school age children get strep throat at some point in their lives. Only when a child has a very episodic course of tics, and/or OCD, and seems to have strep throat shortly before or at the time of a dramatic worsening of symptoms does this indicate the possibility of PANDAS.

What does an elevated anti-streptococcal antibody titer mean? Is this bad for my child?

An elevated anti-strep titer means the child has had a strep infection sometime within the past few months, and his body created antibodies to fight the strep bacteria. This is not bad. In fact, it is a normal, healthy response—all healthy people create antibodies to fight infections. The antibodies stay in the body for some time after the infection is gone, but the amount of time that the antibodies persist varies greatly between different individuals. Some children have positive antibody titers for many months after a single infection. This means that an elevated anti-streptococcal titer may have nothing to do with the present worsening symptoms, but instead indicates a long-since healed strep throat.

Could an adult or teenager have PANDAS?

No. By definition, PANDAS is a pediatric disorder. It is possible that adolescents and adults may have immune mediated OCD, but this is not known. The research studies at the National Institute of Mental Health (NIMH) are restricted to PANDAS.

Will penicillin treat PANDAS?

No. Penicillin and other antibiotics kill streptococcus and other types of bacteria. The antibiotics treat the sore throat or pharyngitis caused by the strep by getting rid of the bacteria. However, in PANDAS, it appears that antibodies produced by the body in response to the strep infection are the cause of the problem, not the bacteria themselves. Therefore, one could not expect antibiotics such as penicillin to treat the symptoms of PANDAS.

Current research at the NIMH has been investigating the use of antibiotics as a form of prophylaxis or prevention of future problems. It is important to note that the success of antibiotic prophylaxis for PANDAS patients has not yet been proven. Until its usefulness is determined, penicillin and other antibiotics should not be used as long-term treatment for OCD and tics.

Will plasma exchange and immunoglobulin (IVIG) treat PANDAS?

The results of the first study of plasma exchange (also known as plasmapheresis) and immunoglobulin (IVIG) for the treatment of children in the PANDAS subgroup was published in *The Lancet*, Vol. 354, October 2, 1999. The study showed that plasma exchange and IVIG were both effective for the treatment of severe, strep-triggered OCD and tics. Further, all of the children participating in the study had clear evidence of a strep infection as the trigger of their OCD and tics, and all were severely ill at the time of treatment. Side-effects of the treatments were common, but not severe and included nausea, vomiting, and headaches with IVIG, and nausea, vomiting, and dizziness with plasma exchange. Follow-up evaluations conducted one year after treatment revealed that all children remained improved, suggesting that the treatments had long-lasting effects. However, only 29 children participated in the study, so it is not clear that plasma exchange and IVIG will be helpful to all children.

Although the results of the preliminary NIMH investigation were encouraging, further research is needed before either IVIG or plasma exchange is used routinely to treat OCD and tics in PANDAS. A separate study was conducted to evaluate the effectiveness of plasma exchange in the treatment of chronic OCD (Nicolson et al: An Open Trial of Plasma Exchange in Childhood Onset Obsessive-Compulsive

Disorder without Poststreptococcal Exacerbations. *J Am Acad Child Adolesc Psychiatry* 2000, 39(10): 1313-1315). None of those children benefited suggesting that plasma exchange or IVIG is not helpful for children who do not have strep-triggered symptoms.

Chapter 55

Pemphigus Diseases

Pemphigus is a group of rare autoimmune blistering diseases of the skin and/or mucous membranes.

Our immune system produces antibodies that normally attack hostile viruses and bacteria in an effort to keep us healthy. In a person with pemphigus, however, the immune system mistakenly perceives the cells in skin and/or mucous membrane as foreign, and attacks them. Antibodies that attack one's own cells are called autoantibodies. The part of the cells that are attacked in pemphigus are proteins called desmogleins. Desmogleins form the glue that attaches adjacent skin cells keeping the skin intact.

When auto-antibodies attack desmogleins, the cells become separated from each other. The skin virtually becomes unglued. This causes burn-like lesions or blisters that do not heal. In some cases, these blisters can cover a significant area of the skin.

Types of Pemphigus

There are three main categories of pemphigus: pemphigus vulgaris, pemphigus foliaceus, and paraneoplastic pemphigus. Pemphigus is not pemphigoid, cicatricial pemphigoid, or benign familial pemphigus, also known as Hailey-Hailey disease.

"What Is Pemphigus?" © 2001 Internation Pemphigus Foundation. All rights reserved. Reprinted with permission.

411

Pemphigus Vulgaris (PV)

The term vulgar means common, and PV is the most frequently diagnosed form of pemphigus. Sores and blisters almost always start in the mouth. Because the skin is an organ, PV is called a one-organ disease. It does not affect any of the internal organs. The blisters can go as far down as the vocal cords, but no further. PV does not cause permanent scars unless there is infection associated with the lesion.

In PV, auto-antibodies attack the protein glue—desmogleins—which holds skin cells together. The lesions are painful. Sometimes there is the Nikolsky effect where just touching the skin can cause it to tear. Before drug treatment, PV was 99% fatal, but today with the current therapies, the mortality rate is only 5 to 15%.

Pemphigus Foliaceus (PF)

In pemphigus foliaceus, blisters and sores do not occur in the mouth. Crusted sores or fragile blisters usually first appear on the face and scalp and later involve the chest and back.

Auto-antibodies are produced by the immune system, but they bind only to desmoglein 1. The blisters are superficial and often itchy, but are not usually as painful as PV.

In PF, disfiguring skin lesions can occur, but the mortality rate from the disease is much lower than in PV.

Paraneoplastic Pemphigus (PNP)

PNP is the most serious form of pemphigus. It occurs most often in someone who has already been diagnosed with a malignancy (cancer). Fortunately, it is also the least common. Painful sores of the mouth, lips, and esophagus are almost always present; and skin lesions of different types occur. PNP can affect the lungs. In some cases, the diagnosis of the disease will prompt doctors to search for a hidden tumor. In some cases, the tumor will be benign, and the disease will improve if the tumor is surgically removed.

It is important to know that this condition is rare and looks different than the other forms of pemphigus. The antibodies in the blood are also different, and the difference can be determined by laboratory tests.

Diagnosis

Because it is rare, pemphigus is often the last disease considered during diagnosis. Consult a dermatologist if there are any persistent skin or mouth lesions. Early diagnosis may permit successful treatment with only low levels of medication.

There are three criteria that must be met for a definite diagnosis:

1. **Proper clinical presentation**—visual examination of skin lesions.

2. **Lesion biopsy**—A sample of the blistered skin is removed and examined under the microscope to determine if the cells are separated in the manner characteristic of pemphigus. Additionally, the layer of skin in which cell-to-cell separation occurs can be determined.

3. **Direct immunofluorescence**—The biopsy skin sample is treated to detect desmoglein antibodies in the skin. The presence of these antibodies indicates pemphigus.

In addition, another diagnostic test that may be used is called indirect immunofluorescence or antibody titer test. This measures desmoglein autoantibodies in the blood serum. It may be used to obtain a more complete understanding of the course of the disease. Also, a serum assay for desmoglein antibodies, known as enzyme-linked immunosorbent assay (ELISA), is available. It is the most accurate, but is not available in all clinical labs.

Treatment

Treatment for pemphigus vulgaris (PV) involves the use of one or more drugs. Initially, PV is treated with a corticosteroid. Other drugs are usually used in conjunction with corticosteroids.

Corticosteroids

Prompt and sufficient doses of corticosteroids, usually prednisone or prednisolone, are required to bring pemphigus under control. Once controlled, the steroid is reduced slowly to minimize side effects. Some patients then go into remission; however, many patients need a small maintenance dose to keep the disease under control.

Immunosuppressants

- Azathioprine (Imuran®)
- Mycophenolate mofetil (CellCept®)

- Cyclophosphamide (Cytoxan®)
- Cyclosporine

Additional Drugs

Other drugs that are used routinely with varying effects are:

- Dapsone®
- Gold injections
- Methotrexate
- Tetracycline, minocycline, or doxycycline combined with niacinamide.

All of these medications can have serious side effects. Patients on these medications must have blood and urine monitored on a regular basis. There is some evidence suggesting that treatment is easier in the early stages of the disease.

Treatment should always be addressed according to the disease activity that is clinically apparent. An indirect immunofluorescence test (antibody titer count) will generally show a high count when the disease is more active, and will be low or undetectable when the disease is in remission. However, this is not always true. The antibody titer test may be most useful with patients on maintenance doses of drugs. If a titer count is low, then it could be reassuring that the flare is controllable and short. A high titer might indicate the need for further treatment.

To date, no studies have shown that alternative, homeopathic, or any other non-traditional method has been successful in treating these diseases. For the best possible results, it is imperative that traditional treatments be administered. However, once the disease is under control, alternative therapies may be useful to help reduce drug side effects.

Who Gets Pemphigus?

To date, definitive statistics on the incidence and prevalence of pemphigus are not available, but estimates of the number of new cases diagnosed each year range from as high as 5 per one hundred thousand to as low as one per million, depending upon the type of pemphigus and the ethnicity of the affected population. It is known to affect people across racial and cultural lines. However, there are certain groups of people (such as eastern European Jews and people of Mediterranean descent) who have a higher incidence of the disease. Men and women are equally affected. Research studies suggest a genetic predisposition to the disease. Although the onset usually occurs in middle-aged and older adults, PV and PF also occur in young adults and children.

Pemphigus is frequently the last disease considered during diagnosis. If you have any persistent skin or mouth lesions, consult your dermatologist. Early diagnosis may permit treatment with low levels of medication.

Pemphigus and Lifestyle

In general, pemphigus can be controlled to the degree that aside from taking some daily medications, the lifestyles of those who live with these diseases are largely unchanged. There are, however, cases where pemphigus can be very debilitating and cause lost time at work, loss of appetite, inability to eat normally, weight loss, loss of sleep, hospitalization, emotional distress, etc. These effects are most often associated with the onset of the disease during the search for a correct diagnosis. If an early diagnosis is made and treatment initiated, it is very common for the patient to return to a fairly normal lifestyle.

Much of the impact on lifestyle comes as a result of side effects caused by prednisone. Type 2 diabetes is a common side effect of prednisone and creates a need for a modified diet. Generally, this type of diabetes will diminish as the dosage of prednisone is reduced and goes away when prednisone is stopped. Many people on prednisone also experience emotional difficulties and mood changes. If these are continual and severe, other medications are often used to help mitigate these side effects. Another commonly reported side effect of prednisone is weight gain. A high protein, low carbohydrate, low fat diet, as well as a regular exercise program is recommended for those taking prednisone. Osteoporosis, glaucoma, and cataracts are also known side effects of prednisone, and regular checkups with your health care providers will enable most people on prednisone to effectively counter these side effects with appropriate therapies and attention.

It is very important to make certain that all physicians, doctors, and specialists involved with a treatment regimen are in contact with one another to avoid conflicting medications and to be sure that treatments are working in harmony. Also, all lab test results should automatically be given to all physicians on a particular case.

Pemphigus and Nutrition

As with lifestyle concerns, many of the nutrition concerns are associated with prednisone. In order to control an outbreak of pemphigus, a prompt response with a large dose of prednisone is generally prescribed. This a glucocorticoid steroid drug which requires a diet high in protein, low in carbohydrates, low in salt, low in fat, with special attention paid to calcium and potassium levels. Calcium with vitamin D supplements are routinely ordered.

Eating a healthy diet is obviously important to health, but it is especially important for pemphigus patients to mitigate the effects of medications, and to give the body all it needs to fight the disease and rebuild the body. Acidophilus, beneficial bacteria found in yogurt as well as in dietary supplements, is recommended for those who frequently use antibiotics. It also helps prevent yeast infections. Be sure to discuss your present diet, medications, and lifestyle with your physician and/or dietitian before making changes to your diet.

It has been documented that some patients have a sensitivity to garlic, onions, and leeks. These foods and possibly others may trigger or worsen flair-ups. Be sensitive to foods that can help or hurt you. Test yourself. If you suspect that eating certain foods causes blisters, then try it a second time, and if it happens again, eliminate that food from your diet.

Pemphigus and Stress

The possible effect of stress on the onset or subsequent flare of pemphigus is not clearly understood. Many people who live with pemphigus report a direct relationship between increased stress and flares in disease activity. Others seem to be unaffected by increased stress.

If you believe stress is related to increased incidence of lesions, it is wise to address and resolve those stress issues. Obviously, many causes of stress are not a matter of choice, but the manner in which an individual deals with the various sources of stress can be modified to minimize the negative impacts of stress. One of the most common and effective ways to help reduce stress is to openly and honestly discuss it with a spouse, friend, or therapist. Having someone in your corner helps.

Another way is take a few irons out of the fire in order to regroup and recover. Focus on getting yourself back to health before you again devote time and energy to other pursuits. Sometimes it is necessary to pull back in some areas and go back to them after you are more able to handle some extras.

Caregiving

Though the concerns of those who live with pemphigus are considerable, the impact on spouses, family members, and caregivers should not be ignored or underestimated. Many caregivers take advantage of an online discussion group not only in behalf of the person for whom they care, but to get information, assistance, and even support from other caregivers in similar circumstances.

Being a caregiver comes with its own set of challenges. The uncertainty of the disease, and the need many caregivers feel to always appear to be strong and positive, often creates stresses and difficulties which make the challenge even greater. One of the most helpful tools in dealing with this issue is to become as informed as possible. When your loved one has questions, it is of great comfort to him or her to be able to hear a good answer. In general, there is very much to be positive about regarding treatment and control of pemphigus. Understanding the basics of the disease, along with general treatment protocol, as well as having a few anecdotal instances gives you and your loved one the assurance that you are not alone, and that what you are experiencing has been experienced and overcome by someone else.

Additional Information

International Pemphigus Foundation
828 San Pablo Ave., Suite 210
Albany, NY 94706
Phone: 510-527-4970
Fax: 510-527-8497
Website: http://www.pemphigus.org
E-mail: pemphigus@pemphigus.org

Chapter 56

Polyarteritis Nodosa

Alternative name: Periarteritis nodosa

Definition: Polyarteritis nodosa is a serious blood vessel disease in which small and medium-sized arteries become swollen and damaged when they are attacked by rogue immune cells.

Causes, Incidence, and Risk Factors

Polyarteritis nodosa is a disease of unknown cause that affects arteries, the blood vessels which carry oxygenated blood to organs and tissues. It occurs when certain immune cells attack the affected arteries.

The condition affects adults more frequently than children. It damages the tissues supplied by the affected arteries because they do not receive enough oxygen and nourishment without a proper blood supply.

In this disease, symptoms result from damage to affected organs, often the skin, heart, kidneys, and nervous system.

Generalized symptoms include fever, fatigue, weakness, loss of appetite, and weight loss. Muscle aches (myalgia) and joint aches (arthralgia) are common. The skin may show rashes, swelling, ulcers, and lumps (nodular lesions).

Nerve involvement may cause sensory changes with numbness, pain, burning, and weakness. Central nervous system involvement may cause strokes or seizures. Kidney involvement can produce varying degrees of renal failure.

Involvement of the arteries of the heart may cause a heart attack (acute myocardial infarction), heart failure, and inflammation of the sack around the heart (pericarditis).

Symptoms

- fatigue
- weakness
- fever
- abdominal pain
- decreased appetite (anorexia)
- weight loss, unintentional
- muscle aches (myalgia)
- joint aches (arthralgia)

Signs and Tests

There are no specific laboratory tests for the diagnosis of polyarteritis nodosa. The diagnosis is generally based upon clinical findings and a few laboratory studies that help to confirm the diagnosis.

- complete blood count (CBC)—may demonstrate an elevated white blood count
- erythrocyte sedimentation rate (ESR)—often elevated
- tissue biopsy—demonstrates inflammation in small arteries (arteritis)
- immunoglobulins—may be increased

Treatment

Treatment involves the use of medications to suppress the immune system, including:

- prednisone
- cyclophosphamide.

Expectations (Prognosis)

Treatment is mandatory for long-term survival. Without treatment, survival is poor. However, with current treatments using steroids and other drugs that suppress the immune system (such as cyclophospha-mide), improvements are seen both in the symptoms as well as in the survival rate. The most serious associated conditions generally involve the kidneys and gastrointestinal tract.

Complications

- stroke
- renal failure
- heart attack
- intestinal necrosis and perforation

Calling Your Health Care Provider

Call your health care provider if you develop symptoms of this dis-order. Early diagnosis and treatment may improve the chance of a good outcome.

Prevention

This disease cannot currently prevented, but early treatment can prevent some damage and symptoms.

Chapter 57

Primary Biliary Cirrhosis

Primary biliary cirrhosis (PBC) is a chronic liver disease that causes slow, progressive destruction of bile ducts in the liver. This destruction interferes with the excretion of bile. Continued liver inflammation causes scarring and eventually leads to cirrhosis. Cirrhosis is present only in the later stage of the disease. In the early stages of the illness, the main problem is the build up of substances (bile acids, cholesterol) in the blood, which are normally excreted into the bile. Ursodeoxycholic acid is a life-saving, safe, and approved therapy.

What are the symptoms?

Women are affected ten times more frequently than men. The disease usually is first diagnosed in people 30 to 60 years old. Many patients have no symptoms of disease and are diagnosed by finding an abnormality on routine liver blood tests. Itching and fatigue are common symptoms. Other signs include jaundice, cholesterol deposits in the skin, fluid accumulation in the ankles and abdomen, and darkening of the skin. Several other disorders are often associated with PBC. The most common is impaired functioning of the tear and salivary glands causing dry eyes or mouth. Arthritis and thyroid problems may also be present. Renal stones and gallstones may develop. Bone softening and fragility leading to fractures can occur in late stages of the disease.

How is PBC diagnosed?

PBC diagnosis is based on several pieces of information. The patient may have symptoms (itching) suggesting bile duct damage. Laboratory tests, such as the alkaline phosphatase activity test, may confirm this. The test for mitochondrial antibodies is particularly useful as it is positive in nearly all patients. Infrequently, the bile ducts are x-rayed to rule out possibilities of other causes of biliary tract disease, such as obstruction. A liver biopsy is useful in confirming the diagnosis and in giving information on the severity and extent of liver damage.

What causes PBC?

Although the cause of the initial bile duct damage in PBC is unknown, there are certain clues that may be important. Strictly speaking, the disease is not inherited, but it is more common among siblings and in families where one member has previously been affected. Multiple disturbances of the immune system have been found in persons with PBC and may be an important factor. Hormones may also play a role given that this illness is so much more common in women.

What is the prognosis for patients?

PBC typically advances slowly. Many patients lead active and productive lives for ten to fifteen years after diagnosis. Patients who show no symptoms at the time of diagnosis often remain symptom-free for years. Jaundice appears to be a sign of diminishing liver reserve and may be an important indication regarding the progression of the disease. The illness is chronic and may lead to life-threatening complications, especially after cirrhosis develops.

How is PBC treated?

Treatment may be useful in several ways. Proper advice will ensure the elimination of potentially harmful drugs, foods, or toxins. If the patient is deficient in vitamin D, then this should be corrected. The thyroid function should be tested and, if low, treated with a thyroid hormone. Symptoms may be successfully relieved. Itching is often reduced by using cholestyramine and rifampin. Salt restriction may be effective in reducing fluid accumulation. The diet should be well-balanced. Corticosteroids have been found ineffective in most patients. The U.S. Food and Drug Administration (FDA) has approved only URSO 250 (manufactured by Axcan Scandipharm) for use in patients with PBC. The recommended dose is 13–15 milligrams/kilo-gram (mg/kg) once a day. Physicians who treat PNC patients often prescribe other ursodiol products off-label—drugs not approved by the FDA to treat this condition. These products include Actigall (manu-factured by Novartis) and various generic formulations.

When is liver transplantation needed?

When medical treatment no longer controls the disease and the patient has severe liver failure, transplantation is indicated. Signs of liver failure include accumulation of fluid in the abdomen, malnutri-tion, gastrointestinal bleeding, intractable itching, jaundice, and bone fractures. Transplantation may be recommended before all these events occur. The outcome for patients with PBC who have undergone transplantation is excellent. The survival rate for two or more years is about 80 percent. The use of new drugs to suppress rejection has made transplantation even more successful. The disease's slow prog-ress makes it possible to plan elective transplant surgery.

What research is underway?

PBC has been known for more than 100 years. This knowledge has led doctors to make earlier diagnoses. Many clues to the cause have been supplied by careful observation of patients over the last 25 years, but the basic cause is unknown.

Research is following two paths:

- Basic investigation of the causes and development of the disease.

- Drug therapy trials, involving a large number of patients around the world, are exploring the potential use of several additional medications to lessen the symptoms and control liver damage.

Additional Information

American Liver Foundation
75 Maiden Lane, Suite 603
New York, NY 10038
Toll-Free: 800-465-4837
Phone: 212-668-1000
Fax: 212-483-8179
Website: http://www.liverfoundation.org
E-mail: info@liverfoundation.org

Chapter 58

Psoriasis

Psoriasis is a chronic (long-lasting) skin disease of scaling and inflammation that affects 2 to 2.6 percent of the United States population, or between 5.8 and 7.5 million people. Although the disease occurs in all age groups, it primarily affects adults. It appears about equally in males and females. Psoriasis occurs when skin cells quickly rise from their origin below the surface of the skin and pile up on the surface before they have a chance to mature. Usually this movement (also called turnover) takes about a month, but in psoriasis it may occur in only a few days. In its typical form, psoriasis results in patches of thick, red (inflamed) skin covered with silvery scales. These patches, which are sometimes referred to as plaques, usually itch or feel sore. They most often occur on the elbows, knees, other parts of the legs, scalp, lower back, face, palms, and soles of the feet, but they can occur on skin anywhere on the body.

The disease may also affect the fingernails, the toenails, and the soft tissues of the genitals and inside the mouth. While it is not unusual for the skin around affected joints to crack, approximately 1 million people with psoriasis experience joint inflammation that produces symptoms of arthritis. This condition is called psoriatic arthritis.

Individuals with psoriasis may experience significant physical discomfort and some disability. Itching and pain can interfere with basic functions, such as self-care, walking, and sleep. Plaques on hands and

"Questions and Answers about Psoriasis," National Institute of Arthritis and Musculoskeletal and Skin Diseases (NIAMS), NIH Publication No. 03–5040, May 2003.

feet can prevent individuals from working at certain occupations, playing some sports, and caring for family members or a home. The frequency of medical care is costly and can interfere with an employment or school schedule. People with moderate to severe psoriasis may feel self-conscious about their appearance and have a poor self-image that stems from fear of public rejection and psychosexual concerns. Psychological distress can lead to significant depression and social isolation.

Causes of Psoriasis

Psoriasis is a skin disorder driven by the immune system, especially involving a type of white blood cell called a T cell. Normally, T cells help protect the body against infection and disease. In the case of psoriasis, T cells are put into action by mistake and become so active that they trigger other immune responses which lead to inflammation and to rapid turnover of skin cells. In about one-third of the cases, there is a family history of psoriasis. Researchers have studied a large number of families affected by psoriasis and identified genes linked to the disease. (Genes govern every bodily function and determine the inherited traits passed from parent to child.) People with psoriasis may notice that there are times when their skin worsens, then improves. Conditions that may cause flare-ups include infections, stress, and changes in climate that dry the skin. Also, certain medicines, including lithium and beta blockers which are prescribed for high blood pressure, may trigger an outbreak or worsen the disease.

Diagnosis

Occasionally, doctors may find it difficult to diagnose psoriasis, because it often looks like other skin diseases. It may be necessary to confirm a diagnosis by examining a small skin sample under a microscope. There are several forms of psoriasis. Some of these include:

- **Plaque psoriasis**—Skin lesions are red at the base and covered by silvery scales.

- **Guttate psoriasis**—Small, drop-shaped lesions appear on the trunk, limbs, and scalp. Guttate psoriasis is most often triggered by upper respiratory infections (for example, a sore throat caused by streptococcal bacteria).

- **Pustular psoriasis**—Blisters of noninfectious pus appear on the skin. Attacks of pustular psoriasis may be triggered by medications, infections, stress, or exposure to certain chemicals.

- **Inverse psoriasis**—Smooth, red patches occur in the folds of the skin near the genitals, under the breasts, or in the armpits. The symptoms may be worsened by friction and sweating.

- **Erythrodermic psoriasis**—Widespread reddening and scaling of the skin may be a reaction to severe sunburn or to taking corticosteroids (cortisone) or other medications. It can also be caused by a prolonged period of increased activity of psoriasis that is poorly controlled.

- **Psoriatic arthritis**—Joint inflammation that produces symptoms of arthritis in patients who have or will develop psoriasis.

Treatment

Doctors generally treat psoriasis in steps based on the severity of the disease, size of the areas involved, type of psoriasis, and the patient's response to initial treatments. This is sometimes called the 1-2-3 approach. In step 1, medicines are applied to the skin (topical treatment). Step 2 uses light treatments (phototherapy). Step 3 involves taking medicines by mouth or injection that treat the whole immune system (called systemic therapy).

Over time, affected skin can become resistant to treatment, especially when topical corticosteroids are used. Also, a treatment that works very well in one person may have little effect in another. Thus, doctors often use a trial-and-error approach to find a treatment that works, and they may switch treatments periodically (for example, every 12 to 24 months) if a treatment does not work or if adverse reactions occur.

Topical Treatment

Treatments applied directly to the skin may improve its condition. Doctors find that some patients respond well to ointment or cream forms of corticosteroids, vitamin D3, retinoids, coal tar, or anthralin. Bath solutions and moisturizers may be soothing, but they are seldom strong enough to improve the condition of the skin. Therefore, they usually are combined with stronger remedies.

Note: Brand names included in this chapter are provided as examples only, and their inclusion does not mean that these products are endorsed by the National Institutes of Health or any other Government agency. Also, if a particular brand name is not mentioned, this does not mean or imply that the product is unsatisfactory.

- **Corticosteroids**—These drugs reduce inflammation and the turnover of skin cells, and they suppress the immune system. Available in different strengths, topical corticosteroids (cortisone) are usually applied to the skin twice a day. Short-term treatment is often effective in improving, but not completely eliminating, psoriasis. Long-term use or overuse of highly potent (strong) corticosteroids can cause thinning of the skin, internal side effects, and resistance to the treatment's benefits. If less than 10 percent of the skin is involved, some doctors will prescribe a high-potency corticosteroid ointment. High-potency corticosteroids may also be prescribed for plaques that do not improve with other treatment, particularly those on the hands or feet. In situations where the objective of treatment is comfort, medium-potency corticosteroids may be prescribed for the broader skin areas of the torso or limbs. Low-potency preparations are used on delicate skin areas. (Note: Brand names for the different strengths of corticosteroids are too numerous to list.)

- **Calcipotriene**—This drug is a synthetic form of vitamin D_3 that can be applied to the skin. Applying calcipotriene ointment (for example, Dovonex) twice a day controls the speed of turnover of skin cells. Because calcipotriene can irritate the skin, it is not recommended for use on the face or genitals. It is sometimes combined with topical corticosteroids to reduce irritation. Use of more than 100 grams of calcipotriene per week may raise the amount of calcium in the body to unhealthy levels.

- **Retinoid**—Topical retinoids are synthetic forms of vitamin A. The retinoid tazarotene (Tazorac) is available as a gel or cream that is applied to the skin. If used alone, this preparation does not act as quickly as topical corticosteroids, but it does not cause thinning of the skin or other side effects associated with steroids. However, it can irritate the skin, particularly in skin folds and the normal skin surrounding a patch of psoriasis. It is less irritating and sometimes more effective when combined with a corticosteroid. Because of the risk of birth defects, women of childbearing age must take measures to prevent pregnancy when using tazarotene.

- **Coal tar**—Preparations containing coal tar (gels and ointments) may be applied directly to the skin, added (as a liquid) to the bath, or used on the scalp as a shampoo. Coal tar products are available in different strengths, and many are sold over the counter (not requiring a prescription). Coal tar is less effective

430

than corticosteroids and many other treatments. It is sometimes combined with ultraviolet B (UVB) phototherapy for a better result. The most potent form of coal tar may irritate the skin, is messy, has a strong odor, and may stain the skin or clothing. Thus, it is not popular with many patients.

- **Anthralin**—Anthralin reduces the increase in skin cells and inflammation. Doctors sometimes prescribe a 15- to 30-minute application of anthralin ointment, cream, or paste once each day to treat chronic psoriasis lesions. Afterward, anthralin must be washed off the skin to prevent irritation. This treatment often fails to adequately improve the skin, and it stains skin, bathtub, sink, and clothing brown or purple. In addition, the risk of skin irritation makes anthralin unsuitable for acute or actively inflamed eruptions.

- **Salicylic acid**—This peeling agent, which is available in many forms, such as ointments, creams, gels, and shampoos, can be applied to reduce scaling of the skin or scalp. Often, it is more effective when combined with topical corticosteroids, anthralin, or coal tar.

- **Clobetasol propionate**—This is a foam topical medication (Olux), which has been approved for the treatment of scalp and body psoriasis. The foam penetrates the skin very well, is easy to use, and is not as messy as many other topical medications.

- **Bath solutions**—People with psoriasis may find that adding oil when bathing, then applying a moisturizer, soothes their skin. Also, individuals can remove scales and reduce itching by soaking for 15 minutes in water containing a coal tar solution, oiled oatmeal, Epsom salts, or Dead Sea salts.

- **Moisturizers**—When applied regularly over a long period, moisturizers have a soothing effect. Preparations that are thick and greasy usually work best because they seal water in the skin, reducing scaling and itching.

Light Therapy

Natural ultraviolet light from the sun and controlled delivery of artificial ultraviolet light are used in treating psoriasis.

- **Sunlight**—Much of sunlight is composed of bands of different wavelengths of ultraviolet (UV) light. When absorbed into the skin, UV light suppresses the process leading to disease, causing activated T cells in the skin to die. This process reduces inflammation and slows the turnover of skin cells that causes scaling. Daily, short, non-burning exposure to sunlight clears or improves psoriasis in many people. Therefore, exposing affected skin to sunlight is one initial treatment for the disease.

- **Ultraviolet B (UVB) phototherapy**—UVB is light with a short wavelength that is absorbed in the skin's epidermis. An artificial source can be used to treat mild and moderate psoriasis. Some physicians will start treating patients with UVB instead of topical agents. A UVB phototherapy, called broadband UVB, can be used for a few small lesions, to treat widespread psoriasis, or for lesions that resist topical treatment. This type of phototherapy is normally given in a doctor's office by using a light panel or light box. Some patients use UVB light boxes at home under a doctor's guidance. A newer type of UVB, called narrowband UVB, emits the part of the ultraviolet light spectrum band that is most helpful for psoriasis. Narrowband UVB treatment is superior to broadband UVB, but it is less effective than psoralen and ultraviolet A (PUVA) treatment. It is gaining in popularity because it does help and is more convenient than PUVA. At first, patients may require several treatments of narrowband UVB spaced close together to improve their skin. Once the skin has shown improvement, a maintenance treatment once each week may be all that is necessary. However, narrowband UVB treatment is not without risk. It can cause more severe and longer lasting burns than broadband treatment.

- **Psoralen and ultraviolet A phototherapy (PUVA)**—This treatment combines oral or topical administration of a medicine called psoralen with exposure to ultraviolet A (UVA) light. UVA has a long wavelength that penetrates deeper into the skin than ultraviolet B (UVB). Psoralen makes the skin more sensitive to this light. PUVA is normally used when more than 10 percent of the skin is affected or when the disease interferes with a person's occupation (for example, when a teacher's face or a salesperson's hands are involved). Compared with broadband UVB treatment, PUVA treatment taken two to three times a week clears psoriasis more consistently and in fewer treatments. However, it is associated with more short-term side effects, including nausea, headache, fatigue, burning, and itching. Care must be taken to avoid sunlight after ingesting psoralen to avoid severe sunburns, and the eyes must be protected for one to two days with UVA-absorbing glasses. Long-term treatment is associated with an increased risk of squamous-cell and, possibly, melanoma skin cancers. Simultaneous use of drugs that suppress the immune system, such as cyclosporine, have little beneficial effect and increase the risk of cancer.

- **Light therapy combined with other therapies**—Studies have shown that combining ultraviolet light treatment and a retinoid, such as acitretin, adds to the effectiveness of UV light for psoriasis. For this reason, if patients are not responding to light therapy, retinoids may be added. UVB phototherapy, for example, may be combined with retinoids and other treatments. One combined therapy program, the Ingram regime, involves a coal tar bath, UVB phototherapy, and application of an anthralin-salicylic acid paste that is left on the skin for 6 to 24 hours. A similar regime, the Goeckerman treatment, combines coal tar ointment with UVB phototherapy. Also, PUVA can be combined with some oral medications (such as retinoids) to increase its effectiveness.

Systemic Treatment

For more severe forms of psoriasis, doctors sometimes prescribe medicines that are taken internally by pill or injection. This is called systemic treatment. Recently, attention has been given to a group of drugs called biologics (for example, alefacept and etanercept), which are made from proteins produced by living cells instead of chemicals. They interfere with specific immune system processes.

- **Methotrexate**—Like cyclosporine, methotrexate slows cell turnover by suppressing the immune system. It can be taken by pill or injection. Patients taking methotrexate must be closely monitored because it can cause liver damage and/or decrease the production of oxygen-carrying red blood cells, infection-fighting white blood cells, and clot enhancing platelets. As a precaution, doctors do not prescribe the drug for people who have had liver disease or anemia (an illness characterized by weakness or tiredness due to a reduction in the number or volume of red blood cells that carry oxygen to the tissues). It is sometimes combined with PUVA or UVB treatments. Methotrexate should not be used by pregnant women, or by women who are planning to get pregnant, because it may cause birth defects.

- **Retinoids**—A retinoid, such as acitretin (Soriatane), is a compound with properties of vitamin A that may be prescribed for severe cases of psoriasis that do not respond to other therapies. Because this treatment also may cause birth defects, women must protect themselves from pregnancy beginning 1 month before through 3 years after treatment with acitretin. Most patients experience a recurrence of psoriasis after these products are discontinued.

- **Cyclosporine**—Taken orally, cyclosporine acts by suppressing the immune system to slow the rapid turnover of skin cells. It may provide quick relief of symptoms, but the improvement stops when treatment is discontinued. The best candidates for this therapy are those with severe psoriasis who have not responded to, or cannot tolerate, other systemic therapies. Its rapid onset of action is helpful in avoiding hospitalization of patients whose psoriasis is rapidly progressing. Cyclosporine may impair kidney function or cause high blood pressure (hypertension). Therefore, patients must be carefully monitored by a doctor. Also, cyclosporine is not recommended for patients who have a weak immune system or those who have had skin cancers as a result of PUVA treatments in the past. It should not be given with phototherapy.

- **6-Thioguanine**—This drug is nearly as effective as methotrexate and cyclosporine. It has fewer side effects, but there is a greater likelihood of anemia. This drug must also be avoided by pregnant women and by women who are planning to become pregnant, because it may cause birth defects.

- **Hydroxyurea (Hydrea)**—Compared with methotrexate and cyclosporine, hydroxyurea is somewhat less effective. It is sometimes combined with PUVA or UVB treatments. Possible side effects include anemia and a decrease in white blood cells and platelets. Like methotrexate and retinoids, hydroxyurea must be avoided by pregnant women or those who are planning to become pregnant because it may cause birth defects.

- **Alefacept (Amevive)**—This is the first biologic drug approved specifically to treat moderate to severe plaque psoriasis. It is administered by a doctor, who injects the drug once a week for 12 weeks. The drug is then stopped for a period of time while changes in the skin are observed and a decision is made regarding the need or further treatment. Because alefacept suppresses the immune system, the skin often improves, but there is also an increased risk of infection or other problems, possibly including cancer. Monitoring by a doctor is required, and a patient's blood must be tested weekly around the time of each injection to make certain that T cells and other immune system cells are not overly depressed.

- **Etanercept (Enbrel)**—This drug is an approved treatment for psoriatic arthritis where the joints swell and become inflamed. Like alefacept, it is a biologic response modifier which after injection blocks interactions between certain cells in the immune system. Etanercept limits the action of a specific protein that is overproduced in the lubricating fluid of the joints and surrounding tissues, causing inflammation. Because this same protein is overproduced in the skin of people with psoriatic arthritis, patients receiving etanercept also may notice an improvement in their skin. Individuals should not receive etanercept treatment if they have an active infection, a history of recurring infections, or an underlying condition, such as diabetes, that increases their risk of infection. Those who have psoriasis and certain neurological conditions, such as multiple sclerosis, cannot be treated with this drug. Added caution is needed for psoriasis patients who have rheumatoid arthritis; these patients should follow the advice of a rheumatologist regarding this treatment.

- **Antibiotics**—These medications are not indicated in routine treatment of psoriasis. However, antibiotics may be employed when an infection, such as that caused by the bacteria *Streptococcus*, triggers an outbreak of psoriasis as in certain cases of guttate psoriasis.

Combination Therapy

There are many approaches for treating psoriasis. Combining various topical, light, and systemic treatments often permits lower doses of each and can result in increased effectiveness. Therefore, doctors are paying more attention to combination therapy.

Psychological Support

Some individuals with moderate to severe psoriasis may benefit from counseling or participation in a support group to reduce self-consciousness about their appearance, or relieve psychological distress resulting from fear of social rejection.

Promising Areas of Research

Significant progress has been made in understanding the inheritance of psoriasis. A number of genes involved in psoriasis are already known or suspected. In a multifactor disease (involving genes, environment, and other factors), variations in one or more genes may produce a greater likelihood of getting the disease. Researchers are continuing to study the genetic aspects of psoriasis. Since discovering that inflammation in psoriasis is triggered by T cells, researchers have been studying new treatments that quiet immune system reactions in the skin. Among these are treatments that block the activity of T cells or block cytokines (proteins that promote inflammation).

Advances in laser technology are making it possible for doctors to experiment with laser light treatment of localized plaques. A UVB laser was recently tested in a study that was conducted at several medical centers. Although improvements in the skin were noted, this treatment is not without possible side effects. In some patients, the skin became inflamed, blistered, or discolored following treatment.

Chapter 59

Sarcoidosis

Sarcoidosis is a disease that causes inflammation of the body's tissues. Inflammation is a basic response of the body to injury and usually causes reddened skin, warmth, swelling, and pain. Inflammation from sarcoidosis is different. In sarcoidosis, the inflammation produces small lumps (also called nodules or granulomas) in the tissues.

The inflammation of sarcoidosis can occur in almost any organ and always affects more than one. Most often, the inflammation starts in either the lungs or the lymph nodes (small bean-shaped organs of the immune system). Once in a while, the inflammation occurs suddenly and symptoms appear quickly, but usually it develops gradually and only later produces symptoms.

Sarcoidosis usually is a mild condition and does not result in lasting harm to tissues. In most patients, the inflammation that causes the granulomas gets better with or without treatment and the lumps go away. In others, however, the lumps do not heal or disappear, and the tissues remain inflamed. If untreated, these tissues can become scarred. The tissue is then called fibrotic. But even those who need treatment can usually lead a normal life. The cause of sarcoidosis is not yet known—there may be several. For instance, an abnormal response from the immune system may be involved. (The immune system normally attacks and eliminates foreign substances, such as bacteria, that enter the body.)

Once thought rare, sarcoidosis is now known to be common and affects persons worldwide. In fact, sarcoidosis is the most common chronic

Excerpted from "Sarcoidosis," National Heart, Lung, and Blood Institute (NHLBI), NIH Publication No. 02–5060, April 2003.

fibrotic interstitial lung disorder. (Chronic illnesses are those that last for some time or recur often; interstitial lung diseases affect the tissue that surrounds the air sacs, blood vessels, and air passageways.)

Incidence

Sarcoidosis occurs worldwide. It affects men and women of all ages and races. However, it occurs most commonly in adults between the ages of 20 and 40, and in those of African (especially women), Asian, German, Irish, Puerto Rican, or Scandinavian origin. In the United States, the disease occurs slightly more often and more severely among African Americans.

Studies also have shown that the disease is more likely to affect certain organs in certain populations. For example, sarcoidosis of the heart and eye appears to be more common in Japan. Painful skin lumps on the legs (erythema nodosum) occur more often in people from Northern Europe. Sarcoidosis may occur in families. In the United States, this happens more often among African Americans.

Environmental factors also may affect the occurrence of sarcoidosis. For example, sarcoidosis occurs more often in nonsmokers than smokers. Several studies have noted higher rates of sarcoidosis among health care workers. Other environmental factors, such as beryllium metal (used in aircraft and weapons manufacture) and organic dust from birds or hay, may cause sarcoidosis type reactions in the lungs. Thus, doctors need to know a person's history of occupational and environmental exposure in trying to diagnose sarcoidosis. Infectious agents have been suspected of causing sarcoidosis, but there is no proof of an infectious cause. More research is needed to better understand the effect of environmental factors on a person's risk of developing sarcoidosis.

Pathology and Course of Sarcoidosis

A normal organ is made of an orderly arrangement of cells. Sarcoidosis upsets this arrangement, eventually causing lumps to form in organs. These lumps get larger and are called granulomas because they look like grains of sugar or sand. These grains are very small and can only be seen with a microscope.

Various other diseases can cause the formation of granulomas. For example, tuberculosis can cause granulomas. However, in other diseases, the granuloma forms around a particle, germ, or other foreign substance. In the case of tuberculosis, for instance, the granuloma forms around the invading organism which is a mycobacterium. The immune system causes granulomas to form so that particles, germs, or other foreign substances can be isolated or eliminated.

In sarcoidosis, there is no such visible enclosed particle or germ. No cause for the granuloma can be seen under the microscope. The immune system appears to be responding to an unknown substance.

When thousands of these microscopic granulomas clump together, they result in a variety of small and large lumps. These lumps can appear on the lungs, skin, or other organs, such as the eyes, mouth, salivary glands, liver, spleen, or lymph nodes in the neck, armpits, and groin. Lymph nodes are small organs of the body's immune system.

The lumps can show up as shadows on x-rays. If many large groups of granulomas form, they can affect the organ's function. This can cause symptoms that need to be treated.

The disease has active and nonactive stages. In the active stage, the immune system is fighting the disease and granulomas form or enlarge. In this stage, symptoms can develop and scar tissue can form. In the nonactive stage, the disease is easing, and the granulomas are stable, shrinking, or have become scars.

The course of the disease varies: In most persons, the sarcoidosis goes away over time. In others, the sarcoidosis does not get worse, but the disease remains and a person can feel well or continue to have symptoms. When treatment is given, it usually shrinks the granulomas, and they may even disappear. Such treatment may last for many months. In still other persons, scars can form in the granulomas. Even with treatment, the scars often remain and symptoms may never go away, the affected organs may continue to function poorly.

Symptoms

Most people with sarcoidosis have no symptoms. Some have only one symptom, while others have many. Symptoms typically depend on which organs the disease affects. General symptoms caused by the disease include weight loss, fatigue, night sweats, fever, and an overall feeling of ill health. Most often, the disease will affect the lungs. Thus, the most common symptoms of the disease are a cough that does not go away and shortness of breath, particularly with exertion.

Symptoms common in sarcoidosis include the following:

General Symptoms

- Uneasiness, feeling sick (malaise)

- Tiredness, fatigue, weakness
- Loss of appetite or weight
- Fever
- Sweating at night during sleep

Lymph Node Symptoms

- Enlarged lymph nodes—most often those of the neck, but also may be those under the chin, in the arm pits, or in the groin

Skin Symptoms

- Skin rash—painful or hot red bumps on the legs or arms, or small brownish and painless bumps on the arms, legs, and/or back

Eye Symptoms

- Burning, itching, tearing, pain
- Red eye
- Sensitivity to light (photophobia)
- Dryness
- Seeing black spots (called floaters)
- Blurred vision

Lungs and Heart Symptoms

- Shortness of breath
- Wheeze
- Cough
- Chest pain
- Irregular heartbeat (palpitations)

Joint Symptoms

- Joint stiffness, swelling—most commonly of the ankles, feet, and hands

Diagnosis

The symptoms of sarcoidosis are like those of other diseases, some are more harmful and even life-threatening. So it is important to properly diagnose the condition.

Someone who is thought to have the disease should see a doctor who specializes in sarcoidosis, usually a lung physician (pulmonologist). The specialist will work with patients and their regular physician to help diagnose the disease and to develop a schedule of treatment and follow-up care.

To make a diagnosis, a doctor will ask for a medical history and do a physical examination. The doctor also may need to take laboratory tests of the blood, a chest x-ray, and breathing tests. Tests and procedures used to help diagnose and monitor sarcoidosis include the following:

- physical examination
- chest x-ray
- blood tests
- pulmonary function tests
- fiberoptic bronchoscopy
- fiberoptic bronchoscopy biopsy
- bronchoalveolar lavage
- computed tomography (CT) scan
- magnetic resonance (MR) scan
- thallium and gallium scans
- eye test

Treatment

The treatment of sarcoidosis depends on a person's symptoms. Often, no treatment is needed—up to 60 percent of those with sarcoidosis receive no therapy. But, for some, intense treatment is required, especially if there is critical organ involvement, such as of the lungs, eyes, heart, or central nervous system. Here are some key points about the use of treatment:

- Treatment is done to control symptoms or to improve the function of organs affected by the disease.

- Treatment may or may not affect the long-term outcome of the disease. One study found that 5–10 years after diagnosis, there was no difference in recovery between those who had received a short course of treatment and those who had not.

- Sarcoidosis granulomas result from a response of the immune system. Thus, most medications used to treat sarcoidosis suppress the immune system. This can leave a person more likely to get sick from an infection, and this risk must be considered in making treatment decisions.

Treatment for sarcoidosis involves the use of medications. A wide variety is available, but most are strong and can cause bad side effects. Different ones will work better for different persons, and sometimes more than one is used. Living with the symptoms of the disease must thus be weighed against the side effects produced by the drugs.

Drugs are either taken by mouth for systemic effects throughout the body, or are applied locally to an affected area. Local therapy is the safest way to treat the disease, since only the affected area is exposed to the drug. Drugs can be applied locally by drop, inhaler, or cream. Drugs used in this way include corticosteroids. However, to use drugs locally, the affected area must be easily reached. For instance, drops and creams help with some eye or skin problems, while inhalers are used to apply steroids to affected lung tissue, especially to ease coughing and wheezing. It does not appear that an inhaled drug can relieve such symptoms when the affected lung tissue is deep within the chest.

The main drugs used to treat sarcoidosis are the following:

• Prednisone
• Hydroxychloroquine
• Methotrexate
• Azathioprine
• Cyclophosphamide

Effects on Organs

Some organs are affected more often than others. Sarcoidosis occurs most often in the lungs. It also commonly affects the skin, eyes, lymph nodes, and liver. Less commonly, it affects the spleen, brain, nerves, heart, tear glands, salivary glands, bones, and joints. Rarely, it affects other organs, such as the thyroid gland, breasts, kidneys, and reproductive organs.

A doctor may not detect sarcoidosis in every organ affected by the disease. Often, the effects of sarcoidosis in an organ are so mild that there are no symptoms and the organ continues to function well. In such cases, identifying the disease in that organ is not necessary and would not change the treatment given.

Follow-Up Tests

Those with sarcoidosis need to have their condition checked during and after treatment. Those who receive no treatment also need regular checkups, since symptoms can develop later. The patient will work with his or her sarcoidosis specialist and regular physician to develop a schedule of periodic examinations and laboratory tests. The

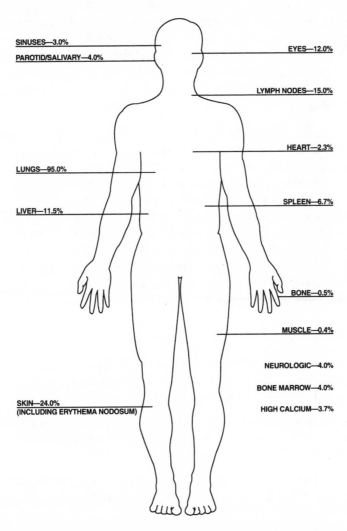

SINUSES—3.0%

PAROTID/SALIVARY—4.0%

EYES—12.0%

LYMPH NODES—15.0%

HEART—2.3%

LUNGS—95.0%

SPLEEN—6.7%

LIVER—11.5%

BONE—0.5%

MUSCLE—0.4%

NEUROLOGIC—4.0%

BONE MARROW—4.0%

SKIN—24.0%
(INCLUDING ERYTHEMA NODOSUM)

HIGH CALCIUM—3.7%

Figure 59.1. *Percent of Cases with Sarcoidosis in Specific Organs According to Data from "A Case Control Etiologic Study of Sarcoidosis."*

follow-up examination usually includes a review of symptoms, a physical examination, a chest x-ray, breathing tests, and laboratory blood tests. How often these examinations and tests are done depends on the severity of the symptoms and the organs affected at diagnosis, the therapy used, and any complications that may develop during treatment.

Routine follow-up care usually lasts for 2–3 years. Whether the specialist or primary doctor oversees this care depends on symptoms during the first year of follow-up. Patients should tell their doctor about any new symptom that lasts for more than a week. They also should see the doctor if symptoms appear and do not go away before the next regularly scheduled follow-up visit. Changes in sarcoidosis occur slowly—usually over months. Except for disturbed heart rhythms, sarcoidosis does not cause sudden illness.

Prognosis

Sarcoidosis affects the body in many ways and the outcome can vary from person to person. But the chance of recovering from the disease is good. Most often, the disease goes away within a few years. About 75 percent of all patients have only the acute form of sarcoidosis—the disease leaves no significant problems for about half of them.

However, sarcoidosis sometimes stays for years and can cause organ damage and significantly reduce physical activity. About 25 percent of all patients have the chronic form of the disease. In these patients, the disease usually leaves scar tissue in the lungs, skin, eyes, or other organs. However, chronic cases can be improved with treatment. Sarcoidosis—whether acute or chronic—rarely results in death.

References

1.   American Thoracic Society. Medical Section of the American Lung Association: statement on sarcoidosis. *Am J Respir Cri Care Med*. 1999;160:736-55.

2.   Askling J, Grunewald J, Eklund A, et al. Increased risk for cancer following sarcoidosis. *Am J Respir Cri Care Med*. 1999;160(5 Pt 1:1668-72).

3.   Baughman RP, Lower EE. Alternatives to corticosteroids in the treatment of sarcoidosis. *Sarcoidosis Vasc and Diffuse Lung Dis*. 1997;14:121-30.

4.   Baughman RP, Winget DB, Lower EE. Methotrexate is steroid sparing in acute sarcoidosis: results of a double blind,

randomized trial. *Sarcoidosis Vasc and Diffuse Lung Dis.* 2000;17:60-6.

5. Costable U. Sarcoidosis: clinical update. *Eur Respir J.* 2001;18(suppl 32):56s-68s.

6. Hunninghake GW, Costable U, Ando M, et al. ATS/ERS/ WASOG statement on sarcoidosis. *Sarcoidosis Vasc and Diffuse Lung Dis.* 1999;16:149-73.

7. McGrath DS, Goh N, Foley PJ, et al. Sarcoidosis: genes and microbes—soil or seed? *Sarcoidosis Vasc and Diffuse Lung Dis.* 2001;18:149-64.

8. Newman LS, Rose CS, Maier LA. Sarcoidosis. *N Engl J Med.* 1997;336(17):1224-34.

9. Paramothayan S, Jones PW. Corticosteroid therapy in pulmonary sarcoidosis: a systematic review. *JAMA.* 2002;287(10): 1301-7.

10. Yee AM, Pochapin MB. Treatment of complicated sarcoidosis with infliximab anti-tumor necrosis factor-a therapy. *Ann Internal Med.* 2001;135(1):27-31.

Additional Information

American Lung Association
61 Broadway, 6ᵗʰ Floor
New York, NY 10006
Toll-Free: 800-548-8252 (to speak to a lung health professional)
Toll-Free: 800-LUNGUSA (586-4872) (to contact the American Lung Association nearest you)
Phone: 212-315-8700
Website: http://www.lungusa.org/site/ pp.asp?c=dvLUK9OOE&b=22542

National Heart, Lung, and Blood Institute Health Information Center
P.O. Box 30105
Bethesda, MD 20824-0105
Phone: 301-592-8573
TTY: 240-629-3255
Fax: 240-629-3246
Website: http://www.nhlbi.nih.gov

National Sarcoidosis Resources Center

P.O. Box 1593
Piscataway, NJ 08855-1593
Phone: 732-699-0733
Fax: 732-699-0882
Website: http://www.nsrc-global.net

Chapter 60

Scleroderma

What Is Scleroderma?

Scleroderma is a chronic, often progressive autoimmune disease in which the body's immune system attacks its own tissues. It falls into the same category as rheumatoid arthritis, lupus, Sjögren syndrome, and multiple sclerosis (MS).

The disease, which literally means hard skin, can cause thickening and tightening of skin, and in some cases serious damage to internal organs including lungs, heart, kidneys, esophagus, and gastrointestinal (GI) tract.

Scleroderma can vary a great deal in terms of severity. For a few individuals it is merely a nuisance; for others it is a life-threatening illness. For most, it is a disease that affects how they live their daily lives. Although medicines can sometimes help treat symptoms, there is no cure yet for scleroderma.

Types of Scleroderma

There are two basic types of scleroderma: the systemic form that affects the internal organs or internal systems of the body, and the localized form, that affects a local area of skin.

Systemic Scleroderma

In systemic scleroderma (also called systemic sclerosis), the immune system causes damage to two main areas: the small blood vessels, and the collagen-producing cells located in the skin and throughout the body.

In systemic scleroderma, the small blood vessels in the fingers tend to narrow, and sometimes the blood channel is completely closed off. As a result, small cuts on the hands are slow to heal, and sometimes ulcers form spontaneously. Due to this decreased blood supply, scleroderma patients are notoriously cold-sensitive. This vascular aspect of the disease is responsible for Raynaud phenomenon (color changes of the fingers upon exposure to cold), which occurs in about 95% of people with systemic sclerosis.

The collagen aspect of the disease is responsible for the thick and tight skin, lung and heart problems, and gastrointestinal (GI) tract features. Under normal conditions, the immune system signals cells to produce collagen to form a scar after an area of injury or infection has been cleared. In scleroderma, this scar tissue is produced for no apparent reason, and builds up in the skin and other organs. Many patients will have trouble only with the GI tract, and have normal lungs, hearts, and kidneys. All combinations of symptoms are seen.

To further complicate matters, systemic scleroderma is divided into two forms: limited and diffuse, referring to the degree of skin involvement. Both forms are associated with internal organ damage, but the limited form tends to have less severe organ problems. Limited scleroderma often is referred to as the CREST form. CREST is an acronym that stands for the following terms:

Calcinosis

Raynaud phenomenon

Esophageal dysfunction

Sclerodactyly

Telangiectasias

Calcinosis refers to calcium deposits in the skin. Raynaud phenomenon refers to color changes (white, purple, or red) in the fingers due to cold exposure. Esophageal dysfunction refers to acid in the esophagus, felt as heartburn. Sclerodactyly means tight and thick skin of the fingers. Telangiectasia is a type of red spots in the skin.

Localized Scleroderma

Localized scleroderma affects the collagen producing cells in just some skin areas and usually spares the internal organs and blood vessels. Localized scleroderma occurs either as patches of thickened skin (morphea), or as linear scleroderma, a line of thickened skin that may extend down an arm or leg. If this line involves the forehead, it is called *en coup de sabre* or cut of the saber.

It is easy to confuse the terms localized scleroderma (which is one of the two main types of scleroderma) and limited scleroderma (one of the two types of systemic scleroderma, also called CREST). However, this terminology is widespread and not likely to change.

Scleroderma-Related Disorders

Scleroderma can also occur in patients with other autoimmune disorders, as part of an overlap syndrome. A variety of drugs and chemicals can also produce lesions similar to those seen in scleroderma.

Who Gets Scleroderma?

Localized scleroderma is more common in children, whereas systemic scleroderma is more common in adults. Overall, female patients outnumber males about 4:1, and the average patient is diagnosed in her 40s. Having said this, it is important to note that scleroderma is a disease of many exceptions.

What Causes Scleroderma?

Although much research is focused on this important question, the cause of scleroderma is not known. Most patients do not have any relatives with scleroderma, nor do their children get scleroderma. Research indicates there is a susceptibility gene which raises the likelihood of getting scleroderma, but does not cause scleroderma by itself.

Diagnosing Scleroderma

An experienced doctor bases a diagnosis of scleroderma primarily on a patient's medical history and a physical examination. The most important finding is hard skin, which gives the disease its name.

- About 98% of scleroderma patients have hardening or thickening of the skin of the fingers—and often of the hands, forearms, and face.

- Raynaud phenomenon is present in 95%.

- A third abnormality found in over 95% of patients is a positive antinuclear antibody (ANA) test.

Treating Scleroderma

At present there is no cure for scleroderma, but many treatments are available for specific symptoms. Because there is so much variation in the type and severity of symptoms, it is important that each patient receive individualized care from a doctor who is knowledgeable about the disease.

Additional Information

Scleroderma Foundation
12 Kent Way, Suite 101
Byfield, MA 01922
Toll-Free: 800-722-4673
Phone: 978-463-5843
Fax: 978-463-5809
Website: http://www.scleroderma.org
E-mail: sfinfo@scleroderma.org

The Scleroderma Foundation's mission is three-fold:

- To help patients and cope with scleroderma mutual support programs, counseling, physician referrals, and educational information.

- To promote public awareness and education through patient and health professional seminars, literature, and publicity campaigns.

- To stimulate and support research to improve treatment and ultimately find the cause and cure of scleroderma and related diseases.

The Scleroderma Foundation provides referrals to health professionals, support group information and a quarterly magazine.

Chapter 61

Sjögren Syndrome

What Is Sjögren Syndrome?

Sjögren syndrome is characterized by malfunction of the tear- and saliva-producing glands and the Bartholin glands in the vagina. The end result is the feeling of dryness of the eyes, mouth, and vagina. Sjögren (Show-gren) syndrome may be primary (not associated with other diseases), or secondary (develop in patients who have rheumatoid arthritis, lupus, or scleroderma).

What causes Sjögren syndrome?

Sjögren syndrome is caused by accumulation of activated lymphocytes in the affected glands and the ducts, which drain the glands. These lymphocytes interfere with the production and flow of tears, saliva, and vaginal secretions.

What are the symptoms of Sjögren syndrome?

Dry eyes: You may notice a gritty or sandy feeling in your eyes. On awakening in the morning you may have increased thick mucus visible in the corners of your eyes nearest the nose. Your eyes may be unusually sensitive to bright light (photophobia).

Dry mouth: You will produce less saliva, which makes moving food in your mouth and speaking more difficult, and reduces your sense of taste. You will crave water or other liquids. You may not be able to eat a dry cracker without water, or eat a meal without frequent sips of water. You may feel the need to take a bottle of water with you wherever you go. Your nose and throat can also be dry, leading to decreased sense of smell, nosebleeds, hoarseness, and dry cough.

Dry vagina: Sjögren syndrome may cause vaginal dryness, which results in irritation and makes sexual intercourse uncomfortable.

Caution to patients: There are many other causes of the listed complaints of dryness. Increased age, other diseases of the eyes and mouth, certain medications, and lack of estrogen in the vagina are common reasons for dryness which may be considered by your physicians.

Other symptoms: You may suffer from fatigue, stiffness, and swelling of the small joints of the hands, swollen lymph glands, muscle pain and/or weakness, Raynaud phenomenon, or numbness, tingling, pins and needles feeling, or burning of the toes and feet.

How is Sjögren syndrome diagnosed?

In addition to your medical history and physical examination, certain tests may be useful.

Eye tests: The Schirmer test is a screening test to measure how much you are able to wet a strip of filter paper placed inside your lower eyelid in 5 minutes. More sophisticated tests can be performed by an ophthalmologist.

Mouth tests: A biopsy of the inside of the lower lip may establish the diagnosis; increased numbers of lymphocytes are seen surrounding the small saliva-producing glands.

Laboratory tests: Half of Sjögren patients have anti-SSA and anti-SSB (Sjögren syndrome A and B) antibodies in their blood.

Once Sjögren syndrome has been diagnosed, your doctor may order other tests to determine the activity of the disease and the extent to which it might have spread beyond glands. Regular physician evaluations should be done to determine the extent of Sjögren syndrome, especially any tendency toward lymphoma. Women with Sjögren syndrome and anti-SSA antibody should consult their rheumatologist and obstetrician before becoming pregnant.

What are the complications of Sjögren syndrome?

Eyes: Eye dryness may cause dry spots or ulcers on the cornea, leading to scarring with reduced vision and inability to wear contact lenses.

Mouth: An increased number of cavities (dental caries) and infection of the gums (gingivitis) with loosening of the teeth may occur. Overgrowth of the common yeast candida results in a mouth infection termed candidiasis (can-di-DYE-ah-sis) or thrush. There may be slow and painless enlargement of the parotid (mumps) glands due to duct blockage. If abrupt, painful enlargement of these glands with intense redness of the overlying skin and fever are also present, this may indicate a bacterial infection of the gland and is a medical emergency.

Nervous system involvement: Lymphocytes may directly injure nerves in the brain, spinal cord, or extremities.

Respiratory tract: There is an increased risk of developing infections of the ears and sinuses, as well as bronchitis and pneumonia. The lung tissue itself may be invaded by lymphocytes.

Vasculitis: A few patients develop vasculitis (inflammation of the walls of small blood vessels). A red spotted rash on the legs and numbness and tingling of the feet and toes results. Vasculitis can affect other organs and is a serious complication.

Kidney: Some patients with Sjögren syndrome develop blood and/ or protein in the urine, and in a few cases, mild kidney failure.

Skin: A characteristic rash may appear in skin areas exposed to ultraviolet light or sunlight (photosensitive rash).

Pregnancy: A woman with Sjögren syndrome and ant-SSA antibody in her blood may pass this antibody across the placenta to her developing fetus. The result may be a transient illness called neonatal lupus. There can also be permanent injury to the fetal heart, leading to a very slow heartbeat (heart block) and other heart abnormalities.

Lymphoma: Rarely, the lymphocytes in Sjögren syndrome patients can become malignant, resulting in a lymphoma.

How is Sjögren syndrome treated?

There is no recognized cure for Sjögren syndrome. Therefore, doctors try to treat the symptoms of the disease to minimize their effects on daily life. The following aids may be recommended.

For Dry Eyes

- Artificial tears, every 2 to 4 hours during the day, or a long-acting pellet in the morning and a lubricating ointment at night.
- Punctal occlusion, a surgical procedure to retain moisture by preventing tears from draining out of the eye and into the nose.

For Dry Mouth

- Sips of water throughout the day or over-the-counter saliva substitutes or gels.
- Sugar-free chewing gum or candies to stimulate saliva flow.
- Treatment for oral candidiasis.
- A saliva-stimulant oral medication containing the active ingredient pilocarpine.
- Good oral hygiene to prevent dental caries: frequent checkups and teeth cleaning; brush and floss teeth regularly and thoroughly, especially after meals; avoid sugar-containing foods and drinks between meals; use mouth rinses containing fluoride.

For Vaginal Dryness

- Specially designed lubricants, but do not use petroleum jelly.

For Other Organs Affected

- Common-sense measures: avoid cigarette smoking; pace activities to avoid fatigue; adequate exercise and sleep.
- Aspirin or non-steroidal anti-inflammatory drugs for arthritis or muscle pain.
- Hydroxychloroquine (Plaquenil®) for arthritis, skin rash, and fatigue.
- Cortisone or immune-system-suppressing drugs for more serious problems such as involvement of the lung, kidney, nervous system, or vasculitis.

How is Sjögren syndrome related to scleroderma?

Over 20% of patients with systemic sclerosis and a few with localized scleroderma suffer from secondary Sjögren syndrome. It is more often detected in persons with the limited skin-thickening form of systemic sclerosis, a category which includes patients with the CREST syndrome. The symptoms and examination findings and methods of diagnosis and treatment are very similar to those in primary Sjögren syndrome.

A special problem for systemic sclerosis patients may be maintaining good oral hygiene because of reduced mouth opening, Raynaud's phenomenon, finger-tip ulcers, and deformities of the fingers.

Summary

Sjögren syndrome is rarely a life-threatening disease. However, dryness is likely to last the rest of your life. By using artificial moisturizing methods, you can minimize the symptoms and prevent local complications.

Questions and Answers about Sjögren Syndrome

Who gets Sjögren syndrome?

Experts believe 1 to 4 million people have the disease. Most—90 percent—are women. It can occur at any age, but it usually is diagnosed after age 40 and can affect people of all races and ethnic backgrounds. It's rare in children, but can occur.

Are other autoimmune diseases common among people with Sjögren syndrome?

Connective tissue is the framework of the body that supports organs and tissues. Examples are joints, muscles, bones, skin, blood vessel walls, and the lining of internal organs. Many connective tissue disorders are autoimmune diseases and several are common among people with Sjögren syndrome. These include the following:

- Polymyositis
- Raynaud phenomenon
- Rheumatoid arthritis (RA)
- Scleroderma
- Systemic lupus erythematosus (SLE)
- Vasculitis
- Autoimmune thyroid disorders

Does Sjögren syndrome cause lymphoma?

About 5 percent of people with Sjögren syndrome develop cancer of the lymph nodes, or lymphoma. The most common symptom of lymphoma is a painless swelling of the lymph nodes in the neck, underarm, or groin. In Sjögren Syndrome, when lymphoma develops, it often involves the salivary glands. Persistent enlargement of the salivary glands should be investigated further. Other symptoms may include the following:

- Unexplained fever
- Night sweats
- Constant fatigue
- Unexplained weight loss
- Itchy skin
- Reddened patches on the skin

These symptoms are not sure signs of lymphoma. They may be caused by other, less serious conditions, such as the flu or an infection. If you have these symptoms, see a doctor so that any illness can be diagnosed and treated as early as possible.

Additional Information

Scleroderma Foundation
12 Kent Way, Suite 101
Byfield, MA 01922
Toll-Free: 800-722-4673
Phone: 978-463-5843
Fax: 978-463-5809
Website: http://www.scleroderma.org
E-mail: sfinfo@scleroderma.org

The Scleroderma Foundation also provides referrals to health professionals, support group information and a quarterly magazine.

Sjögren's Syndrome Foundation, Inc.
8120 Woodmont Ave., Suite 530
Bethesda, MD 20814-1437
Toll-Free: 800-475-6473
Phone: 301-718-0300
Fax: 301-718-0322
Website: http://www.sjogrens.org

Chapter 62

Thyroid Disease

Chapter Contents

Section 62.1

Graves Disease

What Is Graves Disease?

The leading cause of hyperthyroidism, Graves disease, represents a basic defect in the autoimmune system, causing production of immunoglobulins (antibodies) which stimulate and attack the thyroid gland. This causes growth of the gland and overproduction of thyroid hormone. Similar antibodies may also attack the tissues in the eye muscles and in the pretibial skin (the skin on the front of the lower leg).

Facts

• Graves disease occurs in less than ¼ of 1% of the population.
• Graves disease is more prevalent among females than males.
• Graves disease usually occurs in middle age, but also occurs in children and adolescents.
• Graves disease is not curable, but is a completely treatable disease.

Symptoms

• Fatigue
• Weight loss
• Restlessness
• Tachycardia (rapid heart beat)
• Changes in libido (sex drive)
• Muscle weakness
• Heat intolerance

- Tremors
- Enlarged thyroid gland
- Heart palpitations
- Increased sweating
- Blurred or double vision
- Nervousness and irritability
- Eye complaints, such as redness and swelling
- Hair changes
- Restless sleep
- Erratic behavior
- Increased appetite
- Distracted attention span
- Decrease in menstrual cycle
- Increased frequency of stools

Who Develops Graves Disease?

Although Graves disease most frequently occurs in women in the middle decades (8:1 more than men), it also occurs in children and in the elderly. There are several elements contributing to the development of Graves disease. There is a genetic predisposition to autoimmune disorders. Infections and stress play a part. Graves disease may have its onset after a severe external stressor. In other instances, it may follow a viral infection or pregnancy. Many times the exact cause of Graves is simply not known. It is not contagious, although it has been known to occur coincidentally between husbands and wives. Of research importance, the Graves gene in deoxyribonucleic acid (DNA) has not yet been identified.

How Is Graves Disease Treated?

There are three standard ways of treating Graves disease. The choice of treatment varies to some degree from country to country and among particular physicians as well. The decision should be made with the full knowledge and informed consent of the patient, who is the primary member of the treatment team. The selection of treatment will include factors such as age, degree of illness, and personal preferences. Generally speaking, from least invasive to most invasive, the treatments include:

1. Anti-thyroid drugs that either block the production or the conversion of thyroid hormone into its active form in the body. They may be used exclusively or in combination with replacement hormone.

2. Radioactive iodine (I-131), which destroys part or all of the thyroid gland and renders it incapable of overproducing thyroid hormone.

3. Subtotal thyroidectomy in which a surgeon removes most of the thyroid gland and renders it incapable of overproducing thyroid hormone.

The first treatment is about 30–50% effective and the latter two treatments result in about a 90–95% remission rate of the disease. In a few cases, the treatments must be repeated. In all cases, lifetime follow-up laboratory studies must be done; and in almost all cases, lifetime replacement thyroid hormone must be taken.

Are There Any Alternatives to These Treatments of Graves Disease?

There are a number of things you can do to assist your body in healing. However, the state of science as we know it, indicates there is no natural way to cure Graves disease. For instance, although there are no specific foods that will change your thyroid function, the more healthy, nutritionally dense foods you eat, the better your body will be able to fight against infection and further insult. Equally, many treatments like acupuncture, exercise, meditation, and various mind-body therapies may provide comfort measures and relief, but are not a substitute for standard medical treatment. Be sure to consult and collaborate with your physician when embarking on additional therapies. There are many studies of other autoimmune disorders that indicate the more input and control a patient has in their care, the more rapid their recovery will be. It is of interest to all who are hopeful of effective additional treatment models in the future that the National Institutes of Health are trying to adequately research and evaluate the hard data of alternative therapies.

What Are the Complications?

Graves disease usually responds to treatment and, after the initial period of hyperthyroidism, is relatively easy to treat and manage.

There are some exceptions to this and, for some, treatment and subsequent stabilization are much more challenging, both to the patient and the treating team of physicians. The more serious complications of prolonged, untreated, or improperly treated Graves disease includes the possibilities of weakened heart muscle leading to heart failure, osteoporosis, or possible severe emotional disorders.

Additional Information

National Graves' Disease Foundation
P.O. Box 8387
Fleming Island, FL 32006
Phone: 904-278-9488
Website: http://www.ngdf.org

The NGDF is a lay organization that provides patient education and support. Informational bulletins on topics that affect Graves patients and their families are available for a small fee.

The National Graves' Disease Foundation seeks:

- To provide current medical information and referral and resource information to those with Graves disease.

- To provide social and psychological support for those with Graves disease by aiding in the development of locally based support groups.

- To provide public education through the distribution of literature, lectures, and presentations in the media and the community.

- To provide professional education through lectures and forums on the prevalence and treatment of Graves disease.

- To publish a periodic newsletter to share information with the membership.

- To establish liaison relationships with major schools, hospitals, and research institutions both nationally and internationally.

Section 62.2

Hashimoto Disease

"Hashimoto's Thyroiditis," The National Women's Health Information
Center (NWHIC), March 2001.

What is Hashimoto thyroiditis?

Hashimoto thyroiditis is a type of autoimmune thyroid disease in
which the immune system attacks and destroys the thyroid gland. The
thyroid helps set the rate of metabolism—the rate at which the body
uses energy. Hashimoto disease prevents the gland from producing
enough thyroid hormones for the body to work correctly. It is the most
common form of hypothyroidism (underactive thyroid).

What are the symptoms of Hashimoto thyroiditis?

Some patients with Hashimoto thyroiditis may have no symptoms.
However, the common symptoms are fatigue, depression, and sensitivity to cold, weight gain, muscle weakness, coarsening of the skin,
dry or brittle hair, constipation, muscle cramps, increased menstrual
flow, and goiter (enlargement of the thyroid gland).

Is this disease hereditary?

There is some evidence that Hashimoto thyroiditis can have a hereditary link. If autoimmune diseases run in your family, you are at
a higher risk of developing one yourself.

How can I know for sure if I have this disease?

Your doctor will perform a simple blood test that will be able to
tell if your body has the correct amount of thyroid hormones. This test
measures the blood TSH (thyroid stimulating hormone) to determine
if the thyroid hormone levels are in the normal range. The range is
set by your doctor and should be discussed with you. Work with your
doctor to find what level is right for you.

What is the treatment for this disease?

Hashimoto thyroiditis can usually be treated with thyroid hormone replacement. A small pill taken once a day should be able to regulate the thyroid hormone in the body to normal levels. This medication will, in most cases, need to be taken for the rest of the patient's life. When trying to determine the correct hormone dosage, you may have to return to your doctor several times for adjustments in medication. A yearly visit to your health care provider will help keep your levels normal and help maintain normal health. Be aware of the symptoms. If you note any changes or the return of symptoms, return to your doctor to see if you need to have your medication changed.

What would happen without medication to regulate my thyroid function?

If left untreated, Hashimoto thyroiditis can cause further complications, including changes in menstrual cycles, prevention of ovulation, and an increased risk of miscarriage. It is also important to know that too much thyroid replacement hormone can mimic the symptoms of hyperthyroidism. This is a condition that occurs from over-production of thyroid hormones. These symptoms include insomnia, irritability, weight loss without dieting, heat sensitivity, increased perspiration, thinning of your skin, fine or brittle hair, muscular weakness, eye changes, lighter menstrual flow, rapid heart beat, and hand tremors.

Additional Information

National Institute of Diabetes and Digestive and Kidney Diseases (NIDDK)
Information Clearinghouse
5 Information Way
Bethesda, MD 20892-3560
Toll-Free: 800-860-8747
Phone: 301-654-3810
Website: http://www.niddk.nih.gov

Thyroid Foundation of America, Inc.
One Longfellow Place, Suite 1518
Boston, MA 02114
(*Continued on next page*)

Thyroid Foundation of America, Inc. (continued)
Toll-Free: 800-832-8321
Phone: 617-534-1500
Fax: 617-534-1515
Website: http://www.allthyroid.org
E-mail: info@tsh.org

Chapter 63

Uveitis

Alternative names: Iritis; pars planitis; choroiditis; chorioretinitis; anterior uveitis; posterior uveitis.

Definition: Uveitis is an inflammation of the uvea, the layer between the sclera and the retina, which includes the iris, ciliary body, and the choroid.

Causes, Incidence, and Risk Factors

Uveitis is an inflammation inside the eye, affecting the uvea. The uvea provides most of the blood supply to the retina. Causes of uveitis can include autoimmune disorders, infection, or exposure to toxins. However in many cases, the cause remains unknown.

The most common form of uveitis is anterior uveitis, which involves inflammation in the front part of the eye, which is usually isolated to the iris. This condition is often called iritis. The inflammation may be associated with autoimmune diseases such as rheumatoid arthritis or ankylosing spondylitis, but most cases occur in healthy people and do not indicate an underlying disease. The disorder may affect only one eye and is most common in young and middle-aged people. A history of an autoimmune disease is a risk factor.

Pars planitis is inflammation of the pars plana, a narrow area between the iris and the choroid. Pars planitis usually occurs in young men and is not associated with any other disease. It is usually mild.

"Uveitis," © 2005 A.D.A.M., Inc. Reprinted with permission.

Posterior uveitis affects the back portion of the uveal tract and involves primarily the choroid. This is called choroiditis. If the adjacent retina is also involved it is called chorioretinitis. Posterior uveitis may follow a systemic infection or occur in association with an autoimmune disease.

The inflammation causes spotty areas of scarring on the choroid and retina that correspond to areas with vision loss. The degree of vision loss depends on the amount and location of scarring. If the central part of the retina, called the macula is involved, central vision becomes impaired.

Uveitis, affecting one or both eyes, can be associated with any of the following:

- Toxoplasmosis
- Histoplasmosis
- Tuberculosis
- Sarcoidosis
- Syphilis
- Acquired immunodeficiency syndrome (AIDS)
- CMV retinitis or other cytomegalovirus infection
- Sympathetic ophthalmia following trauma
- Ulcerative colitis
- Rheumatoid arthritis
- Kawasaki disease
- Herpes zoster infection
- Ankylosing spondylitis
- Behçet syndrome
- Psoriasis
- Reiter syndrome

Symptoms

- Redness of the eye
- Blurred vision
- Sensitivity to light
- Dark, floating spots in the vision

* Eye pain

Note: Symptoms may develop rapidly.

Signs and Tests

A complete medical history and eye examination should be performed. If there is suspicion of an associated systemic disease, a physical examination and laboratory tests may be needed to look for underlying causes.

Treatment

Iritis is usually mild. Spasm of the pupil constriction muscle causes pain which is relieved by drops to dilate the pupil. Dark glasses may be helpful. Steroid eye drops or ointment may be needed. More severe cases require a search for an underlying cause.

Pars planitis is usually mild and can be followed without medications.

Choroiditis requires determination of the underlying cause, and treatment of the underlying disease. The underlying disease may be serious, and additional specialists in infectious disease or autoimmunity may be needed for such diseases as syphilis, tuberculosis, AIDS, sarcoidosis, or Behçet syndrome.

Treatment is consistent with treatment for the systemic diseases of toxoplasmosis, tuberculosis, sarcoidosis, and so forth. For infectious diseases, corticosteroids are often used along with antibiotic therapy. For autoimmune diseases, various forms of suppression of the immune system may be required.

Expectations (Prognosis)

In anterior uveitis, most attacks last from a few days to weeks with treatment, but relapses are common. In posterior uveitis, the inflammation may last from months to years and may cause permanent vision damage, even with treatment.

Complications

* Glaucoma
* Cataracts
* Fluid within the retina (cystoid macular edema)

* Retinal detachment
* Vision loss

Calling Your Health Care Provider

Call for an appointment with your health care provider if uveitis symptoms are present (if eye pain or reduced vision are present, this condition is more urgent that if symptoms are very mild).

Prevention

Treatment of the causative disorders may help to prevent uveitis for some people with existing systemic diseases.

Chapter 64

Vitiligo

Vitiligo (vit-ill-EYE-go) is a pigmentation disorder in which melanocytes (the cells that make pigment) in the skin, the mucous membranes (tissues that line the inside of the mouth, nose, genital, and rectal areas), and the retina (inner layer of the eyeball) are destroyed. As a result, white patches of skin appear on different parts of the body. The hair that grows in areas affected by vitiligo usually turns white.

The cause of vitiligo is not known, but doctors and researchers have several different theories. One theory is that people develop antibodies that destroy the melanocytes in their own bodies. Another theory is that melanocytes destroy themselves. Finally, some people have reported that a single event, such as sunburn or emotional distress, triggered vitiligo; however, these events have not been scientifically proven to cause vitiligo.

Incidence

About 1 to 2 percent of the world's population, or 40 to 50 million people, have vitiligo. In the United States, 2 to 5 million people have the disorder. Ninety-five percent of people who have vitiligo develop it before their 40th birthday. The disorder affects all races and both sexes equally.

Vitiligo seems to be more common in people with certain autoimmune diseases (diseases in which a person's immune system reacts against

Excerpted from "Questions and Answers about Vitiligo," National Institute of Arthritis and Musculoskeletal and Skin Diseases (NIAMS), NIH Publication No. 01–4909, May 2001.

the body's own organs or tissues). These autoimmune diseases include hyperthyroidism (an overactive thyroid gland), adrenocortical insufficiency (the adrenal gland does not produce enough of the hormone called corticosteroid), alopecia areata (patches of baldness), and pernicious anemia (a low level of red blood cells caused by failure of the body to absorb vitamin B_{12}). Scientists do not know the reason for the association between vitiligo and these autoimmune diseases. However, most people with vitiligo have no other autoimmune disease.

Vitiligo may also be hereditary, that is, it can run in families. Children whose parents have the disorder are more likely to develop vitiligo. However, most children will not get vitiligo even if a parent has it, and most people with vitiligo do not have a family history of the disorder.

Symptoms of Vitiligo

People who develop vitiligo usually first notice white patches (depigmentation) on their skin. These patches are more common in sun-exposed areas, including the hands, feet, arms, face, and lips. Other common areas for white patches to appear are the armpits, groin, mouth, eyes, nostrils, navel, and genitals.

Vitiligo generally appears in one of three patterns. In one pattern (focal pattern), the depigmentation is limited to one or only a few areas. Some people develop depigmented patches on only one side of their bodies (segmental pattern). But for most people who have vitiligo, depigmentation occurs on different parts of the body (generalized pattern). In addition to white patches on the skin, people with vitiligo may have premature graying of the scalp hair, eyelashes, eyebrows, and beard. People with dark skin may notice a loss of color inside their mouths.

There is no way to predict if vitiligo will spread. For some people, the depigmented patches do not spread. The disorder is usually progressive, however, and over time the white patches will spread to other areas of the body. For some people, vitiligo spreads slowly, over many years. For other people, spreading occurs rapidly. Some people have reported additional depigmentation following periods of physical or emotional stress.

Diagnosis

If a doctor suspects that a person has vitiligo, he or she usually begins by asking the person about his or her medical history. Important factors in a person's medical history are a family history of vitiligo; a rash, sunburn, or other skin trauma at the site of vitiligo 2 to

3 months before depigmentation started; stress or physical illness; and premature (before age 35) graying of the hair. In addition, the doctor will need to know whether the patient or anyone in the patient's family has had any autoimmune diseases and whether the patient is very sensitive to the sun. The doctor will then examine the patient to rule out other medical problems. The doctor may take a small sample (biopsy) of the affected skin. He or she may also take a blood sample to check the blood cell count and thyroid function. For some patients, the doctor may recommend an eye examination to check for uveitis (inflammation of part of the eye). A blood test to look for the presence of antinuclear antibodies (a type of autoantibody) may also be done. This test helps determine if the patient has another autoimmune disease.

Emotional and Psychological Aspects of Vitiligo

The change in appearance caused by vitiligo can affect a person's emotional and psychological well-being and may create difficulty in getting or keeping a job. People with this disorder can experience emotional stress, particularly if vitiligo develops on visible areas of the body, such as the face, hands, arms, feet, or genitals. Adolescents, who are often particularly concerned about their appearance, can be devastated by widespread vitiligo. Some people who have vitiligo feel embarrassed, ashamed, depressed, or worried about how others will react.

Several strategies can help a person cope with vitiligo. First, it is important to find a doctor who is knowledgeable about vitiligo and takes the disorder seriously. The doctor should also be a good listener and be able to provide emotional support. Patients need to let their doctors know if they are feeling depressed because doctors and other mental health professionals can help people deal with depression. Patients should also learn as much as possible about the disorder and treatment choices so that they can participate in making important decisions about medical care.

Talking with other people who have vitiligo may also help a person cope. The National Vitiligo Foundation can provide information about vitiligo and refer people to local chapters that have support groups of patients, families, and physicians. Family and friends are another source of support.

Some people with vitiligo have found that cosmetics that cover the white patches improve their appearance and help them feel better about themselves. A person may need to experiment with several brands of concealing cosmetics before finding the product that works best.

What Treatment Options Are Available?

The goal of treating vitiligo is to restore the function of the skin and to improve the patient's appearance. Therapy for vitiligo takes a long time—it usually must be continued for 6 to 18 months. The choice of therapy depends on the number of white patches and how widespread they are and on the patient's preference for treatment. Each patient responds differently to therapy, and a particular treatment may not work for everyone. Current treatment options for vitiligo include medical, surgical, and adjunctive therapies (therapies that can be used along with surgical or medical treatments).

Medical Therapies

- Topical steroid therapy
- Topical psoralen photochemotherapy
- Oral psoralen photochemotherapy
- Depigmentation

Surgical Therapies

- Skin grafts from a person's own tissues (autologous)
- Skin grafts using blisters
- Micropigmentation (tattooing)
- Autologous melanocyte transplants

Adjunctive Therapies

- Sunscreens
- Cosmetics
- Counseling and support

Research

For more than a decade, research on how melanocytes play a role in vitiligo has greatly increased. This includes research on autologous melanocyte transplants. At the University of Colorado, NIAMS supports a large collaborative project involving families with vitiligo in the United States and the United Kingdom. Over 2,400 patients are involved. It is hoped that genetic analysis of these families will uncover the location—and possibly the specific gene or genes—conferring susceptibility to the disease. Doctors and researchers continue to look for the causes of and new treatments for vitiligo.

Part Six

Other Altered
Immune Responses

Chapter 65

Allergies and Asthma

Airborne Allergens

Sneezing is not always the symptom of a cold. Sometimes, it is an allergic reaction to something in the air. Health experts estimate that 35 million Americans suffer from upper respiratory tract symptoms that are allergic reactions to airborne allergens. Pollen allergy, commonly called hay fever, is one of the most common chronic diseases in the United States.

Worldwide, airborne allergens cause the most problems for people with allergies. The respiratory symptoms of asthma, which affect approximately 11 million Americans, are often provoked by airborne allergens. Overall, allergic diseases are among the major causes of illness and disability in the United States, affecting as many as 40 to 50 million Americans.

What is an allergy?

An allergy is a specific reaction of the body's immune system to a normally harmless substance, one that does not bother most people. People who have allergies often are sensitive to more than one

This chapter includes an excerpt from "Airborne Allergens," National Institute of Allergy and Infectious Diseases (NIAID), NIH Publication No. 03–7045, April 2003. Also, "Asthma Basics," NIAID, updated June 18, 2004. Text under the title "Asthma Statistics," is excerpted from "Morbidity and Mortality: 2004 Chart Book on Cardiovascular, Lung, and Blood Diseases," National Heart, Lung, and Blood Institute (NHLBI), May 2004.

substance. Types of allergens that cause allergic reactions include the following:

- Pollens
- House dust mites
- Mold spores
- Food
- Latex rubber
- Insect venom
- Medicines

Why are some people allergic?

Scientists think that some people inherit a tendency to be allergic from one or both parents. This means they are more likely to have allergies. They probably, however, do not inherit a tendency to be allergic to any specific allergen. Children are more likely to develop allergies if one or both parents have allergies. In addition, exposure to allergens at times when the body's defenses are lowered or weakened, such as after a viral infection or during pregnancy, seems to contribute to developing allergies.

What is an allergic reaction?

Normally, the immune system functions as the body's defense against invading germs such as bacteria and viruses. In most allergic reactions, however, the immune system is responding to a false alarm. When an allergic person first comes into contact with an allergen, the immune system treats the allergen as an invader and gets ready to attack.

The immune system does this by generating large amounts of a type of antibody called immunoglobulin E, or IgE. Each IgE antibody is specific for one particular substance. In the case of pollen allergy, each antibody is specific for one type of pollen. For example, the immune system may produce one type of antibody to react against oak pollen and another against ragweed pollen.

The IgE molecules are special because IgE is the only type of antibody that attaches tightly to the body's mast cells which are tissue cells, and to basophils which are blood cells. When the allergen next encounters its specific IgE, it attaches to the antibody like a key fitting into a lock. This action signals the cell to which the IgE is attached to release (and, in some cases, to produce) powerful chemicals like histamine, which cause inflammation. These chemicals act on tissues in various parts of the body, such as the respiratory system, and cause the symptoms of allergy.

What are the symptoms of airborne allergies?

- Sneezing, often with a runny or clogged nose
- Coughing and postnasal drip
- Itching eyes, nose, and throat
- Watering eyes
- Conjunctivitis
- Allergic shiners (dark circles under the eyes caused by increased blood flow near the sinuses)
- Allergic salute (in a child, persistent upward rubbing of the nose that causes a crease mark on the nose)

In people who are not allergic, the mucus in the nasal passages simply moves foreign particles to the throat, where they are swallowed or coughed out. But something different happens in a person who is sensitive to airborne allergens.

In sensitive people, as soon as the allergen lands on the lining inside the nose, a chain reaction occurs that leads the mast cells in these tissues to release histamine and other chemicals. The powerful chemicals contract certain cells that line some small blood vessels in the nose. This allows fluids to escape, which causes the nasal passages to swell—resulting in nasal congestion. Histamine also can cause sneezing, itching, irritation, and excess mucus production which can result in allergic rhinitis. Other chemicals released by mast cells, including cytokines and leukotrienes, also contribute to allergic symptoms.

Some people with allergy develop asthma, which can be a very serious condition. The symptoms of asthma include the following:

- Coughing
- Wheezing
- Shortness of breath

The shortness of breath is due to a narrowing of the airways in the lungs, excess mucus production, and inflammation. Asthma can be disabling and sometimes fatal. If wheezing and shortness of breath accompany allergy symptoms, it is a signal that the airways also have become involved.

Is it an allergy or a cold?

There is no good way to tell the difference between allergy symptoms and cold symptoms. Allergy symptoms, however, may last longer than cold symptoms. Anyone who has any respiratory illness that lasts longer than a week or two should consult a health care provider.

Asthma Basics

What is asthma?

In many people, asthma appears to be an allergic reaction to substances commonly breathed in through the air, such as animal dander, pollen, or dust mite and cockroach waste products. The catch-all name for these substances, allergens, refers to anything that provokes an allergic reaction. Some people have a genetic predisposition to react to certain allergens.

When these people breathe in the allergen, the immune system goes into high gear as if fighting off a harmful parasite. The system produces a molecule called immunoglobulin E (IgE), one of a class of defensive molecules termed antibodies. The IgE antibody is central to the allergic reaction. For example, it causes mast cells, a type of specialized defensive cell, to release chemical weapons into the airways. The airways then become inflamed and constricted, leading to coughing, wheezing, and difficulty breathing—an asthma attack. Without treatment, such as inhaled corticosteroids to reduce the inflammation, asthma attacks can be deadly. The overall death rate for asthma, however, is low.

Why is asthma on the rise?

Although several theories exist about why asthma rates have risen during the last two decades, there probably is no simple answer, says Calman Prussin, M.D., head of the clinical allergy and immunology unit at NIAID. One theory is that people today, especially in developed countries, are spending more time indoors, Dr. Prussin says. We are therefore exposed to more indoor allergens, such as dust mite allergen, that cause asthma. "Our houses are now hermetically sealed to save heating and cooling energy," he notes, "and unfortunately this causes more indoor allergen exposure."

Another reason may be that people today live in cleaner, more sanitary conditions than they did before the industrial revolution, relatively free of disease-causing viruses and bacteria, he says. This clean living affects our immune system. The immune system's defensive white blood cells, called T cells, have two basic settings, he explains. Helper T cells, type 1 (Th1) fight infectious viruses and bacteria. Helper T cells, type 2 (Th2) fight parasites, but are also involved in allergic reactions. "We are exposed to fewer viruses and bacteria than people were 100 years ago, so perhaps our immune systems have not learned to make Th1 cells as well," Dr. Prussin says. "That means we have a greater proportion of Th2 cells in our bodies, which might lead to more allergies and asthma." Other theories point to increased levels of air pollutants, a decline in the amount of exercise people get, or rising obesity as factors in the increase of asthma.

Asthma Statistics

- Between 1980 and the mid-1990s, the prevalence of asthma increased. From 1997 to 2002, asthma attack prevalence increased for persons under 18 and declined for persons 18 and over.[1]

- In 2002, asthma prevalence within racial groups was higher for females than for males 18 or older; for those under 18, it was higher for males than for females. Within sex groups, the prevalence was higher in blacks than in whites for each age group except for ages 65 and over, where it was higher in white than in black males.[1]

- In 2001, 11.3 million physician office visits in the U.S. were for asthma.[2]

- Hospitalizations with asthma as the primary diagnosis remained relatively stable between 1980 and 2002; hospitalizations with asthma as a secondary diagnosis, however, increased significantly from 1990 to 2002.[3]

References

1. National Heart, Lung, and Blood Institute. Unpublished tabulations of the *National Health Interview Survey*. National Center for Health Statistics.

2. National Heart, Lung, and Blood Institute. Unpublished tabulations of the *National Ambulatory Medical Care Survey*. National Center for Health Statistics.

3. National Center for Health Statistics. *National Hospital Discharge Survey: Vital and Health Statistics; series 13.* 1970–2004.

Chapter 66

Serum Sickness

Definition: Serum sickness is a group of symptoms caused by a delayed immune response to certain medications or antiserum (passive immunization with antibodies from an animal or another person).

Causes, Incidence, and Risk Factors

Serum is the clear fluid portion of blood. It does not contain blood cells, but it does contain many proteins, including antibodies, which are formed as part of the immune response to protect against infection.

Antiserum is a preparation of serum that has been removed from a person or animal that has already developed immunity to a particular microorganism. It contains antibodies against that microorganism.

An injection of antiserum (passive immunization) may be used when a person has been exposed to a potentially dangerous microorganism against which the person has not been immunized. It provides immediate, but temporary, protection while the person develops a personal immune response against the toxin or microorganism. Examples include antiserum for tetanus and rabies exposure.

Serum sickness is a hypersensitivity reaction similar to an allergy. The immune system misidentifies a protein in the antiserum as a potentially harmful substance (antigen), and it develops an immune response against the antiserum.

"Serum Sickness," © 2005 A.D.A.M. Inc. Reprinted with permission.

481

Antibodies bind with the antiserum protein to create larger particles (immune complexes). The immune complexes are deposited in various tissues, causing inflammation and various other symptoms.

Because it takes time for the body to produce antibodies to a new antigen, symptoms do not develop until 7 to 21 days after initial exposure to the antiserum. Patients may develop symptoms in 1 to 3 days if they have previously been exposed to the offending agent.

Exposure to certain medications (particularly penicillin) can cause a similar process. Unlike other drug allergies, which occur very soon after receiving the medication for the second (or subsequent) time, serum sickness can develop 7 to 21 days after the first exposure to a medication. Blood products may also induce serum sickness.

Serum sickness is different from anaphylactic shock, which is an immediate reaction with more severe symptoms.

Symptoms

- Skin rash
- Itching
- Hives
- Joint pain
- Fever
- Malaise
- Enlarged lymph nodes

Note: The symptoms develop 1 to 3 weeks after exposure to antiserum or medication.

Signs and Tests

The lymph nodes may be enlarged and tender to the touch. The urine may contain blood or protein. Blood tests may indicate vasculitis, or inflammation of the blood vessels.

Treatment

The goal of treatment is the relief of symptoms.

Topical corticosteroids or other soothing topical (applied to a localized area of the skin) medications may relieve discomfort from itching and rash. Antihistamines may shorten the duration of illness and help to relieve rash and itching.

Nonsteroidal anti-inflammatory drugs (NSAIDs) may relieve joint pain. Corticosteroids such as prednisone may be prescribed for severe cases.

Medications causing the problem should be stopped and future use of the medication or antiserum should be avoided.

Health care providers (such as dentists and hospital personnel) should be advised of drug allergies before treating the patient. Identifying jewelry or cards (such as Medic-Alert or others) may be advised.

Expectations (Prognosis)

The symptoms usually resolve within a few days. The antiserum or medication should be avoided in the future.

Complications

Increased risk of anaphylaxis for future exposures to the substance is a possible complication.

Calling Your Health Care Provider

Call your health care provider if medication or antiserum has been given within the last 2 weeks and symptoms of serum sickness appear.

Prevention

There is no known way to prevent the development of serum sickness. People who have experienced serum sickness, anaphylactic shock, or drug allergy should avoid future use of the antiserum or drug.

Chapter 67

Blood Transfusion Reaction

Definition: Transfusion reaction is a complication of blood transfusion where there is an immune response against the transfused blood cells or other components of the transfusion.

Causes, Incidence, and Risk Factors

The immune response normally protects the body from potentially harmful substances. These substances (antigens) trigger multiple responses, including production of antibodies (immunoglobulins, molecules that attach to a specific antigen and aid in its destruction), and sensitized lymphocytes that recognize a particular antigen and destroy it.

The immune system normally can distinguish its own blood cells from other cells. These foreign proteins (antigens) produce an immune response.

The surface of red blood cells contain several proteins that can be identified by the body as antigens. In 1900, the German pathologist, Karl Landsteiner, identified 2 of these antigenic proteins, which he called A and B.

Blood is classified according to the presence of these antigens, resulting in blood types A, B, AB (contains both antigens), and O (contains neither antigen). Blood plasma contains antibodies against the opposite antigen. A person with type A blood, for example, has antibodies against the B antigen.

In 1940, Dr. Landsteiner discovered another group of antigens. They were named Rhesus factors (Rh factors) because they were discovered during experiments on Rhesus monkeys.

People with Rhesus factors in their blood are classified as Rh positive, while persons without the factors are classified as Rh negative. Rh negative persons form antibodies against the Rh factor if they are exposed to Rh positive blood.

This is of major importance in an Rh negative mother who is pregnant with an Rh positive baby. There are other antigens as well, besides ABO and Rh antigens.

The presence of antibodies against blood antigens results in blood group compatibility or incompatibility. Transfusion of blood between compatible groups (such as O+ to O+) usually causes no problem. Blood transfusion between incompatible groups (such as A+ to O-) causes an immune response against the cells carrying the antigen, resulting in transfusion reaction.

The immune system attacks the donated blood cells, causing them to burst. This may cause serious symptoms, including kidney failure and shock. Antigens also occur on other blood components, including white blood cells, platelets, and plasma proteins.

These components also cause a similar type of transfusion reaction. Alternatively, antibodies in the transfused blood can bind the patient's own blood cells, also causing a reaction.

Today, all blood is carefully screened. Modern lab methods and redundant checks have helped make transfusion reactions extremely rare.

Symptoms

- Fever
- Chills
- Rash
- Flank pain or back pain
- Bloody urine
- Fainting or dizziness

Signs and Tests

Symptoms of transfusion reaction usually appear during or immediately after the transfusion. Occasionally, they may develop after several days (delayed reaction). Symptoms may remain mild or progress to kidney failure, delayed anemia, or shock.

This disease may also alter the results of the following tests:

- Red blood count (RBC)
- Hemoglobin; serum
- Hemoglobin
- Hematocrit
- Haptoglobin
- Fibrin degradation products
- Coombs test, indirect
- Coombs test, direct
- Complete blood count (CBC)
- Bilirubin

Treatment

The goal of treatment is to prevent or treat severe effects of transfusion reaction. If symptoms occur during the transfusion, the transfusion is stopped. Blood samples from the person receiving the transfusion (and from remaining donor blood) may be tested to confirm that symptoms are caused by transfusion reaction.

Mild symptoms may be treated according to the symptom. Antihistamines such as diphenhydramine may reduce itching and rash. Acetaminophen may be recommended to reduce fever and discomfort. Corticosteroids such as prednisone or dexamethasone may be given to reduce the immune response. Intravenous fluids and various medications may be used to treat/prevent kidney failure and shock.

Expectations (Prognosis)

The outcome varies depending on the severity of the reaction. The disorder may disappear completely and without problems. However, it may be severe and life-threatening.

Complications

- Discomfort
- Anemia
- Acute kidney failure
- Shock
- Lung disfunction

Calling Your Health Care Provider

Notify your health care provider if a blood transfusion is planned and previous transfusion reaction has occurred.

Prevention

Typing of donated blood into ABO and Rh groups has reduced the risk of transfusion reaction. Prior to a transfusion, blood is usually crossmatched to further confirm that the blood is compatible. A small amount of donor blood is mixed with a small amount of recipient blood and the mixture is examined under a microscope for signs of antibody reaction.

Chapter 68

Transplant Rejection

Alternative names: Graft rejection; tissue/organ rejection

Definition: Transplant rejection is when a transplant recipient's immune system attacks a transplanted organ or tissue.

Causes, Incidence, and Risk Factors

Your body's immune system protects you from potentially harmful substances, such as microorganisms, toxins, and cancer cells. These harmful substances have proteins called antigens on their surfaces. If your immune system identifies antigens that are foreign (not part of your body), it will attack the substance.

In the same way, foreign blood or tissue can trigger a blood transfusion reaction or transplant rejection. To help prevent this, tissue is typed before the transplant procedure to identify the antigens it contains.

Though tissue typing ensures that the organ or tissue is as similar as possible to the tissues of the recipient, the match is usually not perfect. No two people (except identical twins) have identical tissue antigens.

Immunosuppressive drugs are needed to prevent organ rejection. Otherwise, organ and tissue transplantation would almost always cause an immune response and result in destruction of the foreign tissue.

"Transplant Rejection," © 2005 A.D.A.M., Inc. Reprinted with permission.

There are some exceptions, however. Corneal transplants are rarely rejected because corneas have no blood supply—immune cells and antibodies do not reach the cornea to cause rejection. In addition, transplants from one identical twin to another are almost never rejected.

Symptoms

- The organ does not function properly
- General discomfort, uneasiness, or ill feeling
- Pain or swelling in the location of the organ (rare)
- Fever (rare)

The symptoms vary depending on the transplanted organ or tissue. For example, patients who reject a kidney may have less urine, and patients who reject a heart may have symptoms of heart failure.

Signs and Tests

The doctor will use his or her hands to feel over the organ, and this may feel tender to you (particularly with transplanted kidneys).

There are often signs that the organ is not functioning properly. For example:

- Less urine output with kidney transplants
- Yellow skin color and easy bleeding with liver transplants
- Shortness of breath and less tolerance to exertion with heart transplants

A biopsy of the transplanted organ can confirm that it is being rejected. A routine biopsy is often performed to detect rejection early, before symptoms develop.

When organ rejection is suspected, one or more of the following tests may be performed prior to organ biopsy:

- Lab tests of kidney or liver function
- Kidney ultrasound
- Kidney arteriography
- Abdominal CT scan
- Heart echocardiography
- Chest x-ray

Treatment

The goal of treatment is to make sure the transplanted organ or tissue functions properly, while at the same time suppressing the recipient's immune response. Suppressing the immune response can treat and prevent transplant rejection.

Many different drugs can be used to suppress the immune response. These include azathioprine, cyclosporine, corticosteroids (such as prednisone), and Ortho-Kung T cell (OKT2) monoclonal antibodies. OKT2 monoclonal antibodies specifically reduce the activity of T lymphocytes, which are the main immune system cells responsible for transplant rejection.

The dosage of the medication depends on the patient's status. The dose may be very high while the tissue is actually being rejected, and then reduced to a lower level to prevent it from happening again.

Expectations (Prognosis)

Some organs and tissues are more successfully transplanted than others. If rejection begins, immunosuppressive drugs may stop the rejection. The person must take immunosuppressive drugs for the rest of his or her life. However, immunosuppressive treatment is not always successful.

Complications

- Loss of function of the transplanted organ/tissue
- Infections (because the person's immune system is constantly suppressed)
- Side effects of medications, which may be severe

Calling Your Health Care Provider

Call your health care provider if the transplanted organ or tissue does not seem to be working properly or if other symptoms occur. Also, call your health care provider if medication side effects develop.

Prevention

ABO blood typing and human leukocyte antigens (HLA) tissue antigen typing before transplantation helps to ensure a close match. Suppressing the immune system is usually necessary for the rest of the transplant recipient's life to prevent the tissue from being rejected in the future.

Chapter 69

Anaphylaxis

Alternative names: Anaphylactic reaction; anaphylactic shock; shock—anaphylactic

Definition: Anaphylaxis is a life-threatening type of allergic reaction.

Causes, Incidence, and Risk Factors

Anaphylaxis is a severe, whole-body allergic reaction. After an initial exposure to a substance like bee sting toxin, the person's immune system becomes sensitized to that allergen. On a subsequent exposure, an allergic reaction occurs. This reaction is sudden, severe, and involves the whole body.

Tissues in different parts of the body release histamine and other substances. This causes constriction of the airways, resulting in wheezing, difficulty breathing, and gastrointestinal symptoms such as abdominal pain, cramps, vomiting, and diarrhea.

Histamine causes the blood vessels to dilate (which lowers blood pressure) and fluid to leak from the bloodstream into the tissues (which lowers the blood volume). These effects result in shock. Fluid can leak into the alveoli (air sacs) of the lungs, causing pulmonary edema.

Hives and angioedema (hives on the lips, eyelids, throat, and/or tongue) often occur. Angioedema may be severe enough to block the airway. Prolonged anaphylaxis can cause heart arrhythmias.

Some drugs (polymyxin, morphine, x-ray dye, and others) may cause an anaphylactoid reaction (anaphylactic-like reaction) on the first exposure. This is usually due to a toxic reaction, rather than the immune system mechanism that occurs with true anaphylaxis. The symptoms, risk for complications without treatment, and treatment are the same, however, for both types of reactions.

Anaphylaxis can occur in response to any allergen. Common causes include insect bites/stings, horse serum (used in some vaccines), food allergies, and drug allergies. Pollens and other inhaled allergens rarely cause anaphylaxis. Some people have an anaphylactic reaction with no identifiable cause.

Anaphylaxis occurs infrequently. However, it is life-threatening and can occur at any time. Risks include prior history of any type of allergic reaction.

Symptoms

Symptoms develop rapidly, often within seconds or minutes. They may include the following:

- Difficulty breathing
- Wheezing
- Abnormal (high-pitched) breathing sounds
- Confusion
- Slurred speech
- Rapid or weak pulse
- Blueness of the skin (cyanosis), including the lips or nail beds
- Fainting, light-headedness, dizziness
- Hives and generalized itching
- Anxiety
- Sensation of feeling the heart beat (palpitations)
- Nausea, vomiting
- Diarrhea
- Abdominal pain or cramping
- Skin redness
- Nasal congestion
- Cough

Signs and Tests

Examination of the skin may show hives and swelling of the eyes or face. The skin may be blue from lack of oxygen or may be pale from shock. Angioedema in the throat may be severe enough to block the airway.

Listening to the lungs with a stethoscope may reveal wheezing or indicate fluid (pulmonary edema). The pulse is rapid, and blood pressure may be low. Weakness, pale skin, heart arrhythmias, mental confusion, and other signs may indicate shock.

Testing for the specific allergen that caused anaphylaxis (if the cause is not obvious) is postponed until after treatment.

Treatment

Anaphylaxis is an emergency condition requiring immediate professional medical attention. Assessment of the ABC's (airway, breathing, and circulation) should be done in all suspected anaphylactic reactions.

Cardiopulmonary resuscitation (CPR) should be initiated if needed. People with known severe allergic reactions may carry an Epi-Pen or other allergy kit, and should be assisted if necessary. Emergency interventions by paramedics or physicians may include placing a tube through the nose or mouth into the airway (endotracheal intubation) or emergency surgery to place a tube directly into the trachea (tracheostomy or cricothyrotomy).

Epinephrine should be given by injection without delay. This opens the airways and raises the blood pressure by constricting blood vessels.

Treatment for shock includes intravenous fluids and medications that support the actions of the heart and circulatory system.

Antihistamines, such as diphenhydramine; and corticosteroids, such as prednisone may be given to further reduce symptoms (after lifesaving measures and epinephrine are administered).

Expectations (Prognosis)

Anaphylaxis is a severe disorder which has a poor prognosis without prompt treatment. Symptoms, however, usually resolve with appropriate therapy, underscoring the importance of action.

Complications

- Shock

- Cardiac arrest (no effective heartbeat)
- Respiratory arrest (absence of breathing)
- Airway obstruction

Calling Your Health Care Provider

Go to the emergency room or call the local emergency number (such as 911) if severe symptoms of anaphylaxis develop.

Prevention

Avoid known allergens. Any person experiencing an allergic reaction should be monitored, although monitoring may be done at home in mild cases.

Occasionally, people who have a history of drug allergies may safely be given the offending medication after pretreatment with corticosteroids (prednisone) and antihistamines (diphenhydramine).

People who have a history of allergy to insect bites/stings should be instructed to carry (and use) an emergency kit consisting of injectable epinephrine and chewable antihistamine. They should also wear a Medic-Alert or similar bracelet/necklace stating their allergy.

Part Seven

Treatments for Immune Deficiencies and Diseases

Chapter 70

Immune Globulin Intravenous Injection

Important Warning

Immune globulin intravenous (IGIV) may cause kidney failure. Tell your doctor if you are over 65 years old or if you have or have ever had kidney disease, diabetes, sepsis, plasma cell disease, or volume depletion. Tell your doctor if you are taking amikacin (Amikin), gentamicin (Jenamicin), streptomycin, or other medications that can cause kidney damage. Keep all appointments with your doctor and the laboratory. Your doctor will order certain lab tests to check your response to IGIV. If you experience any of the following symptoms, call your doctor immediately: decreased urination, sudden weight gain, swelling of the legs or ankles, or shortness of breath.

Treatment

Your doctor has ordered IGIV. The drug may be given alone or added to an intravenous fluid that will drip through a needle or catheter placed in your vein for 2–4 hours, once a day for 2–7 days. You will receive another single dose every 10–21 days or every 3–4 weeks, depending on your condition.

"Immune Globulin Intravenous Injection," Medmaster, American Society of Health-System Pharmacists, Bethesda, MD; © 1998, Revised 2003. Reprinted with permission.

IGIV boosts the body's natural response in patients with compromised immune systems [e.g., patients with human immunodeficiency virus (HIV) and premature babies]. It also increases the number of platelets (part of the blood) in patients with idiopathic thrombocytopenic purpura. This medication is sometimes prescribed for other uses; ask your doctor or pharmacist for more information.

Your health care provider (doctor, nurse, or pharmacist) may measure the effectiveness and side effects of your treatment using laboratory tests and physical examinations. It is important to keep all appointments with your doctor and the laboratory. The length of treatment depends on how you respond to the medication.

Precautions

Before administering IGIV:

- Tell your doctor and pharmacist if you are allergic to any drugs.

- Tell your doctor and pharmacist what prescription and non-prescription medications you are taking, especially those listed in the "important warning" section, antibiotics, and vitamins.

- Tell your doctor if you are pregnant, plan to become pregnant, or are breast feeding. If you become pregnant while taking IGIV, call your doctor.

- Tell your doctor if you had a vaccine for measles, mumps, or rubella in the last 3 months.

Administering Your Medication

Before you administer IGIV, look at the solution closely. It should be clear and free of floating material. Gently squeeze the bag or observe the solution container to make sure there are no leaks. Do not use the solution if it is discolored, if it contains particles, or if the bag or container leaks. Use a new solution, but show the damaged one to your health care provider.

It is important that you use your medication exactly as directed. Do not change your dosing schedule without talking to your health care provider. Your health care provider may tell you to stop your infusion if you have a mechanical problem (such as a blockage in the tubing, needle, or catheter); if you have to stop an infusion, call your health care provider immediately so your therapy can continue.

Side Effects

Although side effects from IGIV are not common, they can occur. Tell your health care provider if any of these symptoms are severe or do not go away:

- backache
- headache
- joint or muscle pain
- general feeling of discomfort
- leg cramps
- rash
- pain at the injection site

If you experience any of the following symptoms or those listed in the "important warning" section, call your health care provider immediately:

- hives
- chest tightness
- dizziness
- unusual tiredness or weakness
- chills
- fever
- sweating
- redness of the face
- upset stomach
- vomiting

Storing Your Medication

- Your health care provider probably will give you a 1-day supply of IGIV at a time. Depending on the product you receive, you may be told to store it in the refrigerator.

- If you store IGIV in the refrigerator, take your next dose from the refrigerator 1 hour before using it; place it in a clean, dry area to allow it to warm to room temperature.

- Do not allow IGIV to freeze.

Your health care provider may provide you with directions on how to prepare each dose.

Store your medication only as directed. Make sure you understand what you need to store your medication properly.

Keep your supplies in a clean, dry place when you are not using them, and keep all medications and supplies out of reach of children. Your health care provider will tell you how to throw away used needles, syringes, tubing, and containers to avoid accidental injury.

Signs of Infection

If you are receiving IGIV in your vein or under your skin, you need to know the symptoms of a catheter-related infection (an infection where the needle enters your vein or skin). If you experience any of these effects near your intravenous catheter, tell your health care provider as soon as possible:

- tenderness
- warmth
- irritation
- drainage
- redness
- swelling
- pain

Chapter 71

Plasmapheresis for Autoimmune Disease

Many diseases, including myasthenia gravis, Lambert-Eaton syndrome, Guillain-Barré syndrome and others, are caused by a so-called autoimmune, or self-immune, process. In autoimmune conditions, the body's immune system mistakenly turns against itself, attacking its own tissues. Some of the specialized cells involved in this process can attack tissues directly, while others can produce substances known as antibodies that circulate in the blood and carry out the attack. Antibodies produced against the body's own tissues are known as autoantibodies.

Treatment with medications that suppress the activities of the immune system and/or reduce inflammation of tissues has been the most common approach to autoimmune disease for more than 30 years. Many new immunosuppressants have become available since the 1960s, but all the medications used to treat autoimmune disease have serious side effects when taken in high doses for months or years.

In the 1970s, with the support of the Muscular Dystrophy Association, researchers developed a new approach to the treatment of autoimmune conditions. Instead of trying to change the immune system

Reprinted from "Facts About Plasmapheresis" with permission of the Muscular Dystrophy Association, www.mdausa.org. © 1999 The Muscular Dystrophy Association. For additional information, call the Muscular Dystrophy Association National Headquarters toll-free at 800-572-1717. To find an MDA office in your area, look in your local telephone book, or click on "Clinics and Services" on the MDA website. Reviewed in February 2005 by Dr. David A. Cooke, M.D., Diplomate, American Board of Internal Medicine.

with medication alone, they thought that it might be possible to mechanically remove autoantibodies from the bloodstream in a process similar to that used in an artificial kidney, or dialysis, treatment. The procedure became known as plasmapheresis, meaning plasma separation. It is also known as plasma exchange.

Medications that suppress the immune system or reduce inflammation are often combined with plasmapheresis, but they can usually be given in lower doses than when used alone.

Today, plasmapheresis is widely accepted for the treatment of myasthenia gravis, Lambert-Eaton syndrome, Guillain-Barré syndrome and chronic demyelinating polyneuropathy. Its effectiveness in other conditions, such as multiple sclerosis, polymyositis, and dermatomyositis, is not as well established.

What is plasmapheresis?

Plasmapheresis is a process in which the fluid part of the blood, called plasma, is removed from blood cells by a device known as a cell separator. The separator works either by spinning the blood at high speed to separate the cells from the fluid, or by passing the blood through a membrane with pores so small that only the fluid part of the blood can pass through. The cells are returned to the person undergoing treatment, while the plasma which contains the antibodies, is discarded and replaced with other fluids. Medication to keep the blood from clotting (an anticoagulant) is given through a vein during the procedure.

What's involved in a plasmapheresis treatment?

A plasmapheresis treatment takes several hours and can be done on an outpatient basis. It can be uncomfortable, but normally is not painful. The number of treatments needed varies greatly depending on the particular disease and the person's general condition. An average course of plasma exchanges is six to ten treatments over two to ten weeks. In some centers, treatments are performed once a week, while in others, more than one weekly treatment is done.

A person undergoing plasmapheresis can lie in bed or sit in a reclining chair. A small, thin tube (catheter) is placed in a large vein, usually the one in the crook of the arm, and another tube is placed in the opposite hand or foot (so that at least one arm can move freely during the procedure). Blood is taken to the separator from one tube, while the separated blood cells, combined with replacement fluids, are returned to the patient through the other tube.

The amount of blood outside the body at any one time is much less than the amount ordinarily donated in a blood bank. The procedure takes several hours and can be uncomfortable, although it normally is not painful.

Are there risks associated with plasmapheresis?

Yes, but most can be controlled. Any unusual symptoms should be immediately reported to the doctor or the person in charge of the procedure. Symptoms that may seem trivial sometimes herald the onset of a serious complication.

The most common problem is a drop in blood pressure, which can be experienced as faintness, dizziness, blurred vision, coldness, sweating, or abdominal cramps. A drop in blood pressure is remedied by lowering the patient's head, raising the legs, and giving intravenous fluid.

Bleeding can occasionally occur because of the medications used to keep the blood from clotting during the procedure. Some of these medications can cause other adverse reactions, which begin with tingling around the mouth or in the limbs, muscle cramps, or a metallic taste in the mouth. If allowed to progress, these reactions can lead to an irregular heartbeat or seizures.

An allergic reaction to the solutions used to replace the plasma or to the sterilizing agents used for the tubing can be a true emergency. This type of reaction usually begins with itching, wheezing, or a rash. The plasma exchange must be stopped and the person treated with intravenous medications.

Excessive suppression of the immune system can temporarily occur with plasmapheresis, since the procedure is not selective about which antibodies it removes. In time, the body can replenish its supply of needed antibodies, but some physicians give these intravenously after each plasmapheresis treatment. Outpatients may have to take special precautions against infection.

Medication dosages need careful observation and adjustment in people being treated with plasmapheresis because some drugs can be removed from the blood or changed by the procedure.

How long does it take to see improvement?

Improvement can sometimes occur within days, especially in myasthenia gravis. In other conditions, especially where there is extensive tissue damage, improvement is slower, but can still occur within weeks.

Does MDA pay for plasmapheresis?

MDA supported pioneering research to develop plasmapheresis. However, payment for this procedure is not among the many services included in MDA's program. A number of health insurance plans do cover the procedure.

Where are plasmapheresis treatments offered?

Plasmapheresis is performed at many major medical centers across the country. MDA clinic directors can offer advice about the availability of this treatment and its use for specific conditions.

Additional Information

Muscular Dystrophy Association
3300 E. Sunrise Drive
Tucson, AZ 85718
Toll-Free: 800-572-1717
Website: http://www.mdausa.org
E-mail: mda@mdausa.org

Chapter 72

Gene Therapy

On September 14, 1990, a 4-year-old girl named Ashanthi DeSilva from the suburbs of Cleveland lay on crisp white hospital sheets with a needle stuck in a vein. She did not mind; this happened all the time in her chronically sick childhood. At the other end of the intravenous hookup hung a clear plastic bag of very special cells: her own white blood cells, genetically altered to fix a defect she inherited at birth.

A strikingly thin middle-aged doctor stared anxiously at the tiny figure. W. French Anderson, M.D., and his colleagues R. Michael Blaese, M.D., and Kenneth Culver, M.D., all then working at the National Institutes of Health (NIH), crossed a symbolic threshold with Ashanthi DeSilva that day, becoming the first group to begin a clinical trial in the new frontier of medical treatment: human gene therapy.

The reason for the excitement was simple: Most diseases have a genetic component and gene therapy holds the hope of curing, not merely treating, a broad range of ailments, including inherited diseases like cystic fibrosis and even chronic conditions like cancer and infectious diseases like acquired immunodeficiency syndrome (AIDS).

Ten years from that first genetic treatment on Sept. 14, 1990, the hyperbole exceeded the results. Worldwide, researchers launched more than 400 clinical trials to test gene therapy against a wide array of

Excerpted from "Human Gene Therapy—Harsh Lessons, High Hopes," *FDA Consumer* September-October 2000, U.S. Food and Drug Administration (FDA). Reviewed in February 2005 by Dr. David A. Cooke, M.D., Diplomate, American Board of Internal Medicine.

illnesses. Surprisingly, cancer dominated the research. Even more surprising, little has worked.

"There was initially a great burst of enthusiasm that lasted three, four years where a couple of hundred trials got started all over the world," says Anderson, now at the University of Southern California in Los Angeles. "Then we came to realize that nothing was really working at the clinical level."

Abbey S. Meyers, president of the National Organization for Rare Disorders, Inc., an umbrella organization of patients' groups, is much more blunt. "We haven't even taken one baby step beyond that first clinical experiment," Meyers says. "It has hardly gotten anywhere. Over the last 10 years, I have been very disappointed."

A History of Special Concern

When scientists first learned to clone genes in the mid-1970s, public reaction ranged from antipathy to hostility. Opponents, fearing that genetically engineered bacteria might escape from a laboratory, shut down the research at Harvard University and the Massachusetts Institute of Technology for months. Twenty-five years ago, in response to public concern, American scientists organized a voluntary moratorium on certain types of gene engineering experiments until safety questions could be resolved.

To help assuage public concern, NIH created its Recombinant DNA Advisory Committee, the RAC—which most simply call the rack—to provide a forum for genetic engineering debates to take place in public. As a result, the general opposition subsided.

But the RAC could do little if scientists did not follow the rules. The promise of gene therapy, the glory of being the first to cure human ills, led at least one very smart scientist to make a very questionable decision. In 1980, an ambitious hematologist at the University of California at Los Angeles tested his gene therapy ideas on patients in Israel and Italy after being denied permission to perform the tests in Los Angeles. The experiments, conducted by Martin Cline, M.D., failed to help his subjects, and they violated federal rules designed to protect research subjects, leading to severe censure of the California scientist.

Ethical issues aside, the bigger problem for gene therapy has been basic biology. It is difficult to get new genes into billions of target cells within the body. Once inserted, the new genes need to function. Frequently, the body suppresses gene expression, essentially turning the new genes off, or destroys the transplanted genes. Although techniques have improved, today's scientists still face these challenges. To solve the problems, independent researchers have sometimes devised their own remedies of unknown safety. FDA began paying careful attention to these laboratory constructs when researchers began to request permission to test them in people under Investigational New Drug applications.

"Early investigators were more mom and pop operations," Noguchi says. "They were individual investigators making their own products...Almost all of them went on clinical hold because there was a lack of product information." Before FDA could allow them to proceed, technical questions about safety had to be answered, and that took time.

Typically, scientific questions are answered in laboratory and animal studies, but, with gene therapy, clinicians have been anxious to test their ideas in people. Once the NIH physicians treated their tiny patient in 1990, researchers rushed to get into the game with human trials. At the halfway point in the decade, the field was not progressing well. Then-NIH Director Harold Varmus, M.D., himself critical of the gene therapy trials in people, created a committee to review NIH's investment in the field. Varmus wanted to know whether NIH should continue to invest so heavily in the new technology.

The committee's conclusions were bleak: "While the expectations and the promise of gene therapy are great, clinical efficacy has not been definitively demonstrated at this time in any gene therapy protocol, despite anecdotal claims of successful therapy and the initiation of more than 100 ... approved protocols," concluded the ad hoc committee co-chairmen Stuart H. Orkin, M.D., of Harvard Medical School and Arno G. Motulsky, M.D., of the University of Washington in Seattle in December 1995. While they saw promise, they also saw challenges. "Significant problems remain in all basic aspects of gene therapy. Major difficulties at the basic level include shortcomings in all current gene transfer vectors, and an inadequate understanding of the biological interaction of these vectors with the host."

To transfer a repair gene into a patient, the researchers must go through several steps. First, they must isolate the disease-related gene. Then it must be packaged in a vector, usually a disabled virus that cannot reproduce and cause disease, but that can act like a delivery truck to transport the gene inside the patient's cells. Once inside the body's cells, the new gene can begin to function and restore health.

But building an effective delivery truck has not been easy. Scientists started by using a type of mouse virus as a vector—engineered so that it cannot replicate itself—that could easily infect human cells and integrate the new genes into the cell's chromosomes (structures in the cell that hold the genes). These mouse vectors, however, only infect dividing cells, so researchers switched to adenovirus, a type of human virus that causes the common cold. Because the adenovirus' own genes to self-reproduce have been removed, the remaining viral container is unable to cause an illness. At least, that is the idea.

The Gelsinger Case

When Orkin and Motulsky reported on the technical limitations of gene transfer techniques in 1995, they virtually predicted problems in the clinic. During that same December meeting at which Orkin and Motulsky made their disheartening report, the RAC approved the University of Pennsylvania gene therapy trial for ornithine transcarboxylase deficiency (OTCD). FDA, also allowed the study to proceed.

The treatment idea was fairly straightforward. OTCD occurs when a baby inherits a broken gene that prevents the liver from making an enzyme needed to break down ammonia. With the OTCD gene isolated, the University of Pennsylvania researchers packaged it in a replication-defective adenovirus. To reach the target cells in the liver, the Philadelphia scientists wanted to inject the adenovirus directly into the hepatic artery that leads to that organ. Some members of the NIH RAC objected, fearing that direct delivery to the liver was dangerous. Nonetheless, after a vigorous public discussion with the University of Pennsylvania researchers, the RAC voted for approval of the study.

At age 18, Jesse Gelsinger was in good health, but was not truly a healthy teenager. He had a rare form of OTCD that appeared not to be linked to his parents, but the genetic defect arose spontaneously in his body after birth. During his youth, he had many episodes of hospitalization, including an incident just a year before the OTCD trial in which he nearly died from a coma induced by liver failure. But, a strict diet that allowed only a few grams of protein per day and a pile of pills controlled his disease to the point where he appeared to be a normally active teenager. With the encouragement of his father, Paul Gelsinger, Jesse volunteered for the study, and when he was initially evaluated, his medical condition qualified him to participate.

Gelsinger received the experimental treatment in September 1999. Four days later, he was dead. No one is really sure exactly why the gene therapy treatment caused his death, but it appears that his immune system launched a raging attack on the adenovirus carrier. Then an overwhelming cascade of organ failures occurred, starting with jaundice, and progressing to a blood-clotting disorder, kidney failure, lung failure, and ultimately brain death.

In its investigation, FDA found a series of serious deficiencies in the way that the University of Pennsylvania conducted the OTCD gene therapy trial, some more serious than others. For example, researchers entered Gelsinger into the trial as a substitute for another volunteer who dropped out, but Gelsinger's high ammonia levels at the time of the treatment should have excluded him from the study. Moreover, the university failed to immediately report that two patients had experienced serious side effects from the gene therapy, as required in the study design, and the deaths of monkeys given a similar treatment were never included in the informed consent discussion.

Signs of Progress

Not all the news about gene therapy is bad. It is true that dramatic cures have not been seen to date, but there are tantalizing signs that important advances may be just around the corner.

Ashanthi DeSilva, the girl who received the first credible gene therapy, continues to do well a decade later. She suffered a type of inherited immune disorder called severe combined immune deficiency, or SCID (pronounced skid), that left her susceptible to every passing microorganism. Without gene therapy, DeSilva would be living like David, the "Boy in the Bubble," who had a similar disorder. Instead, the NIH researchers inserted a normal copy of the broken gene into some of her white blood cells, healing them, helping them function normally to restore her immune system. Cynthia Cutshall, the second child to receive gene therapy for the same disorder as DeSilva, also continues to do well.

Scientists, however, have discounted the benefit of the first gene therapies because the girls began receiving a new drug treatment that replaces the missing enzyme just before receiving the genetic therapy. And they continue to receive the drug after the genetic treatment, though gene therapy pioneer Anderson argues that since the drug dose has remained the same while their bodies have grown substantially over the decade, it makes a negligible contribution to their well being.

In April, French scientists reported convincing evidence that they successfully treated a different form of SCID (X-linked severe combined immune deficiency, the type suffered by the boy in the bubble) with gene therapy. Four of the first five babies treated by Alain Fischer,

511

M.D., of the Necker children's hospital in Paris have had "a complete or near complete recovery" of their immune systems after the treatment.

Meanwhile, researchers at Children's Hospital of Philadelphia, Stanford University, and Avigen, Inc., a biotech company in Alameda, California, have reported promising results in hemophilia B patients. The team packaged a gene for factor IX, a blood clotting protein, in a defective adeno-associated virus (AAV). They then used the AAV to insert the gene into patients who suffered abnormal blood clotting because they lack factor IX. Normally, these hemophilia patients needed to inject factor IX to prevent uncontrolled bleeding. In June, the researchers reported treating six patients with the factor IX gene therapy. Even though the dose of the gene therapy was so low that no one expected it to help, it reduced the number of injections of factor IX that these patients used on an ad hoc basis.

"The hemophilia studies are looking promising," says FDA's Noguchi, "but will need further study to know whether it is an effective product."

These two studies suggest the power of genetic treatments.

"We do seem to have turned the corner," says Anderson, "and there are a number of clinical trials that are starting to show success."

Even as FDA increases its scrutiny of the field to ensure patient safety, there is a sense of advancement. "There is good progress being made," Noguchi says. "FDA thinks that gene therapy will work, but we don't know for which disease. The recent events in France show that if you have the right disease, and can insert the right gene, you can obtain good results."

—*Larry Thompson, editor of* FDA Consumer.

Chapter 73

Growing a New Immune System: Stem Cell Transplantation

On the Cutting Edge

When the immune system goes awry and starts to destroy the body it was designed to protect, sometimes the only way to stop its damage is to get a new immune system. Researchers have discovered that a procedure called autologous stem cell transplantation allows people with the most severe and treatment-resistant autoimmune diseases to start growing a healthy new immune system within just a couple of weeks.

As the name suggests, autologous (meaning self) stem cell transplantation, involves transplanting one's own stem cells back into one's own body. Found in the bloodstream and bone marrow, stem cells are primitive, immature cells that have the potential to grow into different types of cells that exist in the various systems of our bodies.

To perform an autologous stem cell transplant, a doctor first removes some of the patient's blood—and occasionally bone marrow— then separates and removes the stem cells, reserving them for later

Excerpted from "On the Cutting Edge," © 2003, reprinted with permission of the Arthritis Foundation and *Arthritis Today*, 1330 W. Peachtree St., Suite 100, Atlanta, GA 30309. To order a free copy of other titles by the Arthritis Foundation, call 800-283-7800 or visit www.arthritis.org. Also, "Rebooting: A Promise for Autoimmune Diseases?" by Robert A. Brodsky, M.D., Johns Hopkins University School of Medicine, *InFocus* Newsletter, January 1995. Copyright © 1995 American Autoimmune Related Diseases Association, Inc. Reprinted with permission. Reviewed in February 2005 by Dr. David A. Cooke, M.D., Diplomate, American Board of Internal Medicine.

use. Meanwhile, the patient receives high doses of the strong immunosuppressive drug cyclophosphamide, which destroys the faulty immune system.

Later, the preserved stem cells are infused back into the bloodstream, where they start to form a new immune system, usually in about 10 days. Within one year, a person could potentially have a healthy new immune system—one that does not attack its own tissue, says Ann Traynor, M.D., of Northwestern University Medical Center's Robert H. Lurie Comprehensive Cancer Center in Chicago. Although the procedure is still too new to tell, the hope is that autoimmune diseases like lupus will not redevelop at all—or at least not for many years, she says.

At press time, 25 people in the United States had undergone stem cell transplants for lupus. Twenty-four children with juvenile rheumatoid arthritis have had the procedure. The majority of stem cell transplant patients are doing well; however, four of the children and two of the lupus patients died due to complications of the procedure. In people with lupus, autologous stem cell transplantation may be a promising way to permanently correct the immune system and produce long-term remissions.

The risk of complications—including serious infection, bleeding, blood clots and the failure of the new immune system to take hold—is a major downside of stem cell transplants. For that reason, doctors currently reserve it for people with the most severe disease that has not responded to any other treatment. For those people, the procedure offers some hope in a situation where there once was little hope.

Rebooting: A Promise for Autoimmune Diseases?

Editor's Note: The therapy described in this section is considered to be experimental, and is not standard therapy.

Johns Hopkins University researchers have developed a new technique in treating autoimmune disease patients which reboots the immune system with results that have cured some patients while dramatically improving the health of others. This is a new approach to the use of stem cells in treating autoimmune disease.

Autoimmunity occurs when the blood's lymphocytes, which are designed to defend the body against infections and foreign agents, actually attack one or more of the body's organs. Researchers in the past have focused on ways to destroy the disease-causing lymphocytes and replace them with normal ones. That attempt has not been successful.

Bone marrow transplantation is now being used by many medical institutions worldwide. One attempt to get rid of the misdirected lymphocytes has been the use of high doses of cyclophosphamide, a chemotherapeutic drug. This method also calls for a blood stem cell transplant since it has been thought, incorrectly, that cyclophosphamide in high doses is destructive to the bone marrow's ability to make new blood cells.

Stem cells, present in both bone marrow and blood, regenerate marrow and blood after chemotherapy. In stem cell transplants, stem cells are harvested before chemotherapy by drawing some of the patient's own blood or bone marrow. After the chemotherapy, the blood or marrow stem cells are returned to the patient's body. However, patients who do go into remission after the procedure usually relapse after a time. This is thought to be the result of the "bad" lymphocytes returning to the patient along with the stem cells. How can pure stem cells be isolated from other blood cells?

Now Johns Hopkins researchers have found a way to circumvent the problem.

According to Robert A. Brodsky, M.D., assistant professor in oncology and medicine at the Johns Hopkins University School of Medicine, "...stem cells contain an enzyme, called aldehyde dehydrogenase, which detoxifies cyclophosphamide. Like most blood cells, lymphocytes have very low levels of this enzyme, so cyclophosphamide destroys them but not the stem cells. That means it is not necessary to do a transplant to preserve the stem cells." He further states, "Studies have shown that after chemotherapy—as the stem cells turn into the specialized blood cells that have been destroyed—those that become lymphocytes are normal and do not attack the body. The immune system has been repaired."

This system was first tried with aplastic anemia patients. Seven out of the first ten patients treated by this method have remained disease-free for 10 years—and, in some cases, more than 20 years. The system was later tried with 27 other patients with autoimmune diseases, the majority of whom were lupus patients. Dr. Brodsky reports, "Most are still in remission, and some are off medications two and three years later." He continues, "All the patients we've studied have, at the very worst, remained stable: Virtually all have had major reductions in their immunosuppression medications." Dr. Brodsky cautions that, before this can be called a cure, the patients must remain disease-free for ten or more years.

Dr. Brodsky offers the comment that "When we have more information about the long-term effects of this treatment, and as more physicians and patients learn about it, the technique could well become standard protocol for autoimmune conditions soon after they are diagnosed and well before the diseases progress or become debilitating."

Excerpted from Johns Hopkins "Health Insider," interview with Robert A. Brodsky, M.D., Johns Hopkins University School of Medicine.

Chapter 74

Primary Immune Deficiency Treatments

Treatment for Primary Immune Deficiency (PID)

Treating PID involves not only curing infections, but also correcting the underlying immunodeficiency. In addition, any associated conditions, such as autoimmune disorders or cancer, need special attention.

Treating Infections

The first goal of treatment is to clear up any current infection. Doctors can prescribe a wide range of infection-fighting antimicrobials. Some are broad-spectrum antibiotics that combat a range of germs. Others zero in on specific germs.

When an infection fails to respond to standard medications, the patient may need to be hospitalized to be treated with antibiotics and other drugs intravenously. For chronic infections, a variety of medicines can help relieve symptoms and prevent complications. These may include drugs like aspirin or ibuprofen to ease fever and general body aches; decongestants to shrink swollen membranes in the nose, sinuses, or throat; and expectorants to thin mucus secretions in the airways.

Excerpted from "Primary Immunodeficiency," National Institute of Child Health and Human Development (NICHD), June 1999. Reviewed in February 2005 by Dr. David A. Cooke, M.D., Diplomate, American Board of Internal Medicine.

People who have chronic respiratory infections may be made more comfortable with a technique known as postural drainage (or bronchial drainage). Developed for persons with cystic fibrosis, postural drainage uses gravity along with light blows to the chest wall to help clear secretions from the lungs.

Bone Marrow Transplantation (BMT)

In bone marrow transplantation (BMT), bone marrow is taken from a healthy person and transferred to the patient. Because bone marrow is the source of all blood cells, including infection-fighting white blood cells, a successful bone marrow transplant amounts to getting a new, working immune system.

BMT usually takes place in the hospital. The donor is put to sleep with a light general anesthesia, and bone marrow is removed through a large needle inserted into the pelvic bone in the lower back. A small amount of marrow is removed from each of several sites.

The bone marrow may be treated to remove mature T cells which could attack the recipient's tissues. It is then given to the patient like an ordinary blood transfusion. Marrow cells travel to the patient's own marrow spaces, inside the bones. There they begin making a complete assortment of healthy blood cells.

Preventing Infections

When the immune defenses are weak, it is essential to avoid germs. Precautions range from common sense practices like good hygiene (using mild soaps to keep the skin clean and brushing teeth twice a day) and good nutrition, to elaborate measures to prevent all contact with infectious agents.

Anyone with an immunodeficiency needs to avoid unnecessary exposure to infectious agents. This means staying away from people with colds or other infections and avoiding large crowds. (On the other hand, it is important not to become overly cautious. Children are encouraged to attend school, to play in small groups, and to participate in sports.)

Antibiotics are important for preventing or controlling infections. If infections threaten to become chronic, the doctor may prescribe continuous long-term, low-dose antibiotics. Such preventive, or prophylactic, therapy may help prevent hearing loss or permanent breathing problems.

When *Pneumocystis* pneumonia is a danger—for instance, in children with a profound T cell deficiency—an appropriate prophylactic

518

treatment may consist of a combination of two drugs, trimethoprim and sulfamethoxazole.

Correcting Immunodeficiencies

Not long ago, little could be done to actually cure an immunodeficiency. Today, researchers have developed several possibilities for replenishing the immune defenses. No single approach works for all immunodeficiencies, or in all cases, but taken together these new treatments have transformed a dismal prognosis into one of hope and promise.

For several life-threatening immunodeficiencies, bone marrow transplantation (BMT) offers the chance of a dramatic, complete, and permanent cure. Since the first BMT was performed in 1968, nearly 1,000 children with PID, including SCID, Wiskott-Aldrich syndrome, leukocyte adhesion defect, and other disorders, have shown a remarkable recovery. They recover from infections, gain weight, and move on to essentially normal lives.

Unfortunately, bone marrow transplants do not work for everyone. To be successful, the transplant needs to come from a donor whose body tissues are a close biological match. That is, the donor's tissues and the recipient's tissues should have identical, or nearly identical, sets of marker molecules (known as human leukocyte antigens [HLA]) that serve as unique tissue identification tags. Without a good match, a reaction known as graft-versus-host disease (GVHD) may occur in which cells in the donor marrow see the recipient's tissues as foreign and react against them.

Because tissue marker molecules come in many varieties, finding a good match is not easy. With new techniques and the availability of large donor banks, however, finding a suitable match is easier. The best matches are likely to be with close relatives, especially brothers or sisters.

Another option is marrow from a close relative—typically a parent—who shares half of the patient's major HLA antigens (and many of the minor antigens as well). Cleansed of mature T cells that could trigger a GVHD, such half-matched transplants have saved the lives of many children.

BMT works especially well for SCID, because children with SCID lack T cells that could attack the bone marrow graft and cause rejection. Anyone with T cells may need to be treated prior to transplantation with radiation or drugs. Although this eliminates the recipient's T cells, it also temporarily wipes out other immune defenses, further increasing the patient's risk of infection.

Even with a good match, BMT does not always succeed. Results are best when the child is young, in fairly good health, and free of serious infection at the time of the transplantation.

Another treatment option, for children with a specific form of SCID who do not have a suitable bone marrow donor, is enzyme replacement therapy. About 15 percent of all cases of SCID are due to lack of the enzyme known as adenosine deaminase (ADA). This type of SCID can be partially treated with regular injections of the missing enzyme. For treatment, ADA is linked to a chemical, polyethylene glycol (PEG), which protects ADA from being quickly eliminated from the bloodstream.

For many people with antibody deficiencies, antibody replacement therapy can be a lifesaver. The patient receives regular infusions or injections of immunoglobulins—or antibodies—that have been removed from the blood of healthy donors and purified. Immunoglobulins from thousands of donors are pooled so that each batch contains antibodies to many different types of germs. Because purification removes most IgM and IgA, the product consists almost entirely of IgG. It is known as gamma globulin, immunoglobulin, or immune serum globulin.

Taken regularly and in large doses, gamma globulins can boost serum immunoglobulins to near normal levels and eliminate most infections. If treatment begins early enough, it can prevent lung damage from pneumonia.

Immunoglobulin is administered either intramuscularly or intravenously. Intravenous immunoglobulin (IVIG) is usually preferred because it can be given in large doses, it is fast-acting, and it avoids the pain associated with large intramuscular injections. Infusions of IVIG take two to four hours and are administered every three or four weeks, either at home or in an outpatient clinic.

Injections of cytokines, which are natural chemicals produced by immune cells, are another new way to treat immune deficiencies. For example, the symptoms of chronic granulomatous disease can be traced to faulty phagocytes; phagocytes can be activated with injections of a natural or synthetic product of immune cells called gamma interferon.

In some immune deficiencies, the numbers of neutrophils may be reduced either because they are under attack, or are not produced in normal numbers. In certain cases, this problem can be offset by the injection of growth factors. These growth factors increase the production of neutrophils. Granulocyte-macrophage colony-stimulating factor (GM-CSF) is a natural chemical that boosts the development of blood cells, including the white blood cells known as granulocytes and macrophages. Another granulocyte colony-stimulating factor (G-CSF), is also helpful in raising levels of granulocytes.

Transplanting Cells from Umbilical Cord Blood

Transplanting cord blood stem cells is even newer and easier than transplanting bone marrow. Stem cells are long-lived parent cells that continually give rise to fresh blood cells. Ordinarily, they live in the bone marrow. Some stem cells circulate in the blood, but they are scarce and difficult to extract. However, stem cells are plentiful in blood in the umbilical cord of healthy infants at the time of birth.

To obtain cord blood stem cells, blood is drained from the umbilical cord and placenta as soon as a healthy baby is born and the cord clamped and cut. The cord blood is typed, frozen, and stored. Later it can be transplanted into a matched recipient with an immunodeficiency.

Doctors have used stem cells from cord blood to treat a variety of blood diseases in children. The cord blood has usually come from cord blood banks. Research suggests that cord blood stem cells may not need to be matched as closely as bone marrow.

Important Precautions

Children with PID diseases, especially those with defective T cells, X-linked agammaglobulinemia, and ataxia-telangiectasia should not receive live virus vaccines, such as the oral polio, measles, and chicken pox (varicella) vaccines. It is not even safe to give live virus vaccines to children suspected of immunodeficiency until a definitive diagnosis is rendered. There is a risk that such vaccines could cause serious illness or even death. Moreover, blood transfusions should not only be free of infectious viruses (e.g., hepatitis or cytomegalovirus), but also—for T cell deficient children—irradiated to incapacitate mature donor T cells that might attack the tissues of the recipient and result in GVHD.

Research

Research on PID is under way on many fronts. Geneticists, immunologists, molecular biologists, microbiologists, and biochemists are working to understand fundamental defects and to devise remedies. New genes are being identified, and scientists are making rapid progress in untangling the intricate connections and pathways that govern immune responses. Clinical scientists are developing new treatments to alleviate symptoms and prevent complications.

Gene Therapy

Gene therapy is one of the most publicized forms of treatment for PID. This revolutionary approach was first used to treat two young girls with SCID due to ADA deficiency.

Gene therapy attempts to cure disease by inserting a healthy version of a missing or malfunctioning gene into a cell to restore normal function. If successful, the newly inserted gene directs the cell to produce the missing protein.

In the pioneering 1990 experiment, some of the girls' T cells were removed, treated to make them more active, and a gene for ADA was introduced. These T cells carrying the new gene were then reinjected into the girls. Meanwhile, these girls still continued to receive their PEG-ADA treatment.

Today, the girls are healthy and free of severe infections. Both of them are attending school and living relatively normal lives. One of the two girls has had an especially good response. She has some T cells that carry the new gene and produce the ADA enzyme. However, since both girls have always received PEG-ADA, it is not clear how much of the credit for their good health can be attributed to the new genes.

Still more recently, doctors have tried gene therapy using stem cells which are much longer-lived than T cells. In three different cases, babies were diagnosed with ADA deficiency before they were born. Their own umbilical cord blood was collected, and stem cells taken from the cord blood had new genes inserted. Each of the babies was then given a transfusion of his/her own genetically-engineered stem cells. These children did well initially. But like the girls given T cell gene therapy, they continue to require other treatments. Currently, gene therapy remains strictly experimental, and not yet used routinely for therapy.

Research Challenges

Since there are many different types of PID, they present a formidable research challenge to the scientific community. However, thanks to the timely and extraordinary advances of genetics, molecular biology, and molecular medicine, the challenge can be met and conquered. Already these exciting new scientific tools have unraveled many of the mysteries behind PID, and have significantly increased our insight and basic understanding of them. Moreover, they have contributed to the development of new and improved approaches and strategies to diagnose, treat, and prevent PID.

A major challenge is to identify the genes that cause PID, and characterize the nature of each genetic defect and its associated immunodeficiency disease. More than 70 PID genes have already been identified and characterized. With more advances in genetic technology and rapid molecular analytical methods, progress on defective gene identification and characterization should accelerate.

Although gamma globulin therapy, bone marrow transplantation, gamma interferon, and PEG-ADA have been effective for treating specific forms of PID, new and emerging opportunities for improving these therapies show great promise. In addition, research into using gene therapy will continue to improve the prognosis of patients with PID. Finally, an important research challenge is to develop new and innovative treatments that are more efficacious, easier to administer, less costly, and that allow the patient to lead a normal lifestyle.

Additional Information

Immune Deficiency Foundation
40 W. Chesapeake Ave., Suite 308
Towson, MD 21204
Toll-Free: 800-296-4433
Website: http://www.primaryimmune.org
E-mail: idf@primaryimmune.org

Jeffrey Modell Foundation
National Primary Immunodeficiency Resource Center
747 Third Ave.
New York, NY 10017
Phone: 212-819-0200
Fax: 212-764-4180
Website: http://www.jmfworld.org/index.cfm
E-mail: info@jmfworld.org

Chapter 75

Treatment of Human Immunodeficiency Virus (HIV) Infection

When acquired immunodeficiency syndrome (AIDS) was first recognized in 1981, patients with the disease were unlikely to live longer than a year or two. Since then, scientists have developed an effective arsenal of drugs that can help many people infected with human immunodeficiency virus (HIV) live longer and healthier lives. The treatment and prevention of HIV is a high priority for the National Institute of Allergy and Infectious Diseases (NIAID).

What drugs have been developed for HIV infection?

Twenty drugs have been approved for treating individuals with HIV infection. They are called antiretroviral drugs because they attack HIV, which is a retrovirus.

Once inside the cell, HIV uses specific enzymes to survive. The first approved classes of antiretroviral drugs that were approved work by interfering with the virus' ability to use these enzymes. They fall into two categories:

- **Reverse transcriptase (RT) inhibitors.** RT inhibitors interfere with an enzyme called reverse transcriptase or RT that HIV needs to make copies of itself. There are two main types of RT inhibitors, and they each work differently.

"Treatment of HIV Infection," Fact Sheet, National Institute of Allergy and Infectious Diseases (NIAID), October 2003.

- Nucleoside/nucleotide drugs provide faulty deoxyribonucleic acid (DNA) building blocks, halting the DNA chain that the virus uses to make copies of itself.

- Non-nucleoside RT inhibitors bind RT so the virus cannot carry out its copying function.

- **Protease Inhibitors (PI).** Protease inhibitors interfere with the protease enzyme that HIV uses to produce infectious viral particles.

The newest class of antiretroviral drugs works by changing the shape of the gp41 envelope protein surrounding HIV. This class of drug is called fusion inhibitors.

- **Fusion inhibitors** interfere with the virus' ability to fuse with and enter the host cell.

Table 75.1. Drugs Approved for HIV Infection

Nucleoside/Nucleotide RT Inhibitors: abacavir, ddC, ddI, d4T, 3TC, ZDV tenofovir

Non-nucleoside RT Inhibitors: delavirdine, nevirapine, efavirenz

Protease Inhibitors: ritonavir, saquinavir, indinavir, amprenavir, nelfinavir, lopinavir, atazanavir, emtricitabine, fosamprenavir calcium

Fusion Inhibitors: pentafuside

Do antiretroviral drugs cure HIV infection?

No, the currently available drugs cannot cure HIV infection. This is because the current drugs can suppress HIV, but are unable to eliminate it from the body. Since HIV can become resistant to any one drug, researchers use a combination of antiretroviral drugs to suppress the virus. By combining both RT inhibitors and protease inhibitors, NIAID-supported research groups and drug companies developed the potent and effective combination therapy called highly active antiretroviral therapy or HAART.

Although the use of HAART has greatly reduced the number of deaths due to AIDS, this powerful combination of drugs cannot suppress the virus indefinitely. In addition, while people with HIV are living longer, new medical problems are surfacing. Even those individuals who take antiretroviral drugs can pass on HIV to others through unprotected sex.

What problems are associated with antiretroviral drug use?

People with HIV must take medicines with complicated regimens, often taking several drugs per day, some of which may require the person to fast. Patients may have difficulty adhering to these complicated regimens, find the food restrictions difficult to deal with, and may experience unpleasant side effects such as nausea and vomiting.

Aside from the complicated dosing regimens, antiretroviral drugs themselves may cause significant medical problems. Metabolic changes occur in people with HIV infection. Some of these changes may be related to the antiretrovirals, and may include abnormal fat distribution, abnormal lipid and glucose metabolism, and bone loss.

Some anti-HIV drugs are toxic to mitochondria, the energy producers in cells. Tissues that require high levels of energy, like muscles and nerves, are most susceptible to the affects of damaged mitochondria. Muscle wasting, heart failure, nerve damage, degeneration of the liver, and inflammation of the pancreas may be associated with mitochondrial damage.

What is NIAID doing to address the complications of anti-HIV drugs?

NIAID supports studies understanding the side effects of drugs or combinations of drugs as well as strategies to reduce exposure to potentially toxic drug regimens, such as:

- Structured treatment interruption (STI) protocols.

- Use of immune-based therapies with HAART.

- Studies to compare different dosing schedules.

- Studies to compare early versus delayed treatment.

NIAID also supports projects evaluating regimens containing agents associated with toxicities. For example, NIAID funded researchers are investigating treatments for some metabolic complications. There are ongoing studies evaluating various treatments of fat redistribution, lipid and glucose abnormalities, and bone loss.

In addition, researchers are studying the metabolic effects of various antiretroviral regimens in pregnant women and their infants, and in HIV-infected children and adolescents, including long-term follow-up of such patients.

How does research ensure safety?

NIAID supports the development and testing of new classes of anti-retroviral compounds or combinations that will be able to continuously suppress the virus with few side effects. Such studies will provide accurate and extensive information about the safety of the new agents and combinations. They will identify potential uncommon, but important, toxicities of newly approved agents. Studies are also underway to assess rare toxicities of older approved agents, especially as a result of long-term use.

Through its Multi-center AIDS Cohort Study (MACS) and the Women's Interagency HIV Study (WIHS), NIAID supports long-term studies of HIV disease in both men and women. Since their inception, these cohort studies have enrolled and collected data on more than 8,000 people. In addition to the information gleaned from this epidemiological gold mine, other studies on the specific metabolic complications of HIV treatment are supported through both the adult and pediatric AIDS Clinical Trials Groups (AACTG and PACTG), as well as through the Terry Beirn Community Programs for Clinical Research on AIDS (CPCRA).

Are any new drugs in the pipeline?

The Pharmaceutical Research and Manufacturers Association lists nearly two dozen new anti-HIV drugs now in development. They include new protease inhibitors and more potent, less toxic RT inhibitors, as well as drugs that interfere with entirely different steps in the virus' life cycle. These new categories of drugs include:

- Entry inhibitors—drugs that interfere with HIV ability to enter cells.

- Integrase inhibitors—drugs that interfere with HIV ability to insert its genes into a cell's normal DNA.

- Assembly and budding inhibitors—drugs that interfere with the final stage of the HIV life cycle, when new virus particles are released into the bloodstream.

- Cellular metabolism modulators—drugs that interfere with the cellular processes needed for HIV replication.

In addition, scientists are learning how immune modulators help boost the immune system's response to the virus and may make the existing anti-HIV drugs more effective. Therapeutic vaccines are also being evaluated for this purpose and could help reduce the number of anti-HIV drugs needed or the duration of treatment.

Chapter 76

Treatments for Rheumatic Conditions

Myth: Arthritis affects only older people.

Fact: Arthritis affects any age, including children. There's no question that the incidence of arthritis increases with age, but nearly three of every five sufferers are under age 65.

Myth: Arthritis is just minor aches and pains.

Fact: Arthritis can be permanently debilitating.

Myth: Arthritis cannot be treated.

Fact: The FDA has approved several treatments for osteoarthritis and rheumatoid arthritis.

These myths keep people from seeking a doctor's help against the number one cause of disability in the United States, according to the national Centers for Disease Control and Prevention (CDC). Arthritis disables more Americans than heart disease and stroke, and the

"Arthritis: Timely Treatments for an Ageless Disease," *FDA Consumer*, May-June 2000, revised in August 2000 and August 2001, U.S. Food and Drug Administration (FDA), Publication No. (FDA) 01-1313. "An Update Regarding Cox-2 Inhibitors and Other NSAIDs," is excerpted from "Questions and Answers on COX-2 Selective and Non-Selective Non-Steroidal Anti-Inflammatory Drugs [NSAIDs]," U.S. Food and Drug Administration, April 7, 2005. The complete text is available at http://www.fda.gov/cder/drug/infopage/COX2/COX2qa.htm.

CDC says it's what Americans don't know about the disease that can hurt them.

"People ignore arthritis both as public and personal health problems because it doesn't kill you," says Chad Helmick, a medical epidemiologist at the CDC. "But what they don't realize is that as Americans work and live longer, arthritis can affect their quality of life and eventually lead to disability." Current costs to the U.S. economy total nearly $65 billion annually—an impact equal to a moderate recession.

And the extent of the suffering is going to get worse. Arthritis already affects more than 42 million Americans in its chronic form, including 300,000 children. By 2020, CDC estimates that 60 million people will be affected, and that more than 12 million will be disabled.

The Arthritis Foundation and the American College of Rheumatology agree that awareness, early diagnosis, and an aggressive treatment plan developed by a doctor are key to stopping arthritis from taking over your life.

What Is Arthritis?

Although the term literally means joint inflammation, arthritis really refers to a group of more than 100 rheumatic diseases and conditions that can cause pain, stiffness, and swelling in the joints. Certain conditions may affect other parts of the body—such as the muscles, bones, and some internal organs—and can result in debilitating, and sometimes life-threatening, complications. If left undiagnosed and untreated, arthritis can cause irreversible damage to the joints.

The two most common forms of the disease, osteoarthritis and rheumatoid arthritis, have the greatest public health implications, according to the Arthritis Foundation.

Osteoarthritis, previously known as degenerative joint disease, results from the wear and tear of life. The pressure of gravity—the load of living—causes physical damage to the joints and surrounding tissues, leading to pain, tenderness, swelling, and decreased function. Initially, osteoarthritis is noninflammatory, and its onset is subtle and gradual usually involving one or only a few joints. The joints most often affected are the knee, hip, and hand. Pain is the earliest symptom, usually made worse by repetitive use. Osteoarthritis affects 21 million people, and the risk of getting it increases with age. Other risk factors include joint trauma, obesity, and repetitive joint use.

Rheumatoid arthritis is an autoimmune disease that occurs when the body's own immune system mistakenly attacks the synovium (cell lining inside the joint). This chronic, potentially disabling disease causes pain, stiffness, swelling, and loss of function in the joints. While the cause remains elusive, doctors suspect that genetic factors are important in rheumatoid arthritis. Studies have begun to tease out the genetic characteristics that can be passed from generation to generation. However, the inherited trait alone does not cause the illness. Researchers think this trait, along with some other unknown factor—probably in the environment—triggers the disease. Rheumatoid arthritis can be difficult to diagnose early because it may begin gradually with subtle symptoms. According to the CDC, this form of arthritis affects more than 2 million people in the United States and two to three times more women are affected than men.

Finding Effective Treatments

For years, the pain and inflammation of arthritis have been treated with varying success, using medications, local steroid injections, and joint replacement. Seldom did the therapies make the pain go away completely or for very long, nor did they affect the underlying joint damage. Now there are some new treatments available, and patients should consult with their doctors to determine which are the most appropriate for their conditions.

Osteoarthritis

When taken regularly and at high doses, traditional nonsteroidal anti-inflammatory drugs (NSAIDs) used for pain relief can cause gastrointestinal (GI) bleeding or ulcers. But a new type of NSAID, cyclooxygenase-2 inhibitors, better known as COX-2 inhibitors, has joined the old standbys. These drugs help suppress arthritis with less stomach irritation.

Cyclooxygenases are enzymes needed for the synthesis of hormone-like substances called prostaglandins. There are two types of cyclooxygenases: the COX-2 enzyme that mediates inflammation and pain, and the COX-1 enzyme that helps maintain other physiological functions in the body. Traditional NSAIDs inhibit both enzymes. The new NSAIDs, however, block mostly the COX-2 enzyme, offering a new treatment option for people who have had difficulty tolerating the old NSAIDs.

"COX-2 inhibitors are just as effective in treating osteoarthritis as other NSAIDs," says Maria Villalba, M.D., a medical officer with the Food and Drug Administration's Center for Drug Evaluation and Research.

The FDA approved the first COX-2 inhibitor, Celebrex (celecoxib), in 1998 to treat rheumatoid arthritis and osteoarthritis. Vioxx (rofecoxib) became the second COX-2 inhibitor to receive approval, in 1999, for the treatment of osteoarthritis, dysmenorrhea (pain with menstrual periods), and the relief of acute pain in adults, such as that caused by dental surgery.

An Update Regarding Cox-2 Inhibitors and Other NSAIDs

Vioxx was voluntarily removed from the market by its manufacturer, Merck, in September 2004. In April 2005, FDA requested the manufacturer of Bextra, Pfizer, Inc., to voluntarily withdraw Bextra from the market.

FDA also requested that manufacturers of all marketed prescription NSAIDs, including Celebrex, a COX-2 selective NSAID, revise the labeling (package insert) for their products to include a boxed warning and a Medication Guide highlighting the potential for increased risk of cardiovascular (CV) events and the well-described, serious, and potentially life-threatening gastrointestinal (GI) bleeding associated with these drugs.

FDA asked manufacturers of non-prescription products containing ibuprofen (Motrin, Advil, Ibu-Tab 200, Medipren, Cap-Profen, Tab-Profen, Profen, Ibuprohm), naproxen (Aleve), and ketoprofen (Orudis, Actron) to revise their labeling to include more specific information about the potential GI and CV risks and information to assist consumers in the safe use of the drug, including instructions about which patients should seek the advice of a physician before using these drugs, stronger reminders about limiting the dose and duration of treatment in accordance with the package instructions unless otherwise advised by a physician, and a warning about potential skin reactions.

Non-Drug Alternatives

Two non-drug alternatives for the treatment of pain in osteoarthritis of the knee were approved by the FDA's Center for Devices and Radiological Health in 1997 for patients who have failed to respond adequately to simple analgesics, such as acetaminophen, and to conservative nonpharmacologic therapy. Hyalgan and Synvisc are viscous solutions composed of hyaluronan (hyaluronic acid, a lubricant found naturally in the joints), and are injected directly into the knee joint. Both are believed to increase the quality of synovial fluid, although the mechanism of action for these products is not well understood. The most common side effects reported from these treatments—injection site pain and knee pain and/or swelling—were found to be temporary. For patients who cannot tolerate oral medications and who are not candidates for surgical knee replacement, these treatments may be an ideal option.

Rheumatoid Arthritis

Typical treatments for rheumatoid arthritis have relied on a combination of NSAIDs, such as ibuprofen or aspirin (which reduce swelling and alleviate pain, but do not change the course of the disease); and disease-modifying anti-rheumatic drugs (DMARDs) such as methotrexate and sulfasalazine, also called slow-acting drugs. DMARDs work to slow inflammation and can alter the course of the disease. Until recently, most doctors reserved the use of DMARDs for patients who failed to respond to other therapies. Now, most physicians use DMARDs early and aggressively in the hope of slowing disease progression and damage to joints and internal organs.

FDA Approves New Therapy for Rheumatoid Arthritis

FDA has approved adalimumab (marketed by Abbott Laboratories as Humira) to treat rheumatoid arthritis (RA). Humira is produced by recombinant DNA technology. It is a human-derived antibody that binds to human tumor necrosis factor alpha (TNF alpha). TNF is naturally produced by the body and is involved with normal inflammatory and immune responses. Individuals with RA have high levels of TNF in the synovial fluid (lubricating fluid in joints). The extra TNF plays an important role in both the pathologic inflammation and the joint destruction that are hallmarks of RA. By working against the inflammatory process, Humira, like other TNF blockers has been shown to be effective in controlling symptoms of the disease. Humira is indicated for reducing signs and symptoms and inhibiting the progression of structural damage in adult patients with moderately to severely active rheumatoid arthritis who have had an inadequate response to one or more disease-modifying anti-rheumatic drugs (DMARDs). Humira can be used alone or in combination with methotrexate or other DMARDs. Humira is administered as a single subcutaneous injection every other week. (Source for this paragraph: *FDA Talk Paper*, U.S. Food and Drug Administration (FDA), December 31, 2002.)

Another approved treatment regimen for rheumatoid arthritis is one that combines the genetically engineered biological drug Remicade (infliximab) with the drug methotrexate. (Not all patients with rheumatoid arthritis can tolerate or respond to methotrexate alone, a standard treatment for the disease.) Remicade is the second in a new class of drugs known as biologic response modifiers, which bind to and block the action of a naturally occurring protein called tumor necrosis factor (TNF), believed to play a role in joint inflammation and damage. Elevated levels of TNF are found in the synovial fluid of rheumatoid arthritis patients. Remicade, which is administered intravenously by a health-care professional in a two-hour outpatient procedure, was approved by the FDA in 1999 to reduce the signs and symptoms in patients who have not experienced significant relief from methotrexate alone.

Approved in 1996, Enbrel (etanercept) is the first biologic response modifier to receive FDA approval for patients with moderate to severe rheumatoid arthritis. Taken twice weekly by injection, Enbrel was shown to decrease pain and morning stiffness and improve joint swelling and tenderness. In 2000, the drug's uses were expanded to include delaying structural damage.

Jeffrey N. Siegel, M.D., a medical officer with FDA's Center for Biologics Evaluation and Research, says that Enbrel is an exciting breakthrough because it helps a majority of patients who have not responded to any of the other commonly used therapies. Although it is injected, the treatment can be administered at home. In addition, Enbrel has been shown to be effective for children with the juvenile form of rheumatoid arthritis. In clinical trials, Enbrel was generally well tolerated, and one of the most common side effects was an injection site reaction.

Both Remicade and Enbrel show promise in treating rheumatoid arthritis, although the long-term risks and benefits of these agents are unknown. In post-marketing reports, serious infections, including fatalities, have been reported with these agents. Caution should be used in patients with a history of recurring infections, or with underlying conditions that may predispose patients to infections.

Arava (leflunomide) is the first oral treatment approved for slowing the progression of rheumatoid arthritis. Although its effects are similar to those of methotrexate, this drug works by a different chemical mechanism that blocks at least one enzyme in certain immune cells called lymphocytes (a type of white blood cell that is part of the immune system), and so retards the progression of the disease.

However, Arava is not a cure for rheumatoid arthritis. It may cause birth defects, and the label carries a special warning for pregnant women and those planning to become pregnant. Liver damage, including deaths, also has been reported. The drug is not recommended for patients with severe immunodeficiency, bone marrow dysplasia, or severe, uncontrolled infections.

The first non-drug alternative for adult patients with moderate to severe rheumatoid arthritis and longstanding disease was approved by the FDA in 1999. The Prosorba column, which was initially approved in 1987 to treat an immune blood disorder, is a single-use medical device, about the size of a coffee mug, containing a material that binds antibodies and antigen-antibody complexes.

In a two-hour process performed in a hospital or specialized treatment center, a patient's blood is removed and passed through a machine that separates the blood cells from the plasma (the liquid portion of the blood). The plasma is then passed through the Prosorba column, recombined with the blood cells, and returned to the patient. Although this filtering process is believed to remove proteins that may inadvertently attack the joint cells, the mechanism of action of the Prosorba column is not well understood. The treatment is given once a week for 12 weeks. The most common side effects include joint pain and/or swelling, fatigue, hypotension (low blood pressure), and anemia.

"For those patients who have failed or are intolerant to DMARDs, including Arava and the anti-TNF agents," says Sahar M. Dawisha, M.D., a medical officer in the FDA's Center for Devices and Radiological Health, "the Prosorba column may be an additional treatment option."

Exercise and Arthritis

Proper exercises performed on a regular basis are an important part of arthritis treatment, according to the Arthritis Foundation. Twenty years ago, doctors advised exactly the opposite, fearing that activity would cause more damage and inflammation. Not exercising causes weak muscles, stiff joints, reduced mobility, and lost vitality, say rheumatologists, who now routinely advise a balance of physical activity and rest.

According to the 1996 Surgeon General's Report on Physical Activity and Health, regular, moderate, physical activity is beneficial in decreasing fatigue, strengthening muscles and bones, increasing flexibility and stamina, and improving the general sense of well-being.

The National Institutes of Health (NIH) advises that the amount and form of exercise should depend on which joints are involved, the amount of inflammation, how stable the joints are, and whether a joint replacement procedure has been done. A skilled physician who is knowledgeable about the medical and rehabilitation needs of people with arthritis, working with a physical therapist, can design an exercise plan for each patient.

Three main types of exercises are recommended:

- **Range-of-motion**—moving a joint as far as it will comfortably go, and then stretching it a little further to increase and maintain joint mobility, decrease pain, and improve joint function. These can be done daily, or at least every other day.

- **Strengthening**—using muscles without moving joints to help increase muscle strength and stabilize weak joints. These can be done daily, or at least every other day, unless there is severe pain or swelling.

- **Endurance**—aerobic exercises such as walking, swimming, and bicycling to strengthen the heart and lungs and increase stamina. These should be done for 20 to 30 minutes, three times a week, unless there is severe pain or swelling.

Unproven Remedies

Many people with arthritis become discouraged with typical treatments because the disease progresses over time and the symptoms worsen. Consequently, they search for alternative therapies aimed at arthritis. But, arthritis patients need to be careful because treatments not shown to be safe and effective through controlled scientific studies may be dangerous. According to the Arthritis Foundation, the benefits of a treatment in controlling arthritis should be greater than the risk of unwanted or harmful effects. Since arthritis symptoms may come and go, a person using an unproven remedy may mistakenly think the remedy worked simply because he or she tried it when symptoms were going into a natural remission.

Two controversial nutritional supplements, not approved by the FDA, have catapulted into the spotlight because of claims that they rebuild joint tissues damaged by osteoarthritis—or halt the disease entirely. But at this time, the use of glucosamine and chondroitin sulfate supplements warrant further in-depth studies on their safety and effectiveness, according to the Arthritis Foundation.

Both glucosamine and chondroitin sulfate occur in the body naturally and are vital to normal cartilage formation, but the Arthritis Foundation says there is no evidence that swallowed chondroitin is absorbed into the body and deposited into the joints. Moreover, no one knows how much glucosamine and chondroitin sulfate are in the bottles since current law does not require dietary supplements to be manufactured under the same good manufacturing practice standards as pharmaceuticals. As reported in the December 1999 University of California-Berkeley Wellness Letter, "It's a hit-or-miss proposition because there's no standardization and no guarantee that you're getting what the label says."

The Arthritis Foundation urges anyone considering using these supplements to become "fully educated about potential positive and negative effects." In addition, people are encouraged to consult their physicians about how the supplements fit within their existing treatment regimens. Above all, do not stop proven treatments and disease-management techniques in favor of the supplements.

The Arthritis Foundation also says that copper bracelets, mineral springs, vibrators, magnets, vinegar and honey, dimethyl sulfoxide, large doses of vitamins, drugs with hidden ingredients (such as steroids), and snake venom are all unproven remedies. And any unproven remedy, no matter how harmless, can become harmful if it stops or delays someone from seeking a prescribed treatment program from a knowledgeable physician.

Prevention Measures

There are ways to help prevent arthritis. Both CDC and the American College of Rheumatology recommend maintaining ideal weight, taking precautions to reduce repetitive joint use and injury on the job, avoiding sports injuries by performing warm-ups and strengthening exercises using weights, and by choosing appropriate sports equipment.

Lyme arthritis may develop after a bacterial infection is transmitted to humans through tick bites. To prevent this type of arthritis, health experts advise people to use insect repellents, wear long-sleeved shirts and pants while walking near wooded areas, and check for and remove ticks to help reduce the risk of getting the disease. CDC also recommends the prompt use of antibiotics for Lyme disease symptoms. In December 1998, FDA approved the first vaccine, Lymerix, to help prevent Lyme disease.

In an efficacy and safety trial, the vaccine's effectiveness in preventing Lyme disease was 49 percent after two injections and 76 percent after three. Vaccination should be considered by people 15 to 70 years old who live in or visit high-risk areas and have frequent or prolonged exposure to ticks. The vaccine has not yet been approved for use in children.

Other Forms of Arthritis and Related Conditions

In addition to rheumatoid and osteoarthritis, there are a number of diseases and conditions that can cause joint pain and stiffness.

Juvenile arthritis is a general term for all types of arthritis that occur in children. Juvenile rheumatoid arthritis is the most prevalent form in children, and there are three major types: polyarticular (affecting many joints), pauciarticular (pertaining to only a few joints), and systemic (affecting the entire body). The signs and symptoms of juvenile rheumatoid arthritis vary from child to child. There is no single test that establishes conclusively a diagnosis of juvenile arthritis, and the condition must be present consistently for six or more consecutive weeks before a correct diagnosis can be made. Heredity is thought to play some part in the development of juvenile arthritis. However, the inherited trait alone does not cause the illness. Researchers think this trait, along with some other unknown factor (probably in the environment), triggers the disease. The Arthritis Foundation says that juvenile arthritis is even more prevalent than juvenile diabetes and cerebral palsy.

Gout is a disease that causes sudden, severe attacks of pain, tenderness, redness, warmth, and swelling in some joints. It usually affects one joint at a time, especially the joint of the big toe. The pain and swelling associated with gout are caused by uric acid crystals that precipitate out of the blood and are deposited in the joint. Factors leading to increased levels of uric acid and then gout include excessive alcohol intake, hypertension, kidney disease, and certain drugs.

Ankylosing spondylitis is a chronic inflammatory disease of the spine that can fuse the vertebrae to produce a rigid spine. Spondylitis is a result of inflammation that usually starts in tissue outside the joint. The most common early symptoms of spondylitis are low back pain and stiffness that continues for months. Although the cause of spondylitis is unknown, scientists have discovered a strong genetic or family link, according to the Arthritis Foundation. Most people with spondylitis have a genetic marker known as HLA-B27. Genetic markers are protein molecules located on the surface of white blood cells that act as a type of name tag. Having this genetic marker does not mean a person will develop spondylitis, but people with the marker are more likely to develop the disease than those without it. Ankylosing spondylitis usually affects men between the ages of 16 and 35, but it also affects women. Other joints besides the spine may be involved.

Systemic lupus erythematosus is an autoimmune disease that can involve the skin, kidneys, blood vessels, joints, nervous system, heart, and other internal organs. Symptoms vary among those affected, but may include a skin rash, arthritis, fever, anemia, hair loss, ulcers in the mouth, and kidney damage. In most cases, the symptoms first appear in women of childbearing age; however, lupus can occur in young children or older people. Studies suggest that there is an inherited tendency to get lupus. Lupus affects women about 9 to 10 times as often as men. It is also more common in African-American women.

Related Arthritis Conditions

Bursitis, tendinitis and myofascial pain are localized, nonsystemic (not affecting the whole body) painful conditions. Bursitis is inflammation of the sac surrounding any joint that contains a lubricating fluid. Tendinitis is inflammation of a tendon, and myofascial pain is a problem that results from the strain or improper use of a muscle. These conditions may start suddenly, and usually stop within a matter of days or weeks.

Carpal tunnel syndrome is a condition in which pressure on the median nerve at the wrist causes tingling and numbness in the fingers. It can begin suddenly or gradually, and can be associated with another disease, such as rheumatoid arthritis, or it may be unrelated to other conditions. If untreated, it can result in permanent nerve and muscle damage. With early diagnosis and treatment, there is an excellent chance of complete recovery.

Fibromyalgia syndrome is a condition with generalized muscular pain, fatigue, and poor sleep that is believed to affect nearly 4 million people. The name fibromyalgia means pain in the muscles, ligaments, and tendons. The condition mainly affects muscles and their attachments to bones. Although it may feel like a joint disease, the Arthritis Foundation says it is not a true form of arthritis and does not cause deformities of the joints. Fibromyalgia is instead a form of soft tissue or muscular rheumatism.

Infectious arthritis is a form of joint inflammation that is caused by bacteria, viruses, or fungi. The diagnosis is made by culturing the organism from the joint. Most infectious arthritis can be cured by antibiotic medications.

Psoriatic arthritis is similar to rheumatoid arthritis. About 5 percent of people with psoriasis, a chronic skin disease, also develop psoriatic arthritis. In psoriatic arthritis, there is inflammation of the joints and sometimes the spine. Fewer joints may be involved than in rheumatoid arthritis, and there is no rheumatoid factor in the blood.

Reiter syndrome (also called reactive arthritis) involves inflammation in the joints, and sometimes where ligaments and tendons attach to bones. This form of arthritis usually develops following an intestinal or a genital/urinary tract infection. People with Reiter syndrome have arthritis and one or more of the following conditions: urethritis, prostatitis, cervicitis, cystitis, eye problems, or skin sores.

Scleroderma is a disease of the body's connective tissue that causes thickening and hardening of the skin. It can also affect joints, blood vessels, and internal organs. There are two types of scleroderma: localized and generalized.

Hope for the Future

Recently approved drugs offer patients new options. As the population ages and arthritis becomes a growing problem, the Arthritis Foundation believes that "more physicians are recognizing the severity of the disease and the need for a broader approach toward treatment."

—by Carol Lewis is a staff writer for FDA Consumer

Chapter 77

Immunotherapy for Allergies

Allergy Shots

Immunotherapy (commonly called allergy shots) is a form of treatment to reduce your allergic reaction to allergens. Allergens are substances to which you are allergic. Research has shown that allergy shots can reduce symptoms of allergic rhinitis (hay fever) and allergic asthma. Remember, not all asthma is due to allergies. Allergy shots can be effective against grass, weed and tree pollens, house dust mites, cat and dog dander, and insect stings. Allergy shots are less effective against molds and are not a useful method for the treatment of food allergy.

Immunotherapy consists of a series of injections (shots) with a solution containing the allergens that cause your symptoms. Treatment usually begins with a weak solution given once or twice a week. The strength of the solution is gradually increased with each dose. Once the strongest dosage is reached, the injections are usually given once a month to control your symptoms. At this point, you have decreased your sensitivity to the allergens and have reached your maintenance level. Allergy shots should always be given at your health care provider's office.

When Is Immunotherapy Recommended?

If you are considering allergy shots, talk to your health care provider about a referral to board certified allergist. A board certified allergist will follow a number of steps to evaluate if allergy shots are appropriate for you.

First, the allergist will ask you questions about your environment and symptoms to determine if skin testing is necessary. Typically, prick skin testing is conducted to identify the specific allergens that are causing your symptoms. Skin testing should only be administered under the supervision of a board certified allergist.

Once an allergy has been identified, the next step is to decrease or eliminate exposure to the allergen. This is called environmental control. Evidence shows that allergy and asthma symptoms may improve over time if the recommended environmental control changes are made. For example, removing furry or feathered pets, or following control measures for house dust mites and cockroaches may decrease symptoms. Preventing contact with grasses, weeds, and tree pollen may be more difficult, but possible by keeping outside doors and windows closed and using air conditioning.

Next, your health care provider may recommend antihistamines and nasal medications as remedies. In general, allergy shots are recommended only for persons with a history of severe or prolonged allergic rhinitis and for persons with allergic asthma when the allergen cannot be avoided. Allergy shots should be prescribed only by a board certified allergist.

How Long Are Allergy Shots Given?

Six months to a year of immunotherapy may be required before you experience any improvement in symptoms. If your symptoms do not improve after this time, your allergist should review your overall treatment program. If the treatment is effective, the shots usually continue three to five years, until the individual is symptom-free or until symptoms can be controlled with mild medications for one year. In general, allergy shots should be stopped if they are not effective within two to three years.

Rush Immunotherapy

Rush immunotherapy is a variation of allergy shots which rushes the initial phase of the treatment. Steadily increasing doses of allergen extract are given every few hours instead of every few days or weeks. There is an increased risk of a reaction with this procedure. Therefore, rush immunotherapy should only be done in a hospital under very close supervision.

Other Therapies

There are a number of alternative treatments which claim to cure allergies. These methods are not supported by scientific studies and are not approved by the American Academy of Allergy and Immunology. Unapproved alternative treatments include the following:

* Desensitization to foods, chemicals, and environmental allergens with sublingual (under the tongue) drops
* High-dose vitamin and mineral therapy
* Urine injections
* Bacterial vaccines
* Exotic diets

It is easy to feel overwhelmed or confused by the many different methods of allergy testing and treatment. Work with a board certified allergist to evaluate and determine what is appropriate for you.

Chapter 78

Asthma Treatment

Questions Used to Assess Patients with Asthma

In the past 2 weeks, how many times have you:

• Had problems with coughing, wheezing (whistling in your chest), shortness of breath, or chest tightness during the day?

• Awakened at night from sleep because of coughing or other asthma symptoms?

• Awakened in the morning with asthma symptoms?

• Had asthma symptoms that did not improve within 15 minutes of inhaling a short-acting ß2-agonist?

• Missed days from work/school?

• Had symptoms while exercising or playing?

Assessing and Monitoring Lung Function

What is your highest and lowest peak flow rate since your last visit?
Has your peak flow dropped below ___Liters/minute (L/min) (80% of personal best) since your last visit?

Excerpted from "Key Clinical Activities for Quality Asthma Care: Recommendations of the National Asthma Education and Prevention Program," National Heart, Lung, and Blood Institute (NHLBI), March 2003.

Table 78.1. Components of Care, Key Clinical Activities, and Action Steps for Providing Quality Asthma Care

Components of care	Key clinical activities	Action steps
Assessment and monitoring	1. Establish asthma diagnosis	Establish a pattern of symptoms and history of recurrent episodes.
		Document reversible airflow using spirometry.
		Rule out other conditions.
	2. Classify severity of asthma	Follow the NAEPP* classification system and recheck at every visit.
	3. Schedule routine follow-up care	See patients at least every 1–6 months according to severity.
		Perform spirometry at least every 1–2 years for the stable patient, more often for the unstable patient.
		Review medication use, care plan, and self-management skills at every visit.
	4. Assess for referral to specialty care	Refer to specialty care when referral criteria are met.
Control of factors contributing to asthma severity	5. Recommend measures to control asthma triggers	Determine exposures and sensitivities, including environmental and occupational triggers.
		Review ways to reduce exposure to allergens and irritants that provoke asthma symptoms.
		Discuss smoking avoidance with every patient who smokes or who is exposed to environmental tobacco smoke.
		Assess for EIB* if symptoms occur during exercise, and provide medication and advice to enable physical activity.
	6. Treat or prevent comorbid conditions	Consider, particularly, rhinitis, sinusitis, GERD,* or COPD.*
		Provide annual influenza vaccination for patients with persistent asthma.

Pharmacotherapy

7. Prescribe medications according to severity
- Reduce inflammation in patients with persistent asthma with antiinflammatory medications.
- Increase medications if necessary; decrease when possible.
- Provide appropriate medication delivery and monitoring devices.
- Recommend spacers, nebulizers, or both if needed and consider PFM* for patients with moderate to severe asthma or a history of severe exacerbations.

8. Monitor use of β2-agonist drugs
- Reevaluate patients using more than one canister per month of short-acting β2-agonist drug.

Education for partnership in care

9. Develop a written asthma management plan
- Agree on therapy goals.
- Outline daily treatment and monitoring measures.
- Prepare an action plan to handle worsening symptoms/exacerbations.

10. Provide routine education on patient self-management
- Teach/review:
- How and why to take long-term control and quick-relief medications.
- Correct technique for inhaler, spacer, PFM,* and nebulizer as indicated.
- Peak flow/symptom monitoring with patients when appropriate.
- Factors that worsen asthma and actions to take.

* NAEPP: National Asthma Education and Prevention Program; EIB: exercise-induced bronchoconstriction; GERD: gastroesophageal reflux disease; COPD: chronic obstructive pulmonary disease; PFM: peak flow meter.

Table 78.2. Medications Used in Different Levels of Asthma Severity*

Classification	Step	Daily medication	Quick relief medication
Severe persistent	4	High-dose inhaled steroids (ICS) and long-acting inhaled β2-agonist If needed, add oral steroids	Short-acting inhaled β2-agonist, as needed; oral steroids may be required
Moderate persistent	3	Low-to-medium-dose ICS and long acting β2-agonist (preferred); **Or** Medium-dose ICS (another preferred option for children aged < 5 years); **Or** Low-to-medium-dose ICS and either leukotriene modifier or theophylline	Short-acting inhaled β2-agonist, as needed; oral steroids may be required
Mild persistent	2	Low-dose inhaled steroids (preferred) **Or** Cromolyn, leukotriene modifier, or (except for children aged < 5 years) nedocromil or sustained release theophylline to serum concentration of 5–15 micrograms/milliliter (µg/mL)	Short-acting inhaled β2-agonist, as needed; oral steroids may be required
Mild Intermittent	1	No daily medicine needed	Short-acting inhaled β2-agonist, as needed; oral steroids may be required

*The medications listed here are appropriate for treating asthma at different levels of severity. The preferred treatments, dosage, and type of medication recommended vary for adults and children and are detailed in the *EPR-Update 2002* stepwise approach to therapy. The stepwise approach emphasizes that therapy should be stepped up as necessary and stepped down when possible to identify the least amount of medication required to achieve goals of therapy. The stepwise approach to care is intended to assist, not replace, the clinical decision making required to meet individual patient needs.

Sources: National Heart, Lung, and Blood Institute, National Asthma Education and Prevention Program. *Expert Panel Report 2: guidelines for the diagnosis and management of asthma.* Bethesda MD: US Department of Health and Human Services, National Institutes of Health, 1997; Pub. No. 97-4051. Available at http://www.nhlbi.nih.gov/guidelines/asthma/asthgdln.pdf. Also, National Heart, Lung, and Blood Institute, National Asthma Education and Prevention Program. *Quick reference for the NAEPP Expert Panel Report: guidelines for the diagnosis and management of asthma—Update on selected topics 2002.* Bethesda MD: US Department of Health and Human Services, National Institutes of Health, 2002; Pub. No. 02-5075. Available at http://www.nhlbi.nih.gov/guidelines/asthma/index.htm

Steps to Reduce Asthma Triggers

Allergens

Reduce or eliminate exposure to allergens to which the patient is sensitive:

- **Animal dander:** Remove animals from the house or, at a minimum, keep animals out of the patient's bedroom; use a filter for the air ducts leading to the bedroom.

- **House dust mites:**

  - Essential: Encase mattress and pillow in an allergen-impermeable cover or wash pillow weekly as an alternative. Wash sheets and blankets from the patient's bed in hot water (greater than 130° F) weekly.

  - Desirable: Reduce indoor humidity to less than 50%. Remove carpets from the bedroom. Avoid sleeping or lying on upholstered furniture. Remove wall-to-wall carpets that are laid on concrete.

- **Cockroaches:** Use poison bait or traps to control. Do not leave food or garbage exposed.

- **Pollens and outdoor molds:** To avoid exposure to outdoor allergens during their active season, persons with asthma should stay indoors with windows closed, especially in the afternoon.

- **Indoor molds:** Fix all leaks and eliminate water sources associated with mold growth; clean moldy surfaces. Consider reducing indoor humidity to <50%.

- **Work environment:** Identify and control exposures to allergens and chemical sensitizers.

Tobacco Smoke

- Patients and others in the home who smoke should stop smoking or smoke outside the home.

- Reduce exposure to other sources of tobacco smoke, such as from childcare providers and the workplace.

Indoor/Outdoor Pollutants and Irritants

Reduce exposure at home and work to the following:

- Wood-burning stoves or fireplaces

- Unvented stoves or heaters

- Other irritants (e.g., perfumes, cleaning agents, sprays, dust, vapors)

Self-Management Skills

- Recognize signs and symptoms of worsening asthma.

- Take medicines appropriately.

- Use peak flow meters appropriately.

- Monitor response to medications.

- Follow a written action plan.

- Seek medical treatment as needed.

Part Eight

Coping with Immune Disease

Chapter 79

Coping with Autoimmunity

When you are diagnosed with a serious chronic autoimmune disease, it is normal to question your well-being and your mental ability to cope with the life changes that are part of living successfully with any serious, chronic illness. A few basic suggestions are crucial for you to consider in order for you to manage your illness better.

- **Understand your illness and the treatment plan established by your physician.** Ask questions of your doctor about your particular condition, especially what changes and symptoms you can expect to encounter.

- **Following the treatment plan designed by your physician is vital.** If you are unsure of the treatment plan, do not be afraid to ask questions or even get a second or third opinion. Ask questions about the side effects of medications and medical tests and the effect or benefit they will have on your condition.

- **Let your doctor know if some new symptom is occurring.** Persons with chronic illness often feel that their doctors are going to think they are chronic complainers if they are honest about how they are feeling. They may worry that their doctors will simply give them more prescriptions, adding to the many medications they are already taking. Another fear patients may have is that if they complain too much, their doctors may not want them as patients. It is much better to discuss what is going on, and how it might be treated, than to worry about what the doctor will think.

- **Do not be intimidated by the medical profession.** Remember, your doctor is your partner in fighting your disease. Be honest with your doctor. You hurt only yourself if you are not up front with your physician. Play a role in your treatment plan. Once satisfied that is right for you, follow it.

- **Fatigue may accompany many of the autoimmune diseases.** Learning how to pace your activity level can put you in control of your illness. It is important to listen to your body and stop before you feel you are tired. Pacing your activity can help you sustain a relatively normal and consistent energy level. Patients often feel guilty if they slow their pace, and therefore rest only when they are not feeling well or are very tired. This forced rest period can last a few days and patients then try to catch up and accomplish all they were unable to do during the time they were resting. The cycle of high activity and prolonged rest periods can interfere with managing of the disease process and, with some autoimmune diseases, create a need for more medication to control the symptoms that accompany those illnesses. By learning to spread out your work load, you will be able to accomplish as much while feeling better both physically and emotionally.

- **If you have an autoimmune disease that requires a special diet, following this diet is very important.** Doing so can play a major role in the management of your illness and your sense of well-being. Learning the ins and outs of nutrition and healthy food preparation puts you in control of your diet and leads to better management of your disease.

- **You can expect to have a variety of emotional responses.** Typically, newly diagnosed patients feel the anger, denial, bargaining, depression, and acceptance cycle identified by Kubler-Ross as a response to coping with a significant loss and major life changes. You may feel isolated from others and experience fear of the unknown future.

- **Understanding these responses and their causes will help you determine what works best for you in overcoming**

them. Be open and forthright with those around you. It is important that you do not blame everything that goes wrong on your illness.

- **Use "I" messages with others.** If you are not feeling well, say "I'm not feeling well, and I could really use your support." "You" messages are usually interpreted defensively, and get in the way of the real issue which is your need for support. It is okay to lean upon your support system.

- **Chronic illness often has so many ups and downs that it can be emotionally draining.** How you handle this emotional roller coaster is very important and personal. Some of the techniques may involve: trying to keep up a normal life-style, pacing yourself and your activities, using relaxation techniques, covering up your pain, and joining support groups. You must find out what works best for you. Understanding that your emotional state, and trying to cope, can be fatiguing in themselves is a step in the right direction.

- **Give yourself and your family time to adjust.** Nobody adjusts overnight to something that may significantly impact on the rest of his or her life. Viewing life with a serious illness as one more of life's challenges is helpful. Understanding that you might experience feelings of worthlessness, depression, anger, and self-pity, and that it is normal to experience these feelings, helps you master coping techniques.

- **Joining a support group for persons with chronic illness is very helpful to many patients.** Professional counseling may be in order if you are unable to cope in spite of every effort to do so.

- **Understand that you did nothing to cause your illness and that life is not always fair.** Bad things do happen to almost everyone at sometime in a lifetime. It is how we deal with these life changes that makes the difference between a life of coping and a life of moping.

- **Dealing with the emotional aspect of having a chronic illness is a challenge.** Often the unpredictability of a serious illness makes you feel out of control of your life and well-being. This can cause anxiety for both you and your family.

Chapter 80

Caring for People with Immune Disorders

Kathy Antilla was very concerned about her son Isaac when he began to battle infection after infection shortly after his birth. No one could tell her why. When Isaac turned five, he was finally diagnosed with common variable immune deficiency (CVID), a rare and chronic immune deficiency disease, which would affect Isaac for the rest of his life. At first Kathy was thrilled that the doctors had a diagnosis; however, she was terrified because she had no idea what this meant for Isaac's future.

Coping with a primary immune deficiency disease or an immune disorder is difficult not only for the person with the illness, but also for the people who love and want to care for that person. It is not always easy to know how best to care for a loved one in a way that will make life enjoyable for the caregiver, the individual, and everyone else involved. An important idea to remember is that with adjustment and time, anybody—a spouse, parent, grandparent, or child—can learn how to become a successful caregiver.

Kathy, along with other caregivers, learned that it was normal to feel scared, overwhelmed, and helpless when Isaac was diagnosed with an immune deficiency. One of the best ways she learned to overcome these feelings was by becoming proactive in understanding the diagnosis and treatment. She began to research the disease in books, on the Internet, and by making a list of questions to ask Isaac's experienced

"Strategies for Caregiving: Developing Coping Mechanisms through Self-Understanding," *IDF Advocate*, Spring 2004. Copyright © 2004 The Immune Deficiency Foundation. Reprinted with permission.

doctors. Kathy also began reading about the Immune Deficiency Foundation. There she found people educated in primary immune deficiency diseases who were able to talk to her about many of her concerns. Through research, caregivers can discover if there are alternative treatments or delivery methods for therapies. Caregivers can also find ways to make the individual feel more comfortable.

Gail Moore, a primary caregiver to her daughter, Kinsey, describes how she and her daughter had fun making art projects and cards for the nurses and doctors in the hospital. For Gail, developing a relationship with her doctors helped her recognize that she was capable of understanding the disease, and that there were people who wanted to help. Developing a good relationship with the person's immunologist and with the nurses administering therapy helps caregivers and those for whom they are giving care feel more comfortable and better equipped to cope with the disease.

Keeping records and staying organized also helps a caregiver to maintain a sense of control. Caregivers often keep a file and update their medical records such as lab results, hospital summaries, and physician summaries. Kathy has kept an extensive binder with all letters, lab results, orthopedic records, and local and regional hospital information since Isaac's birth. She says that it is really important for her to be organized because she can hold doctors and nurses accountable for their actions, and can also provide doctors and nurses with pertinent, up-to-date medical information on her son's history when necessary.

If a patient is undergoing treatment, the best way to track recovery is to keep a log. For example, many caregivers keep an infusion log of the date and time of the last infusion. This log also includes lot numbers of the product, which can be helpful in the event of a product recall. Also, caregivers can manage their finances by tracking medical bills and insurance statements. Kathy hopes that her son will see the work she puts into his disease management, and that one day he will learn to do the same for himself.

By staying organized, caregivers also develop good time management skills. Tools that assist in time management include taking charge, delegating, and prioritizing schedules. They think about what is most important to get done today, what can wait for tomorrow, and they are not afraid to say no. Successful caregivers remember not to sweat the small stuff.

Maintaining a positive attitude is essential to becoming a good caregiver says Melissa Schweitzer, Director of Patient Advocacy at the Immune Deficiency Foundation. Melissa, who also is diagnosed with

CVID, understands that caregivers should concentrate on what they can do instead of what they cannot do, and that they should appreciate their good days. However, sometimes they have to say to themselves, "My body doesn't always do what I want, but my brain is still working and I'm still able to love, and together that helps me have the kind of life I enjoy." Developing a sense of humor and thinking of ways to bring laughter and fun into life is a great idea. Melissa also suggests planning something to look forward to after treatments. For example, going out to dinner or lunch after a doctor or infusion appointment can make managing the disease seem like less of a chore.

Overall, good caregivers must have realistic expectations and strength. When things get tough they need to accept that everyone experiences some sorrow or misfortune in life. Melissa's volunteer work at a Ronald McDonald home and a soup kitchen for the homeless is helpful to her despite her illness. Melissa also advises to think positively about the disease by listing all the positive aspects of taking care of a chronic illness. For example, being a good caregiver gives one a better understanding for others experiencing similar situations or difficulties. It also helps one to build personal strength to help them cope with other difficult challenges that may arise in the future.

Emphasizing the normalities of life, rather than dwelling on the illness, helps those individuals with a primary immune deficiency learn how to lead normal lives. Caregivers can encourage the person to go after their dreams, and help them find ways to successfully achieve those goals. Gail Moore advises other primary caregivers to live for today. As a parent, Gail allows her daughter to lead as much of a normal life as possible. Today, Kinsey is an honor student at her local school and a competitive gymnast. She is also active in church activities, chorus, dance, soccer, and community service.

However, a caregiver also needs to acknowledge that at times, coping with a primary immune deficiency disease or immune disorder is overwhelming and difficult. Once in a while it is okay to give in to the emotions that go along with this, and they should allow themselves to feel this way. Melissa described growing up with CVID and how hard it was for her to miss so much school because her classmates had difficulty understanding that she just was not feeling well. "I had to tell them that yes, I have this disease, and I just can't always do everything they can," she said.

Also, caregivers should not be afraid of getting support from others who want to help or may be dealing with the same illness. Caregivers need to remember that they are not alone. Kathy says that even giving support can be helpful because talking to other people who are dealing with this disease helps her see how far she has come. Caregivers need to give themselves credit for the challenges with which they cope.

Most importantly, caregivers allow some time to relax once in a while so they can re-energize. A caregiver should not get too caught up in taking care of another person. At least once a day they should make plans to get out of the house and exercise, go out for lunch or coffee with a friend, or take a relaxing bath. Caregivers should realize that they must always take care of themselves in order to best care for their loved one.

Primary immune deficiencies and immune disorders are life-long chronic disorders, with unpredictable periods of more acute illness. As a result, caregivers may live with constant stress, punctuated by periods of major illness and disruption. At these times, in particular, it can be very important to have learned skills that enable resilience, or the ability to bounce back from adversity. According to Reginald Nettles, Ph.D., founder of Psychological and Professional Coach Services in Columbia, Maryland, flexibility and balance in one's day-to-day life are key factors in resilience. Dr. Nettles says, "Close relationships with supportive family members and friends, and the ability to experience and express strong emotions are essential. Although it is not healthy to dwell on sadness and grief, it is important to be able to face these feelings honestly when they occur." Joy can arise in life with a chronic illness, but usually not without facing the unhappy feelings when necessary. It should also be noted that professional help can be very beneficial when stress, anxiety, and depression interfere with normal activities.

Each of the individuals mentioned in this chapter describes some of the ways they have managed their lives with primary immune deficiency disease (PIDD) or as caregivers of people with PIDD. No single strategy works for all people. It is therefore essential for caregivers to take time out to develop the self-understanding needed to learn what works for them.

Chapter 81

Students with Chronic Illnesses: Guidance for Families, Schools, and Students

Chronic illnesses affect at least 10 to 15 percent of American children. Responding to the needs of students with chronic conditions, such as asthma, allergies, diabetes, immune disease, and epilepsy (also known as seizure disorders) in the school setting requires a comprehensive, coordinated, and systematic approach. Students with chronic health conditions can function to their maximum potential if their needs are met. The benefits to students can include better attendance; improved alertness and physical stamina; fewer symptoms; fewer restrictions on participation in physical activities and special activities, such as field trips; and fewer medical emergencies. Schools can work together with parents, students, health care providers, and the community to provide a safe and supportive educational environment for students with chronic illnesses and to ensure that students with chronic illnesses have the same educational opportunities as do other students.

Family's Responsibilities

- Notify the school of the student's health management needs and diagnosis when appropriate. Notify schools as early as possible and whenever the student's health needs change.

- Provide a written description of the student's health needs at school, including authorizations for medication administration

"Students with Chronic Illnesses: Guidance for Families, Schools, and Students," National Heart, Lung, and Blood Institute (NHLBI), 2003.

and emergency treatment, signed by the student's health care provider.

- Participate in the development of a school plan to implement the student's health needs:

  - Meet with the school team to develop a plan to accommodate the student's needs in all school settings.

  - Authorize appropriate exchange of information between school health program staff and the student's personal health care providers.

  - Communicate significant changes in the student's needs or health status promptly to appropriate school staff.

- Provide an adequate supply of student's medication in pharmacy-labeled containers and other supplies to the designated school staff, and replace medications and supplies as needed. This supply should remain at school.

- Provide the school with a means of contacting you or another responsible person at all times in case of an emergency or medical problem.

- Educate the student to develop age-appropriate self-care skills.

- Promote good general health, personal care, nutrition, and physical activity.

School District's Responsibilities

- Develop and implement districtwide guidelines and protocols applicable to chronic illnesses generally with specific protocols for asthma, allergies, diabetes, epilepsy (seizure disorders), and other common chronic illnesses of students.

- Guidelines should include safe, coordinated practices (as age and skill level appropriate) that enable the student to successfully manage his or her health in the classroom and at all school-related activities.

- Protocols should be consistent with established standards of care for students with chronic illnesses and Federal laws that provide protection to students with disabilities, including ensuring confidentiality of student health care information and appropriate information sharing.

- Protocols should address education of all members of the school environment about chronic illnesses, including a component addressing the promotion of acceptance and the elimination of stigma surrounding chronic illnesses.

- Develop, coordinate, and implement necessary training programs for staff that will be responsible for chronic illness care tasks at school and school-related activities.

- Monitor schools for compliance with chronic illness care protocols.

- Meet with parents, school personnel, and health care providers to address issues of concern about the provision of care to students with chronic illnesses by school district staff.

School's Responsibilities

- Identify students with chronic conditions, and review their health records as submitted by families and health care providers.

- Arrange a meeting to discuss health accommodations and educational aids and services that the student may need and develop a 504 Plan, Individualized Education Program (IEP), or other school plan, as appropriate. The participants should include the family, student (if appropriate), school health staff, 504/IEP coordinator (as applicable), individuals trained to assist the student, and the teacher who has primary responsibility for the student. Health care provider input may be provided in person or in writing.

- Provide nondiscriminatory opportunities to students with disabilities. Be knowledgeable about and ensure compliance with applicable Federal laws, including Americans with Disabilities Act (ADA), Individuals with Disabilities Education Act (IDEA) Section 504, and Family Educational Rights and Privacy Act of 1974 (FERPA). Be knowledgeable about any State or local laws or district policies that affect the implementation of students' rights under Federal law.

- Clarify the roles and obligations of specific school staff, and provide education and communication systems necessary to ensure that students' health and educational needs are met in a safe and coordinated manner.

- Implement strategies that reduce disruption in the student's school activities, including physical education, recess, offsite events, extracurricular activities, and field trips.

- Communicate with families regularly and as authorized with the student's health care providers.

- Ensure that the student receives prescribed medications in a safe, reliable, and effective manner and has access to needed medication at all times during the school day and at school-related activities.

- Be prepared to handle health needs and emergencies and to ensure that there is a staff member available who is properly trained to administer medications or other immediate care during the school day and at all school-related activities, regardless of time or location.

- Ensure that all staff who interact with the student on a regular basis receive appropriate guidance and training on routine needs, precautions, and emergency actions.

- Provide appropriate health education to students and staff.

- Provide a safe and healthy school environment.

- Ensure that case management is provided as needed.

- Ensure proper record keeping, including appropriate measures to both protect confidentiality and to share information.

- Promote a supportive learning environment that views students with chronic illnesses the same as other students except to respond to health needs.

- Promote good general health, personal care, nutrition, and physical activity.

Student's Responsibilities

- Notify an adult about concerns and needs in managing his or her symptoms or the school environment.

- Participate in the care and management of his or her health as appropriate to his or her developmental level.

Chapter 82

Immunization Recommendations for People with a Weakened Immune System

This chapter summarizes current recommendations by the Advisory Committee on Immunization Practices (ACIP) on the use of active and passive immunization for persons with altered immunocompetence. These recommendations are for use in the United States and its territories and are appropriate for the epidemiologic setting and program priorities of these areas. Other organizations, particularly the Expanded Program on Immunization of the World Health Organization, have made different recommendations, particularly with respect to the use of oral polio vaccine (OPV) and Bacille Calmette-Guérin (BCG) for immunocompromised persons. Those recommendations are appropriate for populations, particularly in developing countries, with higher risks of exposure to wild polio virus infection and tuberculosis.

Summary of Principles for Vaccinating Immunocompromised Persons

The degree to which an individual patient is immunocompromised should be determined by a physician. Severe immunosuppression can

Excerpted from "Recommendations of the Advisory Committee on Immunization Practices (ACIP): Use of Vaccines and Immune Globulins in Persons with Altered Immunocompetence," *Morbidity and Mortality Weekly Report* 1993:42 (No. RR-4), Centers for Disease Control and Prevention (CDC). These recommendations of the Advisory Committee on Immunization Practices are updated as new data dictates and are deemed current by the CDC as of March 2005.

be due to a variety of conditions, including congenital immunodeficiency, human immunodeficiency virus (HIV) infection, leukemia, lymphoma, generalized malignancy, or therapy with alkylating agents, antimetabolites, radiation, or large amounts of corticosteroids. For some of these conditions, all affected persons will be severely immunocompromised; for others, such as HIV infection, the spectrum of disease severity due to disease or treatment stage will determine the degree to which the immune system is compromised. The responsibility for determining whether a patient is severely immunocompromised ultimately lies with the physician.

Killed or inactivated vaccines do not represent a danger to immunocompromised persons and generally should be administered as recommended for healthy persons. For specific immunocompromising conditions (e.g., asplenia), such patients may be at higher risk for certain diseases, and additional vaccines, particularly bacterial polysaccharide vaccines {*Haemophilus influenzae* type b (Hib), pneumococcal, and meningococcal}, are recommended for them. Frequently, the immune response of immunocompromised persons to these vaccine antigens is not as good as that of immunocompetent persons; higher doses or more frequent boosters may be required, although even with these modifications, the immune response may be suboptimal.

Steroid therapy usually does not contraindicate administration of live-virus vaccines when such therapy is short-term (less than 2 weeks); low to moderate dose; long-term, alternate-day treatment with short-acting preparations; maintenance physiologic doses (replacement therapy); or administered topically (skin or eyes), by aerosol, or by intra-articular, bursal, or tendon injection. The exact amount of systemic corticosteroids and the duration of their administration needed to suppress the immune system of an otherwise healthy child are not well defined. The immunosuppressive effects of steroid treatment vary, but many clinicians consider a dose equivalent to either 2 milligrams/kilogram (mg/kg) of body weight or a total of 20 mg/day of prednisone as sufficiently immunosuppressive to raise concern about the safety of immunization with live-virus vaccines. Corticosteroids used in greater than physiologic doses also may reduce the immune response to vaccines. Physicians should wait at least 3 months after discontinuation of therapy before administering a live-virus vaccine to patients who have received high dose, systemic steroids for greater than or equal to 2 weeks.

Specific Immunocompromising Conditions

For practical considerations, persons with immunocompromising conditions may be divided into three groups:

A. Persons who are severely immunocompromised not as a result of HIV infection.

B. Persons with HIV infection.

C. Persons with conditions that cause limited immune deficits (e.g., asplenia, renal failure) that may require use of special vaccines or higher doses of vaccines, but that do not contraindicate use of any particular vaccine.

These groups differ primarily in the recommendations for use of live-virus vaccines, which are contraindicated for all persons in group A, for some vaccines and some persons in group B, and are not contraindicated in group C.

A. Severely Immunocompromised, Not HIV-Infected Persons

Severe immunosuppression not associated with HIV can be the result of congenital immunodeficiency, leukemia, lymphoma, generalized malignancy, or therapy with alkylating agents, antimetabolites, radiation, or large amounts of corticosteroids.[1-3] Virus replication after administration of live, attenuated-virus vaccines can be enhanced in severely immunocompromised persons.[4-6] In general, these patients should not be administered live vaccines, with the exceptions noted later. In addition, OPV should not be administered to any household contact of a severely immunocompromised person. Measles-mumps-rubella (MMR) vaccine is not contraindicated for the close contacts (including health care providers) of immunocompromised persons.

Persons with leukemia in remission who have not received chemotherapy for at least 3 months are not considered severely immunosuppressed for the purpose of receiving live-virus vaccines.[7] When cancer chemotherapy or immunosuppressive therapy is being considered (e.g., for patients with Hodgkin disease or organ transplantation), vaccination ideally should precede the initiation of chemotherapy or immunosuppression by greater than or equal to 2 weeks. Vaccination during chemotherapy or radiation therapy should be avoided because antibody responses are suboptimal. Patients vaccinated while on immunosuppressive therapy or in the 2 weeks before starting therapy should be considered unimmunized and should be revaccinated at least 3 months after discontinuation of therapy.

Passive immunoprophylaxis with immune globulins may be indicated for immunocompromised persons instead of or in addition to vaccination. When exposed to a vaccine-preventable disease such as measles, severely immunocompromised children should be considered susceptible regardless of their history of vaccination.

B. HIV-Infected Persons

In general, persons known to be HIV-infected should not receive live-virus or live-bacteria vaccines. However, evaluation and testing for HIV infection of asymptomatic persons are not necessary before decisions concerning vaccination with live-virus vaccines are made. Limited studies of MMR vaccination among both asymptomatic and symptomatic HIV-infected patients have not documented serious or unusual adverse events.[8] Therefore, MMR vaccination is recommended for all children and for adults when otherwise indicated, regardless of their HIV status. Enhanced inactivated polio vaccine (eIPV) is the preferred polio vaccine for persons known to have HIV infection. Pneumococcal vaccine is indicated for all HIV-infected persons greater than or equal to 2 years of age. Children less than 2 years of age with known HIV infection should receive Hib vaccine according to the routine schedule. Clinicians deciding whether to administer Hib vaccine to HIV-infected persons should take into consideration the individual patient's risk of Hib disease and the effectiveness of the vaccine for these persons. In some settings, the incidence of Hib disease may be higher among HIV-infected adults than adults not HIV-infected,[9, 10] and the disease can be severe in these patients.

In general, symptomatic HIV-infected children and adults have suboptimal immunologic responses to vaccines.[8, 11-15] The response to both live and killed antigens may decrease as the HIV disease progresses. However, the response to higher doses of vaccine and the persistence of antibody in HIV-infected patients have not been systematically evaluated. Although higher doses or more frequent boosters may be considered for these patients, firm recommendations cannot be made at this time.

C. Medical Conditions Associated Only with Special Indications for Vaccines

Certain medical conditions, such as renal failure, diabetes, alcoholic cirrhosis, or asplenia may increase the patient's risk for certain diseases. Some antigens, particularly bacterial polysaccharide vaccines, are recommended for such patients. Frequently, the immune response of these patients to these antigens is not as good as that of immunocompetent persons, and higher doses or more frequent boosters may be required. Persons with these conditions are generally not considered immunosuppressed for the purposes of vaccination and should receive routine vaccinations with both live and inactivated vaccines according to the usual schedules.

Renal Failure

Patients with renal failure have an increased risk of infection with a variety of pathogens, particularly *pneumococcus* and hepatitis B.[16-19] The efficacy of pneumococcal vaccination for some of these patients, including those on dialysis, may be considerably lower than for immunocompetent patients,[20, 21] their antibody levels may be lower,[22] and they may require repeat vaccination,[23, 24] or an increased dose of vaccine. Because secondary antibody responses are less affected than primary antibody responses, immunization strategies should be formulated early in the course of progressive renal disease. This approach is particularly important if transplantation and chronic immunosuppressive therapy are being considered. Nephrotic syndrome is the renal disease most clearly associated with an increased risk for pneumococcal infection.

Diabetes

Although several in vitro tests of immunologic function are known to be abnormal among diabetic patients, these defects may be of little clinical importance. However, because patients with longstanding diabetes mellitus often have cardiovascular, renal, and other organ dysfunction, one-time pneumococcal vaccination and annual influenza vaccination are recommended. Pneumococcal vaccine is safe and effective for these patients and does not interfere with insulin levels or glucose control.[25, 26] Patients receiving either insulin or oral antidiabetic agents respond normally to influenza vaccination without impairment of diabetic control.[27]

Specific Considerations for Live, Attenuated Vaccines

Measles-Mumps-Rubella (MMR, MR, M, R) Vaccine

MMR vaccine should not be administered to severely immuno-compromised persons. For HIV-infected children, MMR should routinely be administered at 15 months of age. MMR should be considered for all symptomatic HIV-infected persons who would otherwise be eligible for measles vaccine, since measles can affect these patients severely.[28] Evaluation and testing for HIV infection of asymptomatic children are not necessary before decisions concerning immunization with live-virus vaccines are made. Limited studies of MMR vaccination among both asymptomatic and symptomatic HIV-infected patients have not documented serious or unusual adverse events.[8] If there is risk of exposure to measles, single-antigen measles vaccine should be administered at 6–11 months of age with a second dose (of MMR) at greater than 12 months of age. Severely immunocompromised patients and symptomatic HIV-infected patients who are exposed to measles should receive immune globulin (IG), regardless of prior vaccination status. The recommended dose of IG for measles prophylaxis of immunocompromised persons is 0.5 mL/kg of body weight (maximum dose, 15 mL). The immunogenicity of measles vaccine is decreased if vaccine is administered less than 6 months after IG.

Oral Polio Vaccine (OPV)

OPV should not be used to immunize immunocompromised patients, their household contacts, or nursing personnel in close contact with such patients; eIPV is recommended for such persons. Immuno-compromised patients may be unable to limit replication of vaccine virus effectively, and administration of OPV to children with congenital immunodeficiency has resulted in severe, progressive neurologic involvement.[29-32] Although a protective immune response to eIPV in the immunocompromised patient cannot be assured, the vaccine is safe and may confer some protection. If OPV is inadvertently administered to a household or intimate contact (regardless of prior immunization status) of an immunocompromised patient, close contact between the patient and the recipient of OPV should be avoided for approximately 1 month after vaccination, the period of maximum excretion of vaccine virus. Because of the possibility of immunodeficiency in other children born to a family in which there has been one such case, OPV should not be administered to a member of a household in which there is a history of inherited immunodeficiency until the immune status of the recipient and other children in the family is documented. Although OPV has not been harmful when administered to asymptomatic HIV-infected children,[8] eIPV is the vaccine of choice for a child who is known to be infected. Evaluation and testing for HIV infection of asymptomatic children are not necessary before decisions concerning immunization with live-virus vaccines are made.

Bacille Calmette-Guérin (BCG)

BCG vaccine is not routinely recommended for use in the United States for prevention of tuberculosis (TB). BCG vaccine is strongly recommended for infants and children with negative tuberculin skin tests who are:

- At high risk of intimate and prolonged exposure to persistently untreated or ineffectively treated patients with infectious pulmonary TB, cannot be removed from the source of exposure, and cannot be placed on long-term preventive therapy.

- Continuously exposed to persons with TB who have bacilli resistant to isoniazid and rifampin. BCG is also recommended for tuberculin-negative infants and children in groups in which the rate of new infections exceeds 1% per year and for whom the usual surveillance and treatment programs have been attempted but are not operationally feasible.

BCG should be administered with caution to persons in groups at high risk for HIV infection or persons known to be severely immunocompromised. Although limited data suggest that the vaccine may be safe for use for asymptomatic children infected with HIV,[33] BCG vaccination is not recommended for HIV-infected adults or for persons with symptomatic disease.[34-36] Until further research can clearly define the risks and benefits of BCG vaccination for this population, vaccination should be restricted to persons at exceptionally high risk for tuberculosis infection. HIV-infected persons thought to be infected with *M. tuberculosis* should be strongly recommended for tuberculosis preventive therapy.

Typhoid Vaccine

Live, attenuated TY21a typhoid vaccine should not be administered to immunocompromised persons, including those known to be infected with HIV. Parenteral inactivated vaccine is a theoretically safer alternative for this group.

Yellow Fever Vaccine

Yellow fever vaccine virus poses a theoretical risk of encephalitis to those with severe immunosuppression or known HIV infection, and such patients should not receive the vaccine. If travel to an area endemic for yellow fever is necessary, patients should be advised of the risk, instructed in methods for avoiding vector mosquitos, and supplied with vaccination waiver letters by their physicians. Persons who are known to be HIV infected and who cannot avoid potential exposure to yellow fever virus should be offered the choice of vaccination. Vaccinees should be monitored for possible adverse effects. Since the vaccination of such persons may be less effective than that for non-HIV-infected persons, it may be desirable to measure their neutralizing antibody responses before travel. (For these tests, contact the appropriate state health department or CDC). Family members of immunosuppressed persons who themselves have no contraindications may receive yellow fever vaccine.

Vaccinia

The only persons for whom vaccinia vaccine is recommended are laboratory personnel working with Orthopoxviruses and certain health care workers involved in clinical trials of vaccinia recombinant vaccines. Vaccinia should not be administered to severely immunocompromised persons or those with symptomatic HIV infection. Disseminated vaccinia has been reported in a military recruit with HIV infection.[37]

Killed or Inactivated Vaccines

Diphtheria-Tetanus-Pertussis (DTP, DTaP, DT, Td)

For children who are severely immunocompromised or who are infected with HIV, DTP vaccine is indicated in the same schedule and dose as for immunocompetent children, including the use of acellular pertussis-containing vaccines (DTaP) as a booster. Although no specific studies with pertussis vaccine are available, if immunosuppressive therapy is to be discontinued shortly it would be reasonable to defer immunization until at least 3 months after the patient last received therapy; otherwise, the patient should be vaccinated while still receiving therapy.

Enhanced Inactivated Polio Vaccine (eIPV)

If polio immunization is indicated, immunocompromised infants, their household members, nursing personnel in close contact, and other close contacts should receive eIPV rather than OPV. For unvaccinated adults at increased risk of exposure to poliovirus, a primary series of enhanced-potency eIPV is recommended. This recommendation applies to both immunologically normal and immunocompromised adults.

Haemophilus influenzae Type B Conjugate Vaccine (Hib)

Immunocompromised children should receive Hib conjugate vaccines in the same dosage and schedule as for immunocompetent children. Unimmunized children greater than or equal to 5 years of age with a chronic illness known to be associated with increased risk of *Haemophilus influenzae* Type b disease, specifically, persons with anatomic or functional asplenia or sickle-cell anemia or those who have undergone splenectomy, should receive Hib vaccine. One dose may be insufficient to induce immunity in children greater than 5 years of age with sickle cell disease, but the data are insufficient to recommend whether persons suffering from this or other immunosuppressive disorders should receive more than one dose. Clinicians deciding whether to administer Hib vaccine to HIV-infected persons should take into consideration the individual patient's risk of Hib disease and the effectiveness of the vaccine for these persons. In some settings, the incidence of Hib disease may be higher among HIV-infected adults than non-HIV-infected adults,[9, 10] and the disease can be severe in these patients. Patients with Hodgkin disease should be vaccinated at least 2 weeks before the initiation of chemotherapy or, if this is not possible, greater than or equal to 3 months after the end of chemotherapy. Hib vaccine can be administered simultaneously with pneumococcal or meningococcal vaccine in separate syringes at different sites.

Influenza Vaccine

Because influenza may result in serious illness and complications for immunocompromised persons, vaccination is recommended and may result in protective antibody levels in many immunocompromised recipients.[38] Influenza vaccine is recommended for children with symptomatic HIV infection. However, the antibody response to vaccine may be low in persons with advanced HIV-related illnesses; a booster dose of vaccine has not been shown to improve the immune response for these persons.[39] There is currently little information regarding the frequency and severity of influenza illness in HIV-infected persons.[40]

Patients with chronic renal failure should receive annual influenza immunization. Uremic patients on chronic hemodialysis may often have an impaired but adequate antibody response to influenza vaccination.[41-43] Antibody response in renal transplant patients after influenza immunization is lower in those receiving cyclosporine A than in those on azathioprine.[44, 45] Amantadine prophylaxis or treatment also should be considered during periods of increased type A influenza activity in the community. However, strict attention must be given to administering reduced doses of amantadine to patients with renal failure.

Pneumococcal Vaccine

Pneumococcal vaccine is recommended for use in persons greater than or equal to 2 years of age with chronic illnesses specifically associated with increased risk of pneumococcal disease or its complications (e.g., anatomic or functional asplenia, including sickle cell disease; nephrotic syndrome; cerebrospinal fluid leaks; and conditions associated with immunosuppression, including HIV infection).[46] Revaccination after 3–5 years should be considered for children with nephrotic syndrome, asplenia, or sickle cell anemia who would be less than or equal to 10 years old at revaccination.

Pneumococcal vaccine is recommended for use in immunocompetent adults who are at increased risk of pneumococcal disease or its complications because of chronic illness (e.g., cardiovascular disease, pulmonary disease, diabetes mellitus, alcoholism, cirrhosis, or cerebrospinal fluid leaks). Vaccination is also recommended for immunocompromised adults at increased risk of pneumococcal disease or its complications (e.g., persons with splenic dysfunction or anatomic asplenia, Hodgkin disease, leukemia, lymphoma, multiple myeloma, chronic renal failure, nephrotic syndrome, or conditions such as organ transplantation associated with immunosuppression). Revaccination should be strongly considered greater than or equal to 6 years after the first dose for those patients at highest risk of fatal pneumococcal infection (e.g., asplenic patients) or for those at highest risk of rapid decline in antibody levels (e.g., those with chronic renal failure, nephrotic syndrome, or transplanted organs).

Hepatitis B Vaccine

Hepatitis B vaccination is recommended for susceptible hemodialysis patients. Although response to hepatitis B vaccine is lower in hemodialysis patients than in healthy persons, for those patients who do respond, hepatitis B vaccine will protect them from hepatitis B virus infection and reduce the necessity for frequent serologic screening.[47] Hepatitis B vaccine is also indicated for patients whose renal disease is likely to lead to dialysis or transplantation. Such patients are at increased risk for hepatitis B because of their need for blood products and hemodialysis. Patients with uremia who were vaccinated before they required dialysis have been shown to have higher seroconversion rates and antibody titers.[48] The response may also be better in children.[49] In addition, periodic booster doses are usually necessary following successful immunization, with their timing determined by serologic testing at 12 month intervals.

For patients undergoing hemodialysis and for other immunosuppressed patients, higher vaccine doses or increased number of doses are required. A special formulation of one vaccine is now available for such persons (Recombivax HB, 40 µg/mL). Persons with HIV infection have an impaired response to hepatitis B vaccine. The immunogenicity of higher doses of vaccine is unknown for this group, and firm recommendations on dosage cannot be made at this time.[50] The antihepatitis B response of such persons should be tested after they are vaccinated, and those who have not responded should be revaccinated with 1–3 additional doses.

Meningococcal Vaccine

Routine immunization with the quadrivalent vaccine is recommended for certain high-risk groups, including persons with terminal complement component deficiencies and those with anatomic or functional asplenia. Persons splenectomized because of trauma or nonlymphoid tumors and those with inherited complement deficiencies have acceptable antibody responses to meningococcal vaccine, although its clinical efficacy has not been documented in these patients.

Rabies Vaccine

Corticosteroids, other immunosuppressive agents, and immunosuppressive illnesses can interfere with the development of active immunity and predispose the patient to developing rabies if exposed.

Immunosuppressive agents should not be administered during post-exposure therapy, unless essential for the treatment of other conditions. When rabies post-exposure prophylaxis is administered to persons receiving steroids or other immunosuppressive therapy, it is especially important that serum be tested for rabies antibody to ensure that an adequate response has developed.

Other Killed Antigens

Other vaccines containing killed antigens, including cholera, plague, and anthrax do not pose a risk to immunocompromised persons and should be used for the same indications as for immunologically normal persons.

Immune Globulin (IG)

Immunocompromised persons may benefit from protection by passive immunization. For immunocompromised persons, IG is indicated to prevent measles following exposure. If immediate protection against measles is required for immunocompromised persons with contraindications to measles vaccination, including exposed infants less than 1 year of age, passive immunization with IG, 0.5 mL/kg of body weight (maximum dose = 15 mL), should be administered intramuscularly as soon as possible after exposure. Exposed symptomatic HIV-infected and other severely immunocompromised persons should receive IG regardless of their previous vaccination status, because measles vaccine may not be effective in such patients and the disease may be severe. For immunocompromised persons, the recommended dose is 0.5 mL/kg of body weight if IG is administered intramuscularly (maximum dose = 15 mL). This corresponds to a dose of protein of approximately 82.5 mg/kg (maximum dose = 2,475 milligrams [mg]). Intramuscular IG may not be necessary if a patient with HIV infection is receiving 100–400 mg/kg IGIV at regular intervals and the last dose was administered within 3 weeks of exposure to measles. Because the amounts of protein administered are similar, high-dose IGIV may be as effective as IG administered intramuscularly. However, no data are available concerning the effectiveness of IGIV in preventing measles.

For immunocompromised persons receiving IG for measles prophylaxis (0.50 mL/kg [82 mg/kg] intramuscularly), measles vaccination should be delayed for 6 months following IG administration. For persons receiving IG for replacement of humoral immune deficiencies

(320 mg/kg intravenously), measles vaccination should be delayed until 8 months following IG administration.

For the prevention of hepatitis A, IG should be administered in the same dose and schedule to both immunocompromised and immunocompetent persons.

Varicella-Zoster Immune Globulin (VZIG)

The most important use of VZIG is for passive immunization of neonates and susceptible, severely immunocompromised persons after significant exposure to chickenpox or zoster. (Significant exposure to a person with varicella is defined to include household contact, close contact indoors of greater than 1 hour, sharing the same two- to four-bed hospital room, or prolonged direct, face-to-face contact such as occurs with nurses or doctors who care for the patient.[51]) Immunocompromised patients who are exposed to varicella and receive VZIG may have lower rates of complications and infections. Varicella-susceptible pregnant women may be at higher risk for serious complications than are adults in general. Of special concern is the risk to the fetus when a woman develops varicella-zoster infection during the first half of pregnancy. Whether the fetus will be protected against development of malformations if VZIG is administered to a pregnant, susceptible woman after exposure is unknown.

When deciding to administer VZIG to an immunocompromised patient, the clinician must determine whether the patient is likely to be susceptible and whether the exposure is likely to result in infection. The risks of VZIG administration appear to be negligible, but the costs of administration can be substantial. A physician should carefully evaluate the susceptibility of patients to varicella before administering VZIG. Both immunocompetent and immunocompromised adults and children who are believed to have had varicella on the basis of a carefully obtained history by an experienced interviewer can be considered immune. Laboratory determination of susceptibility to varicella is often impractical. Modern antibody assays may detect either nonspecific antibody or antibody levels that may not be protective.

Hepatitis B Immune Globulin (HBIG)

Immunocompromised persons should receive HBIG for the same indications (perinatal, needlestick, or sexual exposure to a person positive for hepatitis B surface antigen) and in the same doses as

577

immunocompetent persons. The HB vaccine series should be started concurrently with HBIG treatment.

Vaccinia Immune Globulin (VIG), Tetanus Immune Globulin (TIG), and Human Rabies Immune Globulin (HRIG)

Immunocompromised persons should receive VIG, TIG, and HRIG for the same indications and in the same doses as immunocompetent persons.

References

1. Infections in immunocompromised infants and children, section I. In: *Disorders of host defense*. Patrick CC, ed. New York: Churchill Livingstone, 1992.

2. Hibberd PL, Rubin RH. *Approaches to immunization in the immunocompromised host*. Infectious Disease Clinics of North America 1990; 4:123-42.

3. Vessal S, Kravis LP. Immunologic mechanisms responsible for adverse reactions to routine immunizations in children. *Clin Pediatr* 1976;15:688-96.

4. Mitus A, Holloway A, Evans AE, Enders JF. Attenuated measles vaccine in children with acute leukemia. *Am J Dis Child* 1962;103:243-8.

5. Bellini WJ, Rota JS, Greer PW, Zaki SR. Measles vaccination death in a child with severe combined immunodeficiency: report of a case. *Lab Investig* 1992;66:91A.

6. Mawhinni H, Van Allen I, Beare JM, et al. Dysgammaglobulinemia complicated by disseminated measles. *Br Med J* 1971; 2(758):380-1.

7. Committee on Infectious Diseases, American Academy of Pediatrics. *Report of the Committee on Infectious Diseases, 22nd edition*. Peter G, ed. Elk Grove, IL: American Academy of Pediatrics, 1991, p. 48.

8. Onorato IM, Markowitz LE, Oxtoby MJ. Childhood immunization, vaccine-preventable diseases and infection with human immunodeficiency virus. *Pediatr Infect Dis J* 1988;6:588-95.

9. Farley MM, Stephens DS, Brachman PS Jr, Harvey RC, Smith JD, Wenger JD. Invasive Haemophilus influenzae disease in adults. A prospective, population-based surveillance. CDC meningitis surveillance group. *Ann Intern Med* 1992;116:806-12.

10. Steinhart R, Reingold AL, Taylor F, Anderson G, Wenger JD. Invasive Haemophilus influenzae infections in men with HIV infection. *JAMA* 1992;268:3350-2.

11. Opravil M, Fierz W, Matter L, Blaser J, Luthy R. Poor antibody response after tetanus and pneumococcal vaccination in immunocompromised, HIV-infected patients. *Clin Exp Immunol* 1991;84(2):185-9.

12. Borkowsky W, Steele CJ, Grubman S, et al. Antibody responses to bacterial toxoids in children infected with human immunodeficiency virus. *J Pediatr* 1987;110:563-6.

13. Huang KL, Ruben FL, Rinaldo CR Jr, et al. Antibody responses after influenza and pneumococcal immunization in HIV-infected homosexual men. *JAMA* 1987;257:2047-50.

14. Klein RS, Selwyn PA, Maude D, et al. Responses to pneumococcal vaccine among asymptomatic heterosexual partners of persons with AIDS and intravenous drug users infected with human immunodeficiency virus. *J Infect Dis* 1989;160:826-31.

15. Vardinon N, Handsher R, Burke M, Zacut V, Yust I. Poliovirus vaccination responses in HIV-infected patients: correlation with T4 cell counts. *J Infect Dis* 1990;162:238-41.

16. Schwebke J, Mujais S. Vaccination in hemodialysis patients (editorial). *Int J Artif Organs* 1989;12:481-4.

17. Johnson DW, Fleming SJ. The use of vaccine in renal failure. *Clin Pharmacokin* 1992;22:434-46.

18. Linneman CC Jr, First MR. Risk of pneumococcal infections in renal transplant patients. *JAMA* 1979;241:2619-21.

19. Alter MJ, Farrero MS, Maynard JG. Impact of infection control strategies on the incidence of dialysis-associated hepatitis in the United States. *J Infect Dis* 1986;153:1149-51.

20. Simberkoff MS, Schiffman G, Katz LA, et al. Pneumococcal capsular polysaccharide vaccination in adult chronic hemodialysis patients. *J Lab Clin Med* 1980;96:363-70.

21. Cosio FG, Giebink GS, Le CT, Schiffman G. Pneumococcal vaccination in patients with chronic renal disease and renal allograft recipients. *Kidney Int* 1981;20:254-8.

22. Linneman CC Jr, First MR, Schiffman G. Response to pneumococcal vaccine in renal transplant and hemodialysis patients. *Arch Intern Med* 1981;141:1637-40.

23. Rytel MW, Dailey MP, Schiffman G, Hoffman RG, Piering WF. Pneumococcal vaccine immunization of patients with renal impairment. *Proc Soc Exp Biol Med* 1986;182:468-73.

24. Linneman CC Jr, First MR, Schiffman G. Revaccination of renal transplant and hemodialysis recipients with pneumococcal vaccine. *Arch Intern Med* 1986;146:1554-6.

25. Beam TR Jr, Crigler ED, Goldman JK, Schiffman G. Antibody response to polyvalent pneumococcal polysaccharide vaccine in diabetics. *JAMA* 1980;244:2621-4.

26. Lederman MM, Schiffman G, Rodman HM. Pneumococcal immunization in adult diabetics. *Diabetes* 1981;30:119-21.

27. Feery BJ, Hartman LJ, Hampson AW, Proietto J. Influenza immunization in adults with diabetes mellitus. *Diabetes Care* 1983;6:475-8.

28. Kaplan LJ, Daum RS, Smaron M, McCarthy CA. Severe measles in immunocompromised patients. *JAMA* 1992;267: 1237-41.

29. Sixbey JW. Routine immunization and the immunosuppressed child. *Adv Pediatr Infect Dis* 1987;2:79-114.

30. Wright PF, Hatch MH, Kasselberg AG, et al. Vaccine-associated poliomyelitis in a child with sex-linked agammaglobulinemia. *J Pediatr* 1977;91:408-12.

31. Wyatt HV. Poliomyelitis in hypogammaglobulinemics. *J Infect Dis* 1973;128:802-6.

Immunization Recommendations

32. Davis LE, Bodian D, Price D, Butler IJ, Vickers JH. Chronic progressive poliomyelitis secondary to vaccination of an immunodeficient child. *N Engl J Med* 1977;297:241-5.

33. Bregere P. BCG vaccination and AIDS. *Bull Int Union Tuberc Lung Dis* 1988;63:40-1.

34. Quinn TC. Interactions of the human immunodeficiency virus and tuberculosis and the implications for BCG vaccination. *Rev Infect Dis Suppl* 2, 1989;2:s379-84.

35. CDC. Disseminated Mycobacterium bovis infection from BCG vaccination of a patient with acquired immunodeficiency syndrome. *MMWR* 1985;34:227-8.

36. Ninane J, Grymonprez A, Burtonboy G, Francois A, Cornu G. Disseminated BCG in HIV infection. *Arch Dis Child* 1988;63:1268-9.

37. Redfield RR, Wright DC, James WD, et al. Disseminated vaccinia in a military recruit with human immunodeficiency virus (HIV) disease. *N Engl J Med* 1987;316:673-6.

38. Hodges GR, Davis JW, Lewis HD, et al. Response to influenza A vaccine among high-risk patients. *South Med J* 1979;72:29-32.

39. Gross PA, Lee H, Wolff JA, Hall CB, Minnefore AB, Lazicki ME. Influenza immunization in immunosuppressed children. *J Pediatr* 1978;92:30-5.

40. Safrin S, Rush JD, Mills J. Influenza in patients with human immunodeficiency virus infection. *Chest* 1990;98:33-7.

41. Cappel R, Van Beers D, Liesnard C, Dratwa M. Impaired humoral and cell-mediated immune responses in dialyzed patients after influenza vaccination. *Nephron* 1983;33:21-5.

42. Jordan MC, Rousseau WE, Tegtmeier GE, et al. Immunogenicity of inactivated influenza virus vaccine in chronic renal failure. *Ann Intern Med* 1973;79:790-4.

43. Osanloo EO, Berlin BS, Popli S, et al. Antibody responses to influenza vaccination in patients with chronic renal failure. *Kidney Int* 1978;14:614-8.

44. Huang KL, Armstrong JA, Ho M. Antibody response after influenza immunization in renal transplant patients receiving cyclosporine A or azathioprine. *Infect Immun* 1983;40:421-4.

45. Versluis DJ, Beyer We, Masurel N, Wenting GJ, Weimar W. Impairment of the immune response to influenza vaccination in renal transplant recipients by cyclosporine, but not by azathioprine. *Transplantation* 1986;42:376-9.

46. Landesman SH, Schiffman G. Assessment of the antibody response to pneumococcal vaccine in high-risk populations. *Rev Infect Dis* 1981;3:suppl:s184-97.

47. CDC. Routine screening for viral hepatitis in chronic hemodialysis centers. *Hepatitis surveillance report no. 49.* Atlanta: CDC, 1985:5-6.

48. Seaworth B, Drucker J, Starling J, et al. Hepatitis B vaccine in patients with chronic renal failure before dialysis. *J Infect Dis* 1988;157:332-7.

49. Callis LM, Clanxet J, Fortuny G, et al. Hepatitis B virus infection and vaccination in children undergoing hemodialysis. *Acta Pediatr Scand* 1985;74:213-8.

50. Collier AC, Corey L, Murphy VL, Handsfield HH. Antibody to human immunodeficiency virus (HIV) and suboptimal response to hepatitis B vaccination. *Ann Intern Med* 1988;109:101-5.

51. CDC. Update on adult immunization: recommendations of the Immunization Practices Advisory Committee (ACIP). *MMWR* 1991:41(No. RR-12):49.

Chapter 83

Recommendations for Travelers with Immune System Disorders

International travelers should be advised that some countries serologically screen incoming travelers (primarily those arriving for extended visits, such as for work or study), and deny entry to persons with acquired immunodeficiency syndrome (AIDS), and those whose test results indicate infection with human immunodeficiency virus (HIV). Moreover, travelers carrying antiretroviral medication may be denied entry to some countries. Persons who intend to visit a country for a substantial period or to work or study abroad should be informed of the policies and requirements of the particular country. This information is usually available from the consular officials of the individual nations. An unofficial list by the U.S. Department of State can be found at the following Internet address: http://www.travel.state.gov.

Specific Precautions for HIV-Infected and Severely Immunosuppressed Travelers

Primary-care providers of HIV-infected travelers should advise their patients of the need for advance travel planning. A pre-travel consultation with a travel health practitioner who provides counseling and evaluates the risk-benefit balance of preventive actions such as prophylaxis and vaccinations can minimize the avoidable risks associated with travel.

"General Information Regarding HIV and Travel," Centers for Disease Control and Prevention (CDC), July 2003.

General Concerns for Immunocompromised and HIV-Infected Travelers

- Travel, particularly to developing countries, can carry substantial risks for exposure to opportunistic pathogens for HIV-infected travelers, especially those who are severely immunosuppressed. Discussing the itinerary with a health care provider may identify area- and activity-specific risks that can be addressed.

- Patients should identify sources of medical care in the planned destination before departure and seek medical attention promptly when ill.

- Patients should verify medical insurance coverage and purchase additional travel insurance if necessary, though many policies will not cover pre-existing conditions.

- Because antiretroviral medications are not available in many parts of the world, patients should bring an adequate supply of their medications, along with copies of prescriptions. Attention should be given to refrigeration of medications. For extended visits, travelers should consult with their providers in advance regarding a plan for maintaining appropriate medical follow-up and supplies of medications.

- Avoid changes in the medication regimen shortly before travel, to ensure that no side effects or complications of a new regimen occur while traveling.

Disease Prevention and Treatment

Because immune status is the major factor influencing travel recommendations, patients should have their disease staged before departure.

Food and Waterborne Diseases

During travel to developing countries, immune compromised travelers are at even higher risk for food and waterborne diseases than they are in the United States, and many enteric infections, such as those caused by *Salmonella*, *Campylobacter*, and *Cryptosporidium* can be very severe.

Dietary precautions are the cornerstone of prevention against enteric infections and infections with certain other potential opportunistic

584

pathogens. Food and beverages especially prone to contamination and that pose a greater risk for illness to immune compromised travelers include the following:

- raw or unpeeled fruits and vegetables
- raw or undercooked seafood or meat
- raw or undercooked eggs
- tap water
- ice made with tap water
- unpasteurized dairy products
- items purchased from street vendors

Food and beverages that are generally safe include the following:

- steaming hot foods
- fruits that are peeled by the traveler personally
- bottled (carbonated) beverages
- hot coffee or tea, beer, wine, or water brought to a rolling boil for at least one minute

When local sources of water must be used and boiling is not practical, certain portable water filtration units, when used in conjunction with chlorine or iodine, can increase the safety of water. Some units are available that offer the effects of iodine treatment with filtration in the same unit.

Chemoprophylaxis for HIV-Infected Travelers to Developing Countries

Prophylactic antimicrobial agents against travelers' diarrhea are not recommended routinely because of potential adverse effects and emergence of drug resistance. In certain circumstances (e.g., an important short-term trip to an area where the risk of infection is very high), the health care provider and traveler may decide that prophylactic antibiotics are warranted after the potential risks and benefits are weighed.

When prophylaxis is offered to travelers, fluoroquinolones such as ciprofloxacin (500 milligrams [mg] once a day) are the drugs of choice for nonpregnant adults, although increasing quinolone resistance in *Campylobacter jejuni* has been reported in Thailand and Southeast Asia. Quinolones are not approved for prophylaxis for children and pregnant women. Trimethoprim/sulfamethoxazole (TMP/SMX) (one double-strength tablet daily) was previously an effective prophylactic agent against travelers' diarrhea, but drug resistance is now common in many tropical areas. Travelers already taking TMP/SMX for prophylaxis against *Pneumocystis carinii* pneumonia (PCP) may receive some protection against travelers' diarrhea. However, prescribing TMP/SMX solely for diarrhea prophylaxis to HIV-infected travelers who are not already taking TMP/SMX should be considered carefully because of high rates of drug resistance in tropical areas, high rates of adverse reactions, and potential future need for the agent (e.g., for PCP treatment and prophylaxis). Use of bismuth subsalicylate should be discussed with a travel health practitioner because it confers only moderate protection and has the potential for causing adverse reactions. Total duration of any chemoprophylaxis regimen for travelers' diarrhea should not exceed 3 weeks.

Antimicrobials for Empiric Therapy

All HIV-infected travelers to developing countries should be advised to carry an antimicrobial agent with them for empiric use should diarrhea develop; one appropriate regimen is 500 mg of ciprofloxacin twice a day for 3–7 days. Alternative antibiotics (e.g., TMP/SMX, azithromycin) for empiric treatment of children and pregnant women should be considered on a case-by-case basis. Travelers should be advised to consult a physician if any of the following conditions are present: severe diarrhea that does not respond to empirical therapy, blood in the stool, fever with or without shaking chills, or dehydration. Antiperistaltic agents (e.g., diphenoxylate [Lomotil] and loperamide [Imodium]) can be used to relieve the symptoms of mild diarrhea; however, they should not be used by travelers who have high fever or blood in the stool and should be discontinued if symptoms persist longer than 48 hours. Antiperistaltic agents are not recommended for HIV-infected infants, children, or adolescents.

Other precautions. Travelers should avoid direct skin contact with soil and sand (e.g., by wearing shoes and protective clothing and using towels on beaches) in areas where fecal contamination of soil is likely.

Sexually transmitted diseases. The importance of safe sex practices should be emphasized to the immune compromised travelers to prevent sexually transmitted diseases, avoid transmission of HIV, and prevent acquisition of different HIV strains that may limit therapeutic options (e.g., non-nucleoside reverse transcriptase inhibitors are not active against HIV-2). Bringing a personal supply of condoms may be advisable, as the quality and availability of condoms can be unreliable in parts of the developing world.

Geographical Focal Infections

Health-care providers should identify other area-specific risks and instruct travelers in ways to reduce the risk of infection.

Malaria and other vector-borne diseases. Travelers should be advised to follow standard mosquito precautions, such as using insect repellents, wearing long-sleeved clothing and pants when outdoors, and sleeping in well-screened areas or with a bed net. Malaria chemoprophylaxis for HIV-infected travelers follows the same guidelines as those for seronegative persons. However, potential drug interactions between antimalarials and antiretroviral agents should be considered.

Visceral leishmaniasis (VL). VL, a protozoan infection transmitted by the bite of the sandfly, is an important opportunistic infection in HIV-infected patients. Although over 90% of the world's cases of VL occur in Bangladesh, Brazil, India, Nepal, and Sudan, most cases of VL and HIV co-infection have been reported from the Mediterranean Basin (especially Spain, France, and Italy). Clinical disease usually occurs in patients with a CD4 cell count under 200 cells/µL as a result of reactivation of latent infection, although primary infection has been reported. Treatment of VL with HIV co-infection is difficult, and relapse is common. Travelers, especially those who are immunosuppressed, should be advised to follow precautions against sandfly bites. Cutaneous leishmaniasis has rarely been reported as an opportunistic infection in HIV-infected patients.

Endemic mycoses in certain regions can also pose a substantial risk for immunocompromised and HIV-infected travelers. *Penicillium marneffei* is endemic to Southeast Asia and southern China, and clinical disease may occur after reactivation of latent infection as immunosuppression increases. Penicilliosis has occurred in AIDS patients with a remote history of only brief travel to endemic areas. Although the environmental reservoir is unknown, soil exposure is a known risk factor and should be avoided in those areas, especially during the rainy season.

Coccidioides immitis, Histoplasma capsulatum, **and** *Cryptococcus neoformans*, which cause opportunistic infections in North America, are also present in the tropics. *C. immitis* is endemic to the southwest United States, northern Mexico, and certain areas of Central and South America, while *H. capsulatum* and *C. neoformans* are distributed worldwide. Risk of infection can be minimized by avoiding exposure to disturbed soil in the Americas (*C. immitis*) and avoiding soil or dust exposure in areas likely to be contaminated heavily with bird or bat guano, such as caves or bird roosting sites (*H. capsulatum* and *C. neoformans*).

Tuberculosis. Many tropical and developing areas of the world also have high rates of tuberculosis.

Vaccine Recommendations for Travelers with Altered Immunocompetence, Including HIV

Preparation for travel should include a review and updating of routine vaccinations. At a minimum, HIV-infected adults should be current on the routinely recommended pneumococcal, diphtheria-tetanus, hepatitis B, and influenza vaccines. Influenza is a year-round infection in the tropics; in the Southern Hemisphere the influenza season is April through September. All routine immunizations for infants, children, and adolescents should also be confirmed and administered as appropriate.

In determining the need for other vaccinations, factors to consider include the immune status of the patient, risk for and severity of the disease in the destination region, and type of vaccine. In general, killed or inactivated vaccines (e.g., hepatitis A, rabies, meningococcus, hepatitis B, and Japanese encephalitis vaccines) should be administered to HIV-infected travelers as recommended for non-HIV-infected travelers. When appropriate, the inactivated forms of the polio and typhoid vaccines should be given instead of the live, attenuated forms. Most live virus vaccines are contraindicated, especially if the patient's CD4 cell count is below 200 cells/μL. The measles and yellow fever vaccines, however, are special cases in which live virus vaccination may be warranted.

Measles vaccine is a live virus vaccine that is recommended for most nonimmune travelers, given the increased severity of measles in HIV-infected patients. However, measles vaccine is not recommended for travelers who are severely immunocompromised; immune globulin should be considered for measles-susceptible, severely immunosuppressed travelers who are anticipating travel to measles-endemic countries.

Yellow fever vaccine is a live virus vaccine with uncertain safety and efficacy in HIV-infected patients. Travelers with asymptomatic HIV infection and minimal immunosuppression, as documented by laboratory tests such as CD4 cell count, who cannot avoid potential exposure to yellow fever should be offered the choice of vaccination. If travel to a yellow fever zone is necessary and immunization is not performed, travelers should be advised of the risk, instructed in methods to avoid mosquito bites, and provided a vaccination waiver letter. Patients should also be warned that vaccination waiver documents may not be accepted by some countries.

—by Laura N. Broyles, Jonathan Kaplan, Phyllis Kozarsky

Part Nine

Additional Help
and Information

Chapter 84

Glossary of
Immune System Terms

AIDS (acquired immunodeficiency syndrome): Life-threatening disease caused by the human immunodeficiency virus, which breaks down the body's immune defenses.

Adenoids: See tonsils.

Adrenal gland: A gland located on each kidney that secretes hormones regulating metabolism, sexual function, water balance, and stress.

Allergen: Any substance that causes an allergy.

Allergy: A harmful response of the immune system to normally harmless substances.

Antibodies: Molecules (also called immunoglobulins) produced by a B cell in response to an antigen. When an antibody attaches to an antigen, it helps the body destroy or inactivate the antigen.

Antigen: A substance or molecule that is recognized by the immune system. The molecule can be from foreign material such as bacteria or viruses.

Antiserum: A serum rich in antibodies against a particular microbe.

Appendix: Lymphoid organ in the intestine.

Autoantibodies: Antibodies that react against a person's own tissue.

Excerpted from "Understanding the Immune System: How It Works," National Institute of Allergy and Infectious Diseases (NIAID), NIH Publication No. 03–5423, September 2003.

Autoimmune disease: Disease that results when the immune system mistakenly attacks the body's own tissues. Examples include multiple sclerosis, type I diabetes, rheumatoid arthritis, and systemic lupus erythematosus.

B cells: Small white blood cells crucial to the immune defenses. Also know as B lymphocytes, they come from bone marrow and develop into blood cells called plasma cells, which are the source of antibodies.

Bacteria: Microscopic organisms composed of a single cell. Some cause disease.

Basophils: White blood cells that contribute to inflammatory reactions. Along with mast cells, basophils are responsible for the symptoms of allergy.

Biological response modifiers: Substances, either natural or synthesized, that boost, direct, or restore normal immune defenses. They include interferons, interleukins, thymus hormones, and monoclonal antibodies.

Blood vessels: Arteries, veins, and capillaries that carry blood to and from the heart and body tissues.

Bone marrow: Soft tissue located in the cavities of the bones. Bone marrow is the source of all blood cells.

Chemokines: Certain proteins that stimulate both specific and general immune cells and help coordinate immune responses and inflammation.

Clone: A group of genetically identical cells or organisms descended from a single common ancestor; or, to reproduce identical copies.

Complement: A complex series of blood proteins whose action complements the work of antibodies. Complement destroys bacteria, produces inflammation, and regulates immune reactions.

Complement cascade: A precise sequence of events, usually triggered by antigen antibody complexes, in which each component of the complement system is activated in turn.

Cytokines: Powerful chemical substances secreted by cells that enable the body's cells to communicate with one another. Cytokines include lymphokines produced by lymphocytes and monokine produced by monocytes and macrophages.

Cytotoxic T lymphocytes (CTL): A subset of T cells that carry the CD8 marker and can destroy body cells infected by viruses or transformed by cancer.

DNA (deoxyribonucleic acid): A long molecule found in the cell nucleus; it carries the cell's genetic information.

Enzyme: A protein produced by living cells that promotes the chemical processes of life without itself being altered.

Eosinophils: White blood cells that contain granules filled with chemicals damaging to parasites, and enzymes that affect inflammatory reactions.

Epithelial cells: Cells making up the epithelium, the covering for internal and external body surfaces.

Fungi: Members of a class of relatively primitive vegetable organisms. They include mushrooms, yeasts, rusts, molds, and smuts.

Genes: Units of genetic material (DNA) inherited from a parent. Genes carry the directions a cell uses to perform a specific function.

Graft rejection: An immune response against transplanted tissue.

Graft-versus host disease (GVHD): A life-threatening reaction in which transplanted cells attack the tissues of the recipient.

Granules: Membrane-bound organelles within cells where proteins are stored before secretion.

Granulocytes: Phagocytic white blood cells filled with granules organisms. Neutrophils, eosinophils, basophils, and mast cells are examples of granulocytes.

Growth factors: Chemicals secreted by cells that stimulate proliferation of or changes in the physical properties of other cells.

Helper T cells (Th cells): A subset of T cells that carry the CD4 surface marker and are essential for turning on antibody production, activating cytotoxic T cells, and initiating many other immune functions.

HIV (human immunodeficiency virus): The virus that causes AIDS.

Immune response: Reaction of the immune system to foreign substances.

Immunoglobulins: A family of large protein molecules, also known as antibodies, produced by B cells.

595

Immunosuppressive: Capable of reducing immune responses.

Inflammatory response: Redness, warmth, and swelling produced in response to infection, as the result of increased blood flow and an influx of immune cells and secretions.

Interferons: Proteins produced by cells that stimulate anti-virus immune responses or alter the physical properties of immune cells.

Interleukins: A major group of lymphokines and monokine.

Leukocytes: All white blood cells.

Lymph: A transparent, slightly yellow fluid that carries lymphocytes, bathes the body tissues, and drains into the lymphatic vessels.

Lymph nodes: Small bean-shaped organs of the immune system, distributed widely throughout the body and linked by lymphatic vessels. Lymph nodes are garrisons of B, T, and other immune cells.

Lymphatic vessels: A body-wide network of channels, similar to the blood vessels, which transport lymph to the immune organs and into the bloodstream.

Lymphocytes: Small white blood cells produced in the lymphoid organs and paramount in the immune defenses. B cells and T cells are lymphocytes.

Lymphoid organs: The organs of the immune system, where lymphocytes develop and congregate. They include the bone marrow, thymus, lymph nodes, spleen, and various other clusters of lymphoid tissue. Blood vessels and lymphatic vessels are also lymphoid organs.

Lymphokines: Powerful chemical substances secreted by lymphocytes. These molecules help direct and regulate the immune responses.

Macrophage: A large and versatile immune cell that devours invading pathogens and other intruders. Macrophages stimulate other immune cells by presenting them with small pieces of the invaders.

Major histocompatibility complex (MHC): A group of genes that controls several aspects of the immune response. MHC genes code for self markers on all body cells.

Mast cell: A granulocyte found in tissue. The contents of mast cells, along with those of basophils, are responsible for the symptoms of allergy.

Memory cells: A subset of T cells and B cells that have been exposed to antigens and can then respond more readily when the immune system encounters those same antigens again.

Microbes: Microscopic living organisms, including bacteria, viruses, fungi, and protozoa.

Microorganisms: Microscopic organisms, including bacteria, virus, fungi, plants, and parasites.

Molecule: The smallest amount of a specific chemical substance. Large molecules such as proteins, fats, carbohydrates, and nucleic acids are the building blocks of a cell, and a gene determines how each molecule is produced.

Monoclonal antibodies: Antibodies produced by a single cell or its identical progeny, specific for a given antigen. As tools for binding to specific protein molecules, they are invaluable in research, medicine, and industry.

Monocytes: Large phagocytic white blood cells which, when entering tissue, develop into macrophages.

Monokine: Powerful chemical substance secreted by monocytes and macrophages. These molecules help direct and regulate the immune responses.

Natural killer (NK) cells: Large granule-containing lymphocytes that recognize and kill cells lacking self antigens. Their target recognition molecules are different from T cells.

Neutrophil: White blood cell that is an abundant and important phagocyte.

Organisms: Individual living things.

Parasites: Plants or animals that live, grow, and feed on or within another living organism.

Passive immunity: Immunity resulting from the transfer of antibodies or antiserum produced by another individual.

Pathogen: A disease-causing organism.

Phagocytes: Large white blood cells that contribute to the immune defenses by ingesting microbes or other cells and foreign particles.

Phagocytosis: Process by which one cell engulfs another cell or large particle.

Plasma cells: Large antibody-producing cells that develop from B cells.

Platelet: Cellular fragment critical for blood clotting and sealing off wounds.

Serum: The clear liquid that separates from the blood when it is allowed to clot. This fluid contains the antibodies that were present in the whole blood.

Spleen: A lymphoid organ in the abdominal cavity that is an important center for immune system activities.

Stem cells: Immature cells from which all cells derive. The bone marrow is rich in stem cells, which become specialized blood cells.

T cells: Small white blood cells (also known as T lymphocytes) that recognize antigen fragments bound to cell surfaces by specialized antibody-like receptors. T stands for thymus, where T cells acquire their receptors.

T lymphocytes: See T cells.

Thymus: A primary lymphoid organ, high in the chest, where T lymphocytes proliferate and mature.

Tissue typing: See histocompatibility testing.

Tissues: Groups of similar cells joined to perform the same function.

Tolerance: A state of immune non-responsiveness to a particular antigen or group of antigens.

Tonsils and adenoids: Prominent oval masses of lymphoid tissues on either side of the throat.

Toxins: Agents produced in plants and bacteria, normally very damaging to cells.

Vaccines: Preparations that stimulate an immune response that can prevent an infection or create resistance to an infection. They do not cause disease.

Viruses: Microorganisms composed of a piece of genetic material—RNA or DNA—surrounded by a protein coat. Viruses can reproduce only in living cells.

Chapter 85

Glossary of
Autoimmune Diseases

Autoimmunity plays a role in more than 80 diseases. Following are brief descriptions of some of the many diseases in which autoimmunity may be involved.

Note: Because the specific causes of many diseases are unknown, there is debate among scientists about whether some of these are truly autoimmune diseases. Your own doctor may classify some of these diseases differently.

Alopecia areata: A disorder in which the immune system attacks the hair follicles, causing loss of hair on the scalp, face, and other parts of the body.

Ankylosing spondylitis: A rheumatic disease that causes inflamed joints in the spine and sacroiliac (the joints that connect the spine and the pelvis) and, in some people, inflamed eyes and heart valves.

Arthritis: A general term for more than 100 different diseases that affect the joints. Many forms of arthritis and related conditions are believed to have an autoimmune component.

Autoimmune hemolytic anemia: A condition in which immune system proteins attack the red blood cells, resulting in fewer of these oxygen-transporting cells.

Excerpted from "Questions and Answers about Autoimmunity," National Institute of Arthritis and Musculoskeletal and Skin Diseases (NIAMS), NIH Publication No. 02–4858, January 2002.

Autoimmune hepatitis: A disease in which the body's immune system attacks liver cells, causing inflammation. If not stopped, inflammation can lead to cirrhosis (scarring and hardening) of the liver and eventually liver failure.

Behçet disease: A condition characterized by sores in the mouth and on the genitals and by inflammation in parts of the eye. In some people, the disease also results in inflammation of the joints, digestive tract, brain, and spinal cord.

Crohn disease: An inflammatory disease of the small intestine or colon that causes diarrhea, cramps, and excessive weight loss.

Dermatomyositis: A rare autoimmune disease that causes patchy red rashes around the knuckles, eyes, and other parts of the body along with chronic inflammation of the muscles. It may occur along with other autoimmune diseases such as rheumatoid arthritis or systemic lupus erythematosus.

Diabetes mellitus, type 1: A condition in which the immune system destroys insulin-producing cells of the pancreas, making it impossible for the body to use glucose (blood sugar) for energy. Type 1 diabetes usually occurs in children and young adults.

Glomerulonephritis: Inflammation of the kidney's tiny filtering units, which in severe cases can lead to kidney failure.

Graves disease: An autoimmune disease of the thyroid gland that results in the overproduction of thyroid hormone. This causes such symptoms as nervousness, heat intolerance, heart palpitations, and unexplained weight loss.

Guillain-Barré syndrome: A disorder in which the body's immune system attacks part of the nervous system, leading to numb, weak limbs, and, in severe cases, paralysis.

Inflammatory bowel disease: The general name for diseases that cause inflammation in the intestine, the most common of which are ulcerative colitis and Crohn disease.

Lupus nephritis: Damaging inflammation of the kidneys that can occur in people with lupus. If not controlled, it may lead to total kidney failure.

Multiple sclerosis: A disease in which the immune system attacks the protective coating called myelin around the nerves. The damage affects the brain and/or spinal cord and interferes with the nerve pathways, causing muscular weakness, loss of coordination, and visual and speech problems.

Myasthenia gravis: A disease in which the immune system attacks the nerves and muscles in the neck, causing weakness and problems with seeing, chewing, and/or talking.

Myocarditis: Inflamed and degenerating muscle tissue of the heart that can cause chest pain and shortness of breath. This can lead to congestive heart failure.

Pemphigus/pemphigoid: An autoimmune disease of the skin characterized by itching and blisters.

Pernicious anemia: A deficiency of the oxygen-carrying red blood cells that often occurs in people with autoimmune diseases of the thyroid gland.

Polyarteritis nodosa: An autoimmune disease that causes inflammation of the small and medium-sized arteries. This leads to problems in the muscles, joints, intestines, nerves, kidney, and skin.

Polymyositis: A rare autoimmune disease characterized by inflamed and tender muscles throughout the body, particularly those of the shoulder and hip girdles.

Primary biliary cirrhosis: A disease that slowly destroys the bile ducts in the liver. When the ducts are damaged, bile (a substance that helps digest fat) builds up in the liver and damages liver tissue.

Psoriasis: A chronic skin disease that occurs when cells in the outer layer of the skin reproduce faster than normal and pile up on the skin's surface. This results in scaling and inflammation. An estimated 10 to 30 percent of people with psoriasis develop an associated arthritis called psoriatic arthritis.

Rheumatic fever: A disease that can occur following untreated streptococcus (strep) infection. It most often affects children, causing painful, inflamed joints, and, in some cases, permanent damage to heart valves.

Rheumatoid arthritis: A disease in which the immune system is believed to attack the linings of the joints. This results in joint pain, stiffness, swelling, and destruction.

Sarcoidosis: A disease characterized by granulomas (small growths of blood vessels, cells, and connective tissue) that can lead to problems in the skin, lungs, eyes, joints, and muscles.

Scleroderma: An autoimmune disease characterized by abnormal growth of connective tissue in the skin and blood vessels. In more severe forms, connective tissue can build up in the kidneys, lungs, heart, and gastrointestinal tract, leading in some cases to organ failure.

Sjögren syndrome: A condition in which the immune system targets the body's moisture-producing glands, leading to dryness of the eyes, mouth, and other body tissues.

Systemic lupus erythematosus: An autoimmune disease, primarily of young women, that can affect many parts of the body, including the joints, skin, kidneys, heart, lungs, blood vessels, and brain.

Thyroiditis: An inflammation of the thyroid gland that causes the gland to become underactive. Symptoms include: fatigue, weakness, weight gain, cold intolerance, and muscle aches.

Ulcerative colitis: A disease that causes ulcers in the top layers of the lining of the large intestine. This leads to abdominal pain and diarrhea.

Uveitis: The inflammation of structures of the inner eye, including the iris (the colored tissue that holds the lens of the eye) and the choroid plexus (a network of blood vessels around the eyeball). Uveitis occurs with some rheumatic diseases, including ankylosing spondylitis and juvenile rheumatoid arthritis.

Vitiligo: A disorder in which the immune system destroys pigment-making cells called melanocytes. This results in white patches of skin on different parts of the body.

Wegener's granulomatosis: An autoimmune disease that damages the small and medium-sized blood vessels throughout the body, resulting in disease in the lungs, upper respiratory tract, and kidneys.

Chapter 86

Directory of Organizations with Immune Disorders Information

Government Organizations

National Cancer Institute (NCI)
Suite 3036A, MSC 8322
6116 Executive Blvd.
Bethesda, MD 20892-8322
Toll-Free: 800-4-CANCER
(422-6237)
Toll-Free TTY: 800-332-8615
Website: http://www.cancer.gov
E-mail:
cancergovstaff@mail.nih.gov

National Eye Institute (NEI)
31 Center Dr., MSC 2510
Bethesda, MD 20892-2510
Phone: 301-496-5248
Website: http://www.nei.nih.gov

National Heart, Lung, and Blood Institute (NHLBI)
Health Information Center
P.O. Box 30105
Bethesda, MD 20824-0105
Phone: 301-592-8573
TTY: 240-629-3255
Fax: 240-629-3246
Website: http://
www.nhlbi.nih.gov

National Human Genome Research Institute
Building 31, Room 4B09
31 Center Drive, MSC 2152
9000 Rockville Pike
Bethesda, MD 20892-2152
Phone: 301-402-0911
Fax: 301-402-2218
Website: http://www.genome.gov

The list of resources presented in this chapter was compiled from many sources deemed reliable; contact information was verified and updated in February 2005.

603

National Immunization Program

NIP Public Inquiries
1600 Clifton Rd., N.E., MSE-05
Atlanta, GA 30333
Toll-Free English: 800-232-2522
Toll-Free Spanish: 800-232-0233
Website: http://www.cdc.gov/nip
E-mail: NIPINFO@cdc.gov

National Institute of Allergy and Infectious Diseases (NIAID)

Office of Communications
6610 Rockledge Dr., MSC 6612
Bethesda, MD 20892-6612
Phone: 301-496-5717
Website: http://
www.niaid.nih.gov/publications
Clinical Trials Information:
http://www.niaid.nih.gov/
clintrials/default.htm

National Institute of Arthritis and Musculoskeletal and Skin Diseases (NIAMS)

Information Clearinghouse/NIH
1 AMS Circle
Bethesda, MD 20892-3675
Toll-Free: 877-22-NIAMS
(64267)
Phone: 301-495-4484
TTY: 301-565-2966
Fast Facts: 301-881-2731 (to
receive information by fax)
Website: http://www.nih.gov/
niams/healthinfo
E-mail: niamsinfo@mail.nih.gov

National Institute of Diabetes and Digestive and Kidney Diseases (NIDDK)

Information Clearinghouse
5 Information Way
Bethesda, MD 20892-3560
Toll-Free: 800-860-8747
Phone: 301-654-3810
Website: http://
www.niddk.nih.gov

NIDDK Information Office (Thyroid Diseases)

Bldg. 31, Rm. 9A04
Center Drive, MSC 2560
Bethesda, MD 20892-2560
Phone: 301-496-3583
Website: http://www.niddk.nih.gov

National Institute of Neurological Disorders and Stroke (NINDS)

P.O. Box 5801
Bethesda, MD 20824
Toll-Free: 800-352-9424
Phone: 301-496-5751
TTY: 301-468-5981
Website: http://www.ninds.nih.gov

NIH Clinical Center

Patient Recruitment and
Referral Center (for specific
NIH clinical trials information)
Room 3C01, MSC 7511
6100 Executive Blvd.
Bethesda, MD 20892-7511
Toll-Free: 800-411-1222
Phone: 301-411-1222
Website: http://
clinicalstudies.info.nih.gov/
referring_patient.html

National Kidney and Urologic Diseases Information Clearinghouse
3 Information Way
Bethesda, MD 20892-3580
Toll-Free: 800-891-5390
Phone: 301-654-4415
Fax: 703-738-4929
Website: http://
kidney.niddk.nih.gov
E-mail: nkudic@info.niddk.nih.gov

Office of Rare Diseases, NIH
Room 3B01, MSC 7518
6100 Executive Blvd.
Bethesda, MD 20892
Phone: 301-402-4336
Fax: 301-480-9655
Website: http://
rarediseases.info.nih.gov
E-mail: ord@od.nih.gov

Private Organizations

A-T Children's Project
668 S. Military Trail
Deerfield Beach, FL 33442-3023
Toll-Free: 800-5-HELP-A-T (800-543-5728)
Phone: 954-481-6611
Fax: 954-725-1153
Website: http://www.atcp.org
E-mail: info@atcp.org

American Academy of Dermatology (AAD)
P.O. Box 4014
Schaumberg, IL 60168-4014
Toll-Free: 888-462-3376
Phone: 847-330-0230
Fax: 847-330-0050
Website: http://www.aad.org

American Academy of Orthopaedic Surgeons (AAOS)
6300 N. River Rd.
Rosemont, IL 60018-4262
Toll-Free: 800-346-AAOS (2267)
Phone: 847-823-7186
Fax: 847-823-8125
Website: http://www.aaos.org

American Academy of Physical Medicine and Rehabilitation (AAPMR)
One IBM Plaza, Suite 2500
Chicago, IL 60611
Phone: 312-464-9700
Fax: 312-464-0227
Website: http://www.aapmr.org
E-mail: info@aapmr.org

American Association of Colleges of Osteopathic Medicine (AACOM)
5550 Friendship Blvd., Suite 310
Chevy Chase, MD 20815
Phone: 301-968-4100
Fax: 301-968-4101
Website: http://www.aacom.org

American Autoimmune-Related Diseases Association, Inc. (AARDA)
22100 Gratiot Ave.
East Detroit, MI 48021
Toll-Free: 800-598-4668 (for literature requests)
Phone: 586-776-3900
Fax: 586-776-3903
Website: http://www.aarda.org
E-mail: aarda@aarda.org

American Behçet's Disease Association
P.O. Box 19952
Amarillo, TX 79114
Toll-Free: 800-723-4238
Website: http://www.behcets.com

American Celiac Society
P.O. Box 23455
New Orleans, LA 70183-0455
Phone: 504-737-3293
E-mail:
amerceliacsoc@onebox.com

American College of Rheumatology (ACR)
1800 Century Pl., Suite 250
Atlanta, GA 30345
Phone: 404-633-3777
Fax: 404-633-1870
Website: http://
www.rheumatology.org
E-mail: acr@rheumatology.org

American Diabetes Association
1701 N. Beauregard St.
Alexandria, VA 22311
Toll-Free: 800-DIABETES (342-2383)
Website: http://www.diabetes.org
E-mail: AskADA@diabetes.org

American Dietetic Association
120 S. Riverside Plaza, Suite 2000
Chicago, IL 60606-6995
Toll-Free: 800-877-1600
Website: http://
www.eatright.org/Public
E-mail: hotline@eatright.org

American Federation for Medical Research (AFMR)
900 Cummings Center
Suite 221-U
Beverly, MA 01915
Phone: 978-927-8330
Fax: 978-524-8890
Website: http://www.afmr.org
E-mail: admin@afmr.org

American Juvenile Arthritis Organization (AJAO)
P.O. Box 7669
Atlanta, GA 30357-0669
Toll-Free: 800-568-4045
Phone: 404-965-7888
Website: http://www.arthritis.org
E-mail: help@arthritis.org

American Liver Foundation
75 Maiden Lane, Suite 603
New York, NY 10038
Toll-Free: 800-465-4837
Phone: 212-668-1000
Fax: 212-483-8179
Website: http://
www.liverfoundation.org
E-mail: info@liverfoundation.org

American Lung Association
61 Broadway
6th Floor
New York, NY 10006
Toll-Free: 800-548-8252 (to speak to a lung health professional)
Toll-Free: 800-LUNGUSA (586-4872) (to contact the American Lung Association nearest you)
Phone: 212-315-8700
Website: http://www.lungusa.org

American Skin Association (ASA)
346 Park Ave. S., 4ᵗʰ Floor
New York, NY 10010
Toll-Free: 800-499-SKIN (7546)
Phone: 212-889-4858
Fax: 212-889-4959
Website: http://www.americanskin.org
E-mail: info@americanskin.org

American Thyroid Association
6066 Leesburg Pike, Suite 550
Falls Church, VA 22041
Phone: 703-998-8890
Fax: 703-998-8893
Website: http://www.thyroid.org
E-mail: admin@thyroid.org

Arthritis Foundation
P.O. Box 7660
Atlanta, GA 30357-0669
Toll-Free: 800-568-4045
Phone: 404-965-7888
Website: http://www.arthritis.org
E-mail: help@arthritis.org

Celiac Disease Foundation
13251 Ventura Blvd., #1
Studio City, CA 91604
Phone: 818-990-2354
Fax: 818-990-2379
Website: http://www.celiac.org
E-mail: cdf@celiac.org

Celiac Sprue Association/ USA Inc.
P.O. Box 31700
Omaha, NE 68131-0700
Toll-Free: 877-CSA-4CSA (272-4272)
Phone: 402-558-0600
Fax: 402-558-1347
Website: http://www.csaceliacs.org
E-mail: celiacs@csaceliacs.org

Chediak-Higashi Syndrome Association
One South Road
Oyster Bay, NY 11771
Toll-Free: 800-789-9477
Phone: 516-922-4022
Website: http://www.chediak-higashi.org
E-mail: dappell@hpsnetwork.org

Crohn's and Colitis Foundation of America
386 Park Ave. S., 17ᵗʰ Floor
New York, NY 10016-8804
Toll-Free: 800-932-2423
Website: http://www.ccfa.org
E-mail: info@ccfa.org

Gluten Intolerance Group (GIG) of North America
15110 10ᵗʰ Ave. S.W., Suite A
Seattle, WA 98166
Phone: 206-246-6652
Fax: 206-246-6531
Website: http://www.gluten.net
E-mail: info@gluten.net

Guillain-Barré Syndrome Foundation International
P.O. Box 262
Wynnewood, PA 19096
Phone: 610-667-0131
Fax: 610-667-7036
Website:
http://www.guillain-barre.com
E-mail: info@gbsfi.com

Immune Deficiency Foundation
40 W. Chesapeake Ave., Suite 308
Towson, MD 21204
Toll-Free: 800-296-4433
Website: http://
www.primaryimmune.org
E-mail: idf@primaryimmune.org

International Pemphigus Foundation
828 San Pablo Ave., Suite 210
Albany, NY 94706
Phone: 510-527-4970
Fax: 510-527-8497
Website: http://
www.pemphigus.org
E-mail:
pemphigus@pemphigus.org

Jeffrey Modell Foundation
National Primary
Immunodeficiency Resource
Center
747 Third Ave.
New York, NY 10017
Phone: 212-819-0200
Fax: 212-764-4180
Website: http://
www.jmfworld.org/index.cfm
E-mail: info@jmfworld.org

Juvenile Diabetes Research Foundation International
1400 K St. N.W., Suite 1212
Washington, DC 20005
Toll-Free: 800-JDF-CURE (533-1868)
Phone: 202-371-9746
Fax: 202-371-2760
Website: http://www.jdf.org
E-mail: info@jdrf.org

Lupus Foundation of America, Inc.
2000 L Street N.W., Suite 710
Washington, DC 20036
Toll-Free: 800-558-0121
Phone: 202-349-1155
Fax: 202-349-1156
Website: http://www.lupus.org
E-mail: lupusinfo@lupus.org

Multiple Sclerosis Foundation
6350 N. Andrews Ave.
Ft. Lauderdale, FL 33309-2130
Toll-Free: 888-MSFOCUS (673-6287)
Phone: 954-776-6805
Fax: 954-351-0630
Website: http://www.msfocus.org
E-mail: support@msfocus.org

Muscular Dystrophy Association
3300 E. Sunrise Drive
Tucson, AZ 85718
Toll-Free: 800-572-1717
Website: http://www.mdausa.org
E-mail: mda@mdausa.org

Myasthenia Gravis Foundation of America
1821 University Ave. W.
Suite S256
St. Paul, MN 55104
Toll-Free: 800-541-5454
Phone: 651-917-6256
Fax: 651-917-1835
Website: http://
www.myasthenia.org
E-mail: mgfa@myasthenia.org

Myositis Association
1233 20th St. N.W., Suite 402
Washington, DC 20036
Phone: 202-887-0088
Fax: 202-466-8940
Website: http://www.myositis.org
E-mail: tma@myositis.org

National Academy of Sciences
500 Fifth St. N.W.
Washington, DC 20001
Toll-Free: 800-624-6242
Phone: 202-334-2000
Website: http://national-academies.org

National Adrenal Diseases Foundation
505 Northern Blvd.
Great Neck, NY 11021
Phone: 516-487-4992
Website: http://
www.medhelp.org/nadf
E-mail: nadfmail@aol.com

National Alopecia Areata Foundation (NAAF)
P.O. Box 150760
San Rafael, CA 94915-0760
Phone: 415-472-3780
Fax: 415-472-5343
Website: http://www.naaf.org
E-mail: info@naaf.org

National Graves' Disease Foundation
P.O. Box 8387
Fleming Island, FL 32006
Phone: 904-278-9488
Website: http://www.ngdf.org

National Kidney Foundation
30 East 33rd St.
New York, NY 10016
Toll-Free: 800-622-9010
Phone: 212-889-2210
Website: http://www.kidney.org
E-mail: info@kidney.org

National Multiple Sclerosis Society
733 Third Ave., 6th Floor
New York, NY 10017-3288
Toll-Free: 800-344-4867
Phone: 212-986-3240
Fax: 212-986-7981
Website: http://www.nmss.org
E-mail: info@nmss.org

National Organization for Rare Disorders (NORD)
55 Kansas Ave.
P.O. Box 1968
Danbury, CT 06813-1968
Toll-Free: 800-999-6673
Phone: 203-744-0100
TDD: 203-797-9590
Website: http://
www.rarediseases.org
E-mail:
orphan@rarediseases.org

National Psoriasis Foundation (NPF)
6600 S.W. 92nd Ave., Suite 300
Portland, OR 97223-7195
Toll-Free: 800-723-9166
Phone: 503-244-7404
Fax: 503-245-0626
Website: http://
www.psoriasis.org
E-mail: getinfo@npfusa.org

National Sarcoidosis Resources Center
P.O. Box 1593
Piscataway, NJ 08855-1593
Phone: 732-699-0733
Fax: 732-699-0882
Website: http://www.nsrc-global.net

National Sjögren's Syndrome Association
P.O. Box 22066
Beachwood, OH 44122
Toll-Free: 800-395-NSSA (6772)
Phone: 216-292-3866
Fax: 216-292-4955
Website: http://
www.sjogrenssyndrome.org

National Vitiligo Foundation, Inc. (NVF)
700 Olympic Plaza Circle
Suite 404
Tyler, TX 75701
Phone: 903-595-3713
Fax: 903-593-1545
Website: http://www.nvfi.org
E-mail: info@nvfi.org

Platelet Disorder Support Association
P.O. Box 61533
Potomac, MD 20859
Toll-Free: 87-PLATELET (877-528-3538)
Phone: 301-770-6636
Fax: 301-770-6638
Website: http://
www.itppeople.com
E-mail: pdsa@pdsa.org

Scleroderma Foundation
12 Kent Way, Suite 101
Byfield, MA 01922
Toll-Free: 800-722-4673
Phone: 978-463-5843
Fax: 978-463-5809
Website: http://
www.scleroderma.org
E-mail: sfinfo@scleroderma.org

Scleroderma Research Foundation
220 Montgomery St., Suite 1411
San Francisco, CA 94104
Toll-Free: 800-441-CURE (2873)
Phone: 415-834-9444
Fax: 415-834-9177
Website: http://www.srfcure.org
E-mail: srf@srfcure.org

*Sjögren's Syndrome
Foundation, Inc.*
8120 Woodmont Ave., Suite 530
Bethesda, MD 20814-1437
Toll-Free: 800-475-6473
Phone: 301-718-0300
Fax: 301-718-0322
Website: http://
www.sjogrens.org

*Society for Investigative
Dermatology (SID)*
820 W. Superior Ave., 7th floor
Cleveland, OH 44113-1800
Phone: 216-579-9300
Fax: 216-579-9333
Website: http://www.sidnet.org
E-mail: sid@sidnet.org

*Spondylitis Association of
America (SAA)*
P.O. Box 5872
Sherman Oaks, CA 91413
Toll-Free: 800-777-8189
Phone: 818-981-1616
Website: http://
www.spondylitis.org
E-mail: info@spondylitis.org

SLE Lupus Foundation, Inc.
149 Madison Ave., Suite 205
New York, NY 10016
Toll-Free: 800-74-LUPUS (58787)
Phone: 212-685-4118
Fax: 212-545-1843
Website: http://www.lupusny.org
E-mail: lupus@lupusny.org

*Thyroid Foundation of
America, Inc.*
One Longfellow Place, Suite 1518
Boston, MA 02114
Toll-Free: 800-832-8321
Phone: 617-534-1500
Fax: 617-534-1515
Website: http://
www.allthyroid.org
E-mail: info@tsh.org

Wegener's Association
P.O. Box 28660
Kansas City, MO 64188-8668
Toll-Free: 800-277-9474
Phone/Fax: 816-436-8211
Website: http://
www.wgassociation.org
E-mail: wga@wgassociation.org

Index

Index

Page numbers followed by 'n' indicate a footnote. Page numbers in *italics* indicate a table or illustration.

A

A.D.A.M., Inc., publications, *continued*
  myocarditis 401n
  nephelometry 86n
  pernicious anemia 258n
  polyarteritis nodosa 419n
  serum sickness 481n
  transplant rejection 489n
  uveitis 465n
adaptive immunity, described 17
  see also immune response
Addison disease, overview 239–46
addisonian crisis, described 241–42
"Addison's Disease: Adrenal
  Insufficiency" (NIDDK) 239n
adenoids
  defined 598
  lymphoid tissue 5
  see also tonsils
adrenal corticotropic hormone
  (ACTH)
  Addison disease 240, 242–43
  alcohol use 42
adrenal glands, defined 593
adrenocortical insufficiency, vitiligo
  470
Advil (ibuprofen) 532
AFMR *see* American Federation for
  Medical Research
age factor
  Behçet disease 301
  inclusion body myositis 366
  myasthenia gravis 397
  pernicious anemia 259
  polymyositis 365
  primary immune deficiency 110, *120*
  psoriasis 427
  ulcerative colitis 353
Agenerase (amprenavir) 201
AIDS *see* acquired immune deficiency
  syndrome
AIDSinfo, contact information 203
"Airborne Allergens" (NIAID) 475n
AJAO *see* American Juvenile Arthritis
  Organization
alcohol, immune response 39–50
Aldomet (methyldopa) 78
aldosterone 240
alefacept 434–35
Aleve (naproxen) 532

allergens
  anaphylaxis 494
  asthma 549
  defined 593
  described 4, 475
allergic diseases, described 35
allergic reaction, described 476–77
allergies
  defined 593
  immune system disorders 17
  immunotherapy 541–43
  mast cells 11
  overview 475–78
  selective immunoglobulin A
    deficiency 159, 161
allergy shots *see* immunotherapy
allergy tests, overview 97–99
"Allergy Test: The Test, Common
  Questions" (American Association
  for Clinical Chemistry) 97n
alopecia areata
  defined 599
  overview 247–54
  vitiligo 470
ALPS *see* autoimmune
  lymphoproliferative syndrome
alternative therapies
  alopecia areata 251
  Graves disease 460
  juvenile rheumatoid arthritis 273–74
  rheumatoid arthritis 284
American Academy of Dermatology
  (AAD), contact information 252–53,
  309, 605
American Academy of Family
  Physicians (AAFP), idiopathic
  thrombocytopenic purpura
  publication 341n
American Academy of Orthopaedic
  Surgeons (AAOS), contact
  information 605
American Academy of Physical
  Medicine and Rehabilitation
  (AAPMR), contact information 605
American Association for Clinical
  Chemistry, publications
  allergy tests 97n
  antibody tests 68n
  antinuclear antibody test 71n

bismuth subsalicylate 586
Blaese, R. Michael 507
blood cells
  bone marrow 4
  tests 101–2
blood clots, Behçet disease 304
blood platelets, described 11
blood tests
  antibodies 67–88
  immune function 61–65
blood transfusion reaction, overview
  485–88
blood types, described 485–86
blood vessels
  autoimmune diseases 224
  defined 594
B lymphocytes
  blood tests 63
  selective immunoglobulin A
    deficiency 158
  Wiskott-Aldrich syndrome 171
  X-linked agammaglobulinemia 180
  see also B cells
bone marrow
  defined 594
  described 4
  immune cells 7
  severe combined immunodeficiency
    disease 164
bone marrow transplantation
  Chediak-Higashi syndrome 135
  primary immune deficiency 518–21
  severe combined immunodeficiency
    disease 165–66
  Wiskott-Aldrich syndrome 176
booster shots, vaccines 29
bradykinin, inflammation 16
brain, autoimmune diseases 225–26
branched chain deoxyribonucleic acid
  (bDNA), blood tests 64
breast cancer, alcohol use 39
breast milk
  antibodies 14
  celiac disease 312
Brodsky, Robert A. 513n, 515
Broyles, Laura N. 589
Bruton, Ogden 179
bubble boy disease *see* severe combined
  immunodeficiency disease

budding inhibitors, described 528
budesonide 352, 358
bursitis 539

C

calcinosis, scleroderma 448
calcipotriene 430
cancer
  ataxia-telangiectasia 128
  gene therapy 52
  immune system 38
Cap-Profen (ibuprofen) 532
cardiopulmonary resuscitation
  (CPR), anaphylaxis 495
caregivers
  autoimmune diseases 557–60
  pemphigus diseases 417
carpal tunnel syndrome 539
carrier testing, genes 92–93
CBC *see* complete blood count
CD4 positive T cells, HIV infections
  198–200
CDC *see* Centers for Disease
  Control and Prevention
Celebrex (celecoxib) 532
celecoxib 532
"Celiac Disease" (NIDDK) 311n
Celiac Disease Foundation, contact
  information 318, 607
Celiac Sprue Association/USA
  Inc., contact information 318,
  607
CellCept (mycophenolate mofetil)
  413
cell fragments, described 11
cells, immune system 3–12
cellular immunity *see* immune
  response
cellular metabolism modulators,
  described 528
cellulitis, children 113
Centers for Disease Control and
  Prevention (CDC), publications
  HIV infection, travel 583n
  immunization recommendations
  565n
  vaccines 25n

620

immunizations
electrophoresis 85
infants 32–34
recommendations 565–82
severe combined immunodeficiency
disease 166
see also vaccines
immunodeficiency disorders
ataxia-telangiectasia 128
described 37–38
heredity 111–13
immune system failure 17
treatment 519–21
immunofixation electrophoresis,
overview 83–85
immunoglobulin (Ig)
blood tests 63, 86–88
defined 595
described 8–9
Guillain-Barré syndrome
337–38
immunoglobulin A (IgA)
antibody tests 68
described 9, 63
immune response 22–23
test results 88
see also selective
immunoglobulin A deficiency
immunoglobulin D (IgD)
antibody tests 68
described 9, 63
immunoglobulin E (IgE)
allergic diseases *36*
allergy tests 97–98
antibody tests 68–70
described 9, 63
immunoglobulin G (IgG)
antibody tests 68–70
described 8
test results 87
immunoglobulin M (IgM)
antibody tests 68–70
described 8, 63
test results 87–88
see also hyper-immunoglobulin M
syndrome
immunomodulatory medications,
ulcerative colitis 357
immunosuppressive, defined 596

immunosuppressive medications
autoimmune disease 503
Behçet disease 306
lupus 377–78
immunotherapy
allergies 541–43
multiple sclerosis 390
"Immunotherapy (Allergy Shots)"
(National Jewish Medical and
Research Center) 541n
Imuran (azathioprine) 257, 297, 377,
413
inactivated vaccines, described 29, *31*
"Inclusion-Body Myositis" (Myositis
Association) 366n
inclusion body myositis, overview
366–67
indinavir 201
infants
immune systems 14
passive immunity 17
vaccines 32–34
infections
ataxia-telangiectasia 128
blood tests 62
Chediak-Higashi syndrome 134–35
chronic granulomatous disease 140
cytokines 12
described 22–23
Guillain-Barré syndrome 336–37
hyper-immunoglobulin M syndrome
154
primary immune deficiency 110,
116–17, 517–18
selective immunoglobulin A deficiency 158–59
severe combined immunodeficiency
disease 164–65
Wiskott-Aldrich syndrome 173
X-linked agammaglobulinemia 180–
81
infectious arthritis, described 540
infectious diseases
immune response 21
vaccines 15
inflammation
antibody tests 74–75
Crohn disease 346
erythrocyte sedimentation rate 76

National Sarcoidosis Resources
Center, contact information 446, 610
National Sjögren's Syndrome
Association, contact information 610
National Vitiligo Foundation, Inc.
(NVF), contact information 610
National Women's Health
Information Center (NWHIC),
publications
Hashimoto thyroiditis 462n
lupus 373n
natural immunity, sources *14*
natural killer cells (NK cells)
blood tests 62, 64
defined 597
described 10
see also T cells
Nebert, Daniel W. 209n
NEI *see* National Eye Institute
nelfinavir 201
neomycin 85
neonatal lupus 375
neonatal myasthenia gravis 397
nephelometry, overview 86–88
nephrologists, described 228
nerve impulse conduction therapy,
multiple sclerosis 390
nerves, autoimmune diseases 225–26
nervous system, Guillain-Barré
syndrome 335
Neupogen 62
neurologists
Behçet disease 305
described 228
neutropenia, described 62
neutrophils
blood tests 62
defined 597
depicted *11*
described 11
immune response 40
see also white blood cells
nevirapine 201
newborn screening, genetic testing
94–95
"News: Infant Immunizations Not
Shown to Be Harmful to Children's
Immune Systems" (National
Academy of Sciences) 25n

NGDF *see* National Graves' Disease
Foundation, Inc.
NHGRI *see* National Genome
Research Institute
NIAAA *see* National Institute on
Alcohol Abuse and Alcoholism
niacinamide 414
NIAID *see* National Institute of
Allergy and Infectious Diseases
NIAMS *see* National Institute of
Arthritis and Musculoskeletal and
Skin Diseases
NICHD *see* National Institute
of Child Health and Human
Development
nicotine, ulcerative colitis 359
NIDDK Information Office, contact
information 604
NIH *see* National Institutes of Health
NIH Clinical Center, contact
information 299, 604
NINDS *see* National Institute of
Neurological Disorders and Stroke
NK cells *see* natural killer cells
non-self cells, described 4
nonsteroidal anti-inflammatory drugs
(NSAID)
juvenile rheumatoid arthritis 272
lupus 377
serum sickness 483
NORD *see* National Organization for
Rare Disorders
Norvir (ritonavir) 201
NPF *see* National Psoriasis
Foundation
NSAID *see* nonsteroidal
anti-inflammatory drugs
nucleoside/nucleotide medications,
HIV infection 526
NVF *see* National Vitiligo
Foundation, Inc.
nystagmus, Chediak-Higashi
syndrome 133–34

O

oculocutaneous albinism, Chediak-
Higashi syndrome 133

Health Reference Series
COMPLETE CATALOG

Adolescent Health Sourcebook

Basic Consumer Health Information about Common Medical, Mental, and Emotional Concerns in Adolescents, Including Facts about Acne, Body Piercing, Mononucleosis, Nutrition, Eating Disorders, Stress, Depression, Behavior Problems, Peer Pressure, Violence, Gangs, Drug Use, Puberty, Sexuality, Pregnancy, Learning Disabilities, and More

Along with a Glossary of Terms and Other Resources for Further Help and Information

Edited by Chad T. Kimball. 658 pages. 2002. 0-7808-0248-9. $78.

"It is written in clear, nontechnical language aimed at general readers. . . . Recommended for public libraries, community colleges, and other agencies serving health care consumers."
— American Reference Books Annual, 2003

"Recommended for school and public libraries. Parents and professionals dealing with teens will appreciate the easy-to-follow format and the clearly written text. This could become a 'must have' for every high school teacher." — E-Streams, Jan '03

"A good starting point for information related to common medical, mental, and emotional concerns of adolescents." — School Library Journal, Nov '02

"This book provides accurate information in an easy to access format. It addresses topics that parents and caregivers might not be aware of and provides practical, useable information." — Doody's Health Sciences Book Review Journal, Sep-Oct '02

"Recommended reference source."
— Booklist, American Library Association, Sep '02

AIDS Sourcebook, 3rd Edition

Basic Consumer Health Information about Acquired Immune Deficiency Syndrome (AIDS) and Human Immunodeficiency Virus (HIV) Infection, Including Facts about Transmission, Prevention, Diagnosis, Treatment, Opportunistic Infections, and Other Complications, with a Section for Women and Children, Including Details about Associated Gynecological Concerns, Pregnancy, and Pediatric Care

Along with Updated Statistical Information, Reports on Current Research Initiatives, a Glossary, and Directories of Internet, Hotline, and Other Resources

Edited by Dawn D. Matthews. 664 pages. 2003. 0-7808-0631-X. $78.

ALSO AVAILABLE: AIDS Sourcebook, 1st Edition. Edited by Karen Bellenir and Peter D. Dresser. 831 pages. 1995. 0-7808-0031-1. $78.

AIDS Sourcebook, 2nd Edition. Edited by Karen Bellenir. 751 pages. 1999. 0-7808-0225-X. $78.

"The 3rd edition of the AIDS Sourcebook, part of Omnigraphics' Health Reference Series, is a welcome update. . . . This resource is highly recommended for academic and public libraries."
— American Reference Books Annual, 2004

"Excellent sourcebook. This continues to be a highly recommended book. There is no other book that provides as much information as this book provides."
— AIDS Book Review Journal, Dec-Jan 2000

"Recommended reference source."
— Booklist, American Library Association, Dec '99

"A solid text for college-level health libraries."
— The Bookwatch, Aug '99

Cited in Reference Sources for Small and Medium-Sized Libraries, American Library Association, 1999

Alcoholism Sourcebook

Basic Consumer Health Information about the Physical and Mental Consequences of Alcohol Abuse, Including Liver Disease, Pancreatitis, Wernicke-Korsakoff Syndrome (Alcoholic Dementia), Fetal Alcohol Syndrome, Heart Disease, Kidney Disorders, Gastrointestinal Problems, and Immune System Compromise and Featuring Facts about Addiction, Detoxification, Alcohol Withdrawal, Recovery, and the Maintenance of Sobriety

Along with a Glossary and Directories of Resources for Further Help and Information

Edited by Karen Bellenir. 613 pages. 2000. 0-7808-0325-6. $78.

"This title is one of the few reference works on alcoholism for general readers. For some readers this will be a welcome complement to the many self-help books on the market. Recommended for collections serving general readers and consumer health collections."
— E-Streams, Mar '01

"This book is an excellent choice for public and academic libraries."
— American Reference Books Annual, 2001

"Recommended reference source."
— Booklist, American Library Association, Dec '00

"Presents a wealth of information on alcohol use and abuse and its effects on the body and mind, treatment, and prevention." — SciTech Book News, Dec '00

"Important new health guide which packs in the latest consumer information about the problems of alcoholism." — Reviewer's Bookwatch, Nov '00

SEE ALSO Drug Abuse Sourcebook, Substance Abuse Sourcebook

Allergies Sourcebook, 2nd Edition

Basic Consumer Health Information about Allergic Disorders, Triggers, Reactions, and Related Symptoms, Including Anaphylaxis, Rhinitis, Sinusitis, Asthma, Dermatitis, Conjunctivitis, and Multiple Chemical Sensitivity

Along with Tips on Diagnosis, Prevention, and Treatment, Statistical Data, a Glossary, and a Directory of Sources for Further Help and Information

Edited by Annemarie S. Muth. 598 pages. 2002. 0-7808-0376-0. $78.

ALSO AVAILABLE: Allergies Sourcebook, 1st Edition. Edited by Allan R. Cook. 611 pages. 1997. 0-7808-0036-2. $78.

"This book brings a great deal of useful material together. . . . This is an excellent addition to public and consumer health library collections."
— *American Reference Books Annual, 2003*

"This second edition would be useful to laypersons with little or advanced knowledge of the subject matter. This book would also serve as a resource for nursing and other health care professions students. It would be useful in public, academic, and hospital libraries with consumer health collections."   — *E-Streams, Jul '02*

■

Alternative Medicine Sourcebook, 2nd Edition

Basic Consumer Health Information about Alternative and Complementary Medical Practices, Including Acupuncture, Chiropractic, Herbal Medicine, Homeopathy, Naturopathic Medicine, Mind-Body Interventions, Ayurveda, and Other Non-Western Medical Traditions

Along with Facts about such Specific Therapies as Massage Therapy, Aromatherapy, Qigong, Hypnosis, Prayer, Dance, and Art Therapies, a Glossary, and Resources for Further Information

Edited by Dawn D. Matthews. 618 pages. 2002. 0-7808-0605-0. $78.

ALSO AVAILABLE: Alternative Medicine Sourcebook, 1st Edition. Edited by Allan R. Cook. 737 pages. 1999. 0-7808-0200-4. $78.

"Recommended for public, high school, and academic libraries that have consumer health collections. Hospital libraries that also serve the public will find this to be a useful resource."   — *E-Streams, Feb '03*

"Recommended reference source."
— *Booklist, American Library Association, Jan '03*

"An important alternate health reference."
— *MBR Bookwatch, Oct '02*

"A great addition to the reference collection of every type of library." — *American Reference Books Annual, 2000*

Alzheimer's Disease Sourcebook, 3rd Edition

Basic Consumer Health Information about Alzheimer's Disease, Other Dementias, and Related Disorders, Including Multi-Infarct Dementia, AIDS Dementia Complex, Dementia with Lewy Bodies, Huntington's Disease, Wernicke-Korsakoff Syndrome (Alcohol-Reated Dementia), Delirium, and Confusional States

Along with Information for People Newly Diagnosed with Alzheimer's Disease and Caregivers, Reports Detailing Current Research Efforts in Prevention, Diagnosis, and Treatment, Facts about Long-Term Care Issues, and Listings of Sources for Additional Information

Edited by Karen Bellenir. 645 pages. 2003. 0-7808-0666-2. $78.

ALSO AVAILABLE: Alzheimer's, Stroke & 29 Other Neurological Disorders Sourcebook, 1st Edition. Edited by Frank E. Bair. 579 pages. 1993. 1-55888-748-2. $78.

ALSO AVAILABLE: Alzheimer's Disease Sourcebook, 2nd Edition. Edited by Karen Bellenir. 524 pages. 1999. 0-7808-0223-3. $78.

"This very informative and valuable tool will be a great addition to any library serving consumers, students and health care workers."
— *American Reference Books Annual, 2004*

"This is a valuable resource for people affected by dementias such as Alzheimer's. It is easy to navigate and includes important information and resources."
— *Doody's Review Service, Feb. 2004*

"Recommended reference source."
— *Booklist, American Library Association, Oct '99*

SEE ALSO Brain Disorders Sourcebook

■

Arthritis Sourcebook, 2nd Edition

Basic Consumer Health Information about Osteoarthritis, Rheumatoid Arthritis, Other Rheumatic Disorders, Infectious Forms of Arthritis, and Diseases with Symptoms Linked to Arthritis, Featuring Facts about Diagnosis, Pain Management, and Surgical Therapies

Along with Coping Strategies, Research Updates, a Glossary, and Resources for Additional Help and Information

Edited by Amy L. Sutton. 593 pages. 2004. 0-7808-0667-0. $78.

ALSO AVAILABLE: Arthritis Sourcebook, 1st Edition. Edited by Allan R. Cook. 550 pages. 1998. 0-7808-0201-2. $78.

". . . accessible to the layperson."
— *Reference and Research Book News, Feb '99*

Asthma Sourcebook

Basic Consumer Health Information about Asthma, Including Symptoms, Traditional and Nontraditional Remedies, Treatment Advances, Quality-of-Life Aids, Medical Research Updates, and the Role of Allergies, Exercise, Age, the Environment, and Genetics in the Development of Asthma

Along with Statistical Data, a Glossary, and Directories of Support Groups, and Other Resources for Further Information

Edited by Annemarie S. Muth. 628 pages. 2000. 0-7808-0381-7. $78.

"A worthwhile reference acquisition for public libraries and academic medical libraries whose readers desire a quick introduction to the wide range of asthma information." — *Choice, Association of College & Research Libraries, Jun '01*

"Recommended reference source." — *Booklist, American Library Association, Feb '01*

"Highly recommended." — *The Bookwatch, Jan '01*

"There is much good information for patients and their families who deal with asthma daily." — *American Medical Writers Association Journal, Winter '01*

"This informative text is recommended for consumer health collections in public, secondary school, and community college libraries and the libraries of universities with a large undergraduate population." — *American Reference Books Annual, 2001*

■

Attention Deficit Disorder Sourcebook

Basic Consumer Health Information about Attention Deficit/Hyperactivity Disorder in Children and Adults, Including Facts about Causes, Symptoms, Diagnostic Criteria, and Treatment Options Such as Medications, Behavior Therapy, Coaching, and Homeopathy

Along with Reports on Current Research Initiatives, Legal Issues, and Government Regulations, and Featuring a Glossary of Related Terms, Internet Resources, and a List of Additional Reading Material

Edited by Dawn D. Matthews. 470 pages. 2002. 0-7808-0624-7. $78.

"Recommended reference source." — *Booklist, American Library Association, Jan '03*

"This book is recommended for all school libraries and the reference or consumer health sections of public libraries." — *American Reference Books Annual, 2003*

■

Back & Neck Sourcebook, 2nd Edition

Basic Consumer Health Information about Spinal Pain, Spinal Cord Injuries, and Related Disorders, Such as Degenerative Disk Disease, Osteoarthritis, Scoliosis, Sciatica, Spina Bifida, and Spinal Stenosis, and Featuring Facts about Maintaining Spinal Health, Self-Care, Pain Management, Rehabilitative Care, Chiro-

practic Care, Spinal Surgeries, and Complementary Therapies

Along with Suggestions for Preventing Back and Neck Pain, a Glossary of Related Terms, and a Directory of Resources

Edited by Amy L. Sutton. 633 pages. 2004. 0-7808-0738-3 $78.

ALSO AVAILABLE: Back & Neck Disorders Sourcebook, 1st Edition. Edited by Karen Bellenir. 548 pages. 1997. 0-7808-0202-0. $78.

"The strength of this work is its basic, easy-to-read format. Recommended." — *Reference and User Services Quarterly, American Library Association, Winter '97*

■

Blood & Circulatory Disorders Sourcebook, 2nd Edition

Basic Consumer Health Information about the Blood and Circulatory System and Related Disorders, Such as Anemia and Other Hemoglobin Diseases, Cancer of the Blood and Associated Bone Marrow Disorders, Clotting and Bleeding Problems, and Conditions That Affect the Veins, Blood Vessels, and Arteries, Including Facts about the Donation and Transplantation of Bone Marrow, Stem Cells, and Blood and Tips for Keeping the Blood and Circulatory System Healthy

Along with a Glossary of Related Terms and Resources for Additional Help and Information

Edited by Amy L. Sutton. 659 pages. 2005. 0-7808-0746-4. $78.

ALSO AVAILABLE: Blood and Circulatory Disorders Sourcebook, 1st Edition. Edited by Karen Bellenir and Linda M. Shin. 554 pages. 1998. 0-7808-0203-9. $78.

"Recommended reference source." — *Booklist, American Library Association, Feb '99*

"An important reference sourcebook written in simple language for everyday, non-technical users. " — *Reviewer's Bookwatch, Jan '99*

■

Brain Disorders Sourcebook, 2nd Edition

Basic Consumer Health Information about Acquired and Traumatic Brain Injuries, Infections of the Brain, Epilepsy and Seizure Disorders, Cerebral Palsy, and Degenerative Neurological Disorders, Including Amyotrophic Lateral Sclerosis (ALS), Dementias, Multiple Sclerosis, and More

Along with Information on the Brain's Structure and Function, Treatment and Rehabilitation Options, Reports on Current Research Initiatives, a Glossary of Terms Related to Brain Disorders and Injuries, and a Directory of Sources for Further Help and Information

Edited by Sandra J. Judd. 625 pages. 2005. 0-7808-0744-8. $78.

ALSO AVAILABLE: Brain Disorders Sourcebook, 1st Edition. Edited by Karen Bellenir. 481 pages. 1999. 0-7808-0229-2. $78.

SEE ALSO Alzheimer's Disease Sourcebook

■

Breast Cancer Sourcebook, 2nd Edition

Basic Consumer Health Information about Breast Cancer, Including Facts about Risk Factors, Prevention, Screening and Diagnostic Methods, Treatment Options, Complementary and Alternative Therapies, Post-Treatment Concerns, Clinical Trials, Special Risk Populations, and New Developments in Breast Cancer Research

Along with Breast Cancer Statistics, a Glossary of Related Terms, and a Directory of Resources for Additional Help and Information

Edited by Sandra J. Judd. 595 pages. 2004. 0-7808-0668-9. $78.

ALSO AVAILABLE: Breast Cancer Sourcebook, 1st Edition. Edited by Edward J. Prucha and Karen Bellenir. 580 pages. 2001. 0-7808-0244-6. $78.

SEE ALSO Cancer Sourcebook for Women, Women's Health Concerns Sourcebook

■

Breastfeeding Sourcebook

Basic Consumer Health Information about the Benefits of Breastmilk, Preparing to Breastfeed, Breastfeeding as a Baby Grows, Nutrition, and More, Including Information on Special Situations and Concerns Such as Mastitis, Illness, Medications, Allergies, Multiple Births, Prematurity, Special Needs, and Adoption

Along with a Glossary and Resources for Additional Help and Information

Edited by Jenni Lynn Colson. 388 pages. 2002. 0-7808-0332-9. $78.

SEE ALSO Pregnancy & Birth Sourcebook

■

Burns Sourcebook

Basic Consumer Health Information about Various Types of Burns and Scalds, Including Flame, Heat, Cold, Electrical, Chemical, and Sun Burns

Along with Information on Short-Term and Long-Term Treatments, Tissue Reconstruction, Plastic Surgery, Prevention Suggestions, and First Aid

Edited by Allan R. Cook. 604 pages. 1999. 0-7808-0204-7. $78.

SEE ALSO Skin Disorders Sourcebook

■

Cancer Sourcebook, 4th Edition

Basic Consumer Health Information about Major Forms and Stages of Cancer, Featuring Facts about Head and Neck Cancers, Lung Cancers, Gastrointestinal Cancers, Genitourinary Cancers, Lymphomas, Blood Cell Cancers, Endocrine Cancers, Skin Cancers, Bone Cancers, Sarcomas, and Others, and Including Information about Cancer Treatments and Therapies, Identifying and Reducing Cancer Risks, and Strategies for Coping with Cancer and the Side Effects of Treatment

Along with a Cancer Glossary, Statistical and Demographic Data, and a Directory of Sources for Additional Help and Information

Edited by Karen Bellenir. 1,119 pages. 2003. 0-7808-0633-6. $78.

ALSO AVAILABLE: Cancer Sourcebook, 1st Edition. Edited by Frank E. Bair. 932 pages. 1990. 1-55888-888-8. $78.

New Cancer Sourcebook, 2nd Edition. Edited by Allan R. Cook. 1,313 pages. 1996. 0-7808-0041-9. $78.

Cancer Sourcebook, 3rd Edition. Edited by Edward J. Prucha. 1,069 pages. 2000. 0-7808-0227-6. $78.

"With cancer being the second leading cause of death for Americans, a prodigious work such as this one, which locates centrally so much cancer-related information, is clearly an asset to this nation's citizens and others." — *Journal of the National Medical Association, 2004*

"This title is recommended for health sciences and public libraries with consumer health collections." — *E-Streams, Feb '01*

". . . can be effectively used by cancer patients and their families who are looking for answers in a language they can understand. Public and hospital libraries should have it on their shelves." — *American Reference Books Annual, 2001*

"Recommended reference source." — *Booklist, American Library Association, Dec '00*

Cited in *Reference Sources for Small and Medium-Sized Libraries, American Library Association, 1999*

"The amount of factual and useful information is extensive. The writing is very clear, geared to general readers. Recommended for all levels." — *Choice, Association of College & Research Libraries, Jan '97*

SEE ALSO *Breast Cancer Sourcebook, Cancer Sourcebook for Women, Pediatric Cancer Sourcebook, Prostate Cancer Sourcebook*

■

Cancer Sourcebook for Women, 2nd Edition

Basic Consumer Health Information about Gynecologic Cancers and Related Concerns, Including Cervical Cancer, Endometrial Cancer, Gestational Trophoblastic Tumor, Ovarian Cancer, Uterine Cancer, Vaginal Cancer, Vulvar Cancer, Breast Cancer, and Common Non-Cancerous Uterine Conditions, with Facts about Cancer Risk Factors, Screening and Prevention, Treatment Options, and Reports on Current Research Initiatives

Along with a Glossary of Cancer Terms and a Directory of Resources for Additional Help and Information

Edited by Karen Bellenir. 604 pages. 2002. 0-7808-0226-8. $78.

ALSO AVAILABLE: *Cancer Sourcebook for Women, 1st Edition.* Edited by Allan R. Cook and Peter D. Dresser. 524 pages. 1996. 0-7808-0076-1. $78.

"An excellent addition to collections in public, consumer health, and women's health libraries." — *American Reference Books Annual, 2003*

"Overall, the information is excellent, and complex topics are clearly explained. As a reference book for the consumer it is a valuable resource to assist them to make informed decisions about cancer and its treatments." — *Cancer Forum, Nov '02*

"Highly recommended for academic and medical reference collections." — *Library Bookwatch, Sep '02*

"This is a highly recommended book for any public or consumer library, being reader friendly and containing accurate and helpful information." — *E-Streams, Aug '02*

"Recommended reference source." — *Booklist, American Library Association, Jul '02*

SEE ALSO *Breast Cancer Sourcebook, Women's Health Concerns Sourcebook*

■

Cardiovascular Diseases & Disorders Sourcebook, 3rd Edition

Basic Consumer Health Information about Heart and Vascular Diseases and Disorders, Such as Angina, Heart Attacks, Arrhythmias, Cardiomyopathy, Valve Disease, Atherosclerosis, and Aneurysms, with Information about Managing Cardiovascular Risk Factors and Maintaining Heart Health, Medications and Procedures Used to Treat Cardiovascular Disorders, and Concerns of Special Significance to Women

long with Reports on Current Research Initiatives, a Glossary of Related Medical Terms, and a Directory of Sources for Further Help and Information

Edited by Sandra J. Judd. 713 pages. 2005. 0-7808-0739-1. $78.

ALSO AVAILABLE: *Heart Diseases & Disorders Sourcebook, 2nd Edition.* Edited by Karen Bellenir. 612 pages. 2000. 0-7808-0238-1. $78.

Cardiovascular Diseases & Disorders Sourcebook, 1st Edition. Edited by Karen Bellenir and Peter D. Dresser. 683 pages. 1995. 0-7808-0032-X. $78.

"This work stands out as an imminently accessible resource for the general public. It is recommended for the reference and circulating shelves of school, public, and academic libraries." — *American Reference Books Annual, 2001*

"Recommended reference source." — *Booklist, American Library Association, Dec '00*

"Provides comprehensive coverage of matters related to the heart. This title is recommended for health sciences and public libraries with consumer health collections." — *E-Streams, Oct '00*

SEE ALSO *Healthy Heart Sourcebook for Women*

■

Caregiving Sourcebook

Basic Consumer Health Information for Caregivers, Including a Profile of Caregivers, Caregiving Responsibilities and Concerns, Tips for Specific Conditions, Care Environments, and the Effects of Caregiving

Along with Facts about Legal Issues, Financial Information, and Future Planning, a Glossary, and a Listing of Additional Resources

Edited by Joyce Brennfleck Shannon. 600 pages. 2001. 0-7808-0331-0. $78.

∎

Child Abuse Sourcebook

Basic Consumer Health Information about the Physical, Sexual, and Emotional Abuse of Children, with Additional Facts about Neglect, Munchausen Syndrome by Proxy (MSBP), Shaken Baby Syndrome, and Controversial Issues Related to Child Abuse, Such as Withholding Medical Care, Corporal Punishment, and Child Maltreatment in Youth Sports, and Featuring Facts about Child Protective Services, Foster Care, Adoption, Parenting Challenges, and Other Abuse Prevention Efforts

Along with a Glossary of Related Terms and Resources for Additional Help and Information

Edited by Dawn D. Matthews. 620 pages. 2004. 0-7808-0705-7. $78.

∎

Childhood Diseases & Disorders Sourcebook

Basic Consumer Health Information about Medical Problems Often Encountered in Pre-Adolescent Children, Including Respiratory Tract Ailments, Ear Infections, Sore Throats, Disorders of the Skin and Scalp, Digestive and Genitourinary Diseases, Infectious Diseases, Inflammatory Disorders, Chronic Physical and Developmental Disorders, Allergies, and More

Along with Information about Diagnostic Tests, Common Childhood Surgeries, and Frequently Used Medications, with a Glossary of Important Terms and Resource Directory

Edited by Chad T. Kimball. 662 pages. 2003. 0-7808-0458-9. $78.

∎

Colds, Flu & Other Common Ailments Sourcebook

Basic Consumer Health Information about Common Ailments and Injuries, Including Colds, Coughs, the Flu, Sinus Problems, Headaches, Fever, Nausea and Vomiting, Menstrual Cramps, Diarrhea, Constipation, Hemorrhoids, Back Pain, Dandruff, Dry and Itchy Skin, Cuts, Scrapes, Sprains, Bruises, and More

Along with Information about Prevention, Self-Care, Choosing a Doctor, Over-the-Counter Medications, Folk Remedies, and Alternative Therapies, and Including a Glossary of Important Terms and a Directory of Resources for Further Help and Information

Edited by Chad T. Kimball. 638 pages. 2001. 0-7808-0435-X. $78.

∎

Communication Disorders Sourcebook

Basic Information about Deafness and Hearing Loss, Speech and Language Disorders, Voice Disorders, Balance and Vestibular Disorders, and Disorders of Smell, Taste, and Touch

Edited by Linda M. Ross. 533 pages. 1996. 0-7808-0077-X. $78.

∎

Congenital Disorders Sourcebook

Basic Information about Disorders Acquired during Gestation, Including Spina Bifida, Hydrocephalus, Cerebral Palsy, Heart Defects, Craniofacial Abnormalities, Fetal Alcohol Syndrome, and More

Along with Current Treatment Options and Statistical Data

Edited by Karen Bellenir. 607 pages. 1997. 0-7808-0205-5. $78.

SEE ALSO Pregnancy & Birth Sourcebook

∎

Consumer Issues in Health Care Sourcebook

Basic Information about Health Care Fundamentals and Related Consumer Issues, Including Exams and Screening Tests, Physician Specialties, Choosing a Doctor, Using Prescription and Over-the-Counter Medications Safely, Avoiding Health Scams, Managing Common Health Risks in the Home, Care Options for Chronically or Terminally Ill Patients, and a List of Resources for Obtaining Help and Further Information

Edited by Karen Bellenir. 618 pages. 1998. 0-7808-0221-7. $78.

Contagious Diseases Sourcebook

Basic Consumer Health Information about Infectious Diseases Spread by Person-to-Person Contact through Direct Touch, Airborne Transmission, Sexual Contact, or Contact with Blood or Other Body Fluids, Including Hepatitis, Herpes, Influenza, Lice, Measles, Mumps, Pinworm, Ringworm, Severe Acute Respiratory Syndrome (SARS), Streptococcal Infections, Tuberculosis, and Others

Along with Facts about Disease Transmission, Antimicrobial Resistance, and Vaccines, with a Glossary and Directories of Resources for More Information

Edited by Karen Bellenir. 643 pages. 2004. 0-7808-0736-7. $78.

Contagious & Non-Contagious Infectious Diseases Sourcebook

Basic Information about Contagious Diseases like Measles, Polio, Hepatitis B, and Infectious Mononucleosis, and Non-Contagious Infectious Diseases like Tetanus and Toxic Shock Syndrome, and Diseases Occurring as Secondary Infections Such as Shingles and Reye Syndrome

Along with Vaccination, Prevention, and Treatment Information, and a Section Describing Emerging Infectious Disease Threats

Edited by Karen Bellenir and Peter D. Dresser. 566 pages. 1996. 0-7808-0075-3. $78.

Death & Dying Sourcebook

Basic Consumer Health Information for the Layperson about End-of-Life Care and Related Ethical and Legal Issues, Including Chief Causes of Death, Autopsies, Pain Management for the Terminally Ill, Life Support Systems, Insurance, Euthanasia, Assisted Suicide, Hospice Programs, Living Wills, Funeral Planning, Counseling, Mourning, Organ Donation, and Physician Training

Along with Statistical Data, a Glossary, and Listings of Sources for Further Help and Information

Edited by Annemarie S. Muth. 641 pages. 1999. 0-7808-0230-6. $78.

Dental Care & Oral Health Sourcebook, 2nd Edition

Basic Consumer Health Information about Dental Care, Including Oral Hygiene, Dental Visits, Pain Management, Cavities, Crowns, Bridges, Dental Implants, and Fillings, and Other Oral Health Concerns, Such as Gum Disease, Bad Breath, Dry Mouth, Genetic and Developmental Abnormalities, Oral Cancers, Orthodontics, and Temporomandibular Disorders

Along with Updates on Current Research in Oral Health, a Glossary, a Directory of Dental and Oral Health Organizations, and Resources for People with Dental and Oral Health Disorders

Edited by Amy L. Sutton. 609 pages. 2003. 0-7808-0634-4. $78.

ALSO AVAILABLE: *Oral Health Sourcebook, 1st Edition.* Edited by Allan R. Cook. 558 pages. 1997. 0-7808-0082-6. $78.

Depression Sourcebook

Basic Consumer Health Information about Unipolar Depression, Bipolar Disorder, Postpartum Depression, Seasonal Affective Disorder, and Other Types of Depression in Children, Adolescents, Women, Men, the Elderly, and Other Selected Populations

Along with Facts about Causes, Risk Factors, Diagnostic Criteria, Treatment Options, Coping Strategies, Suicide Prevention, a Glossary, and a Directory of Sources for Additional Help and Information

Edited by Karen Belleni. 602 pages. 2002. 0-7808-0611-5. $78.

651

"Depression Sourcebook is of a very high standard. Its purpose, which is to serve as a reference source to the lay reader, is very well served."
— *Journal of the National Medical Association, 2004*

"Invaluable reference for public and school library collections alike." — *Library Bookwatch, Apr '03*

"Recommended for purchase."
— *American Reference Books Annual, 2003*

■

Diabetes Sourcebook, 3rd Edition

Basic Consumer Health Information about Type 1 Diabetes (Insulin-Dependent or Juvenile-Onset Diabetes), Type 2 Diabetes (Noninsulin-Dependent or Adult-Onset Diabetes), Gestational Diabetes, Impaired Glucose Tolerance (IGT), and Related Complications, Such as Amputation, Eye Disease, Gum Disease, Nerve Damage, and End-Stage Renal Disease, Including Facts about Insulin, Oral Diabetes Medications, Blood Sugar Testing, and the Role of Exercise and Nutrition in the Control of Diabetes

Along with a Glossary and Resources for Further Help and Information

Edited by Dawn D. Matthews. 622 pages. 2003. 0-7808-0629-8. $78.

ALSO AVAILABLE: *Diabetes Sourcebook, 1st Edition.* Edited by Karen Bellenir and Peter D. Dresser. 827 pages. 1994. 1-55888-751-2. $78.

Diabetes Sourcebook, 2nd Edition. Edited by Karen Bellenir. 688 pages. 1998. 0-7808-0224-1. $78.

"This edition is even more helpful than earlier versions. . . . It is a truly valuable tool for anyone seeking readable and authoritative information on diabetes."
— *American Reference Books Annual, 2004*

"An invaluable reference." — *Library Journal, May '00*

Selected as one of the 250 "Best Health Sciences Books of 1999." — *Doody's Rating Service, Mar-Apr 2000*

"Provides useful information for the general public."
— *Healthlines, University of Michigan Health Management Research Center, Sep/Oct '99*

". . . provides reliable mainstream medical information . . . belongs on the shelves of any library with a consumer health collection." — *E-Streams, Sep '99*

"Recommended reference source."
— *Booklist, American Library Association, Feb '99*

■

Diet & Nutrition Sourcebook, 2nd Edition

Basic Consumer Health Information about Dietary Guidelines, Recommended Daily Intake Values, Vitamins, Minerals, Fiber, Fat, Weight Control, Dietary Supplements, and Food Additives

Along with Special Sections on Nutrition Needs throughout Life and Nutrition for People with Such Specific Medical Concerns as Allergies, High Blood Cholesterol, Hypertension, Diabetes, Celiac Disease, Seizure Disorders, Phenylketonuria (PKU), Cancer, and

Eating Disorders, and Including Reports on Current Nutrition Research and Source Listings for Additional Help and Information

Edited by Karen Bellenir. 650 pages. 1999. 0-7808-0228-4. $78.

ALSO AVAILABLE: *Diet & Nutrition Sourcebook, 1st Edition.* Edited by Dan R. Harris. 662 pages. 1996. 0-7808-0084-2. $78.

"This book is an excellent source of basic diet and nutrition information." — *Booklist Health Sciences Supplement, American Library Association, Dec '00*

"This reference document should be in any public library, but it would be a very good guide for beginning students in the health sciences. If the other books in this publisher's series are as good as this, they should all be in the health sciences collections."
— *American Reference Books Annual, 2000*

"This book is an excellent general nutrition reference for consumers who desire to take an active role in their health care for prevention. Consumers of all ages who select this book can feel confident they are receiving current and accurate information." — *Journal of Nutrition for the Elderly, Vol. 19, No. 4, '00*

"Recommended reference source."
— *Booklist, American Library Association, Dec '99*

SEE ALSO *Digestive Diseases & Disorders Sourcebook, Eating Disorders Sourcebook, Gastrointestinal Diseases & Disorders Sourcebook, Vegetarian Sourcebook*

■

Digestive Diseases & Disorders Sourcebook

Basic Consumer Health Information about Diseases and Disorders that Impact the Upper and Lower Digestive System, Including Celiac Disease, Constipation, Crohn's Disease, Cyclic Vomiting Syndrome, Diarrhea, Diverticulosis and Diverticulitis, Gallstones, Heartburn, Hemorrhoids, Hernias, Indigestion (Dyspepsia), Irritable Bowel Syndrome, Lactose Intolerance, Ulcers, and More

Along with Information about Medications and Other Treatments, Tips for Maintaining a Healthy Digestive Tract, a Glossary, and Directory of Digestive Diseases Organizations

Edited by Karen Bellenir. 335 pages. 2000. 0-7808-0327-2. $78.

"This title would be an excellent addition to all public or patient-research libraries."
— *American Reference Books Annual, 2001*

"This title is recommended for public, hospital, and health sciences libraries with consumer health collections." — *E-Streams, Jul-Aug '00*

"Recommended reference source."
— *Booklist, American Library Association, May '00*

SEE ALSO *Diet & Nutrition Sourcebook, Eating Disorders Sourcebook, Gastrointestinal Diseases & Disorders Sourcebook*

Disabilities Sourcebook

Basic Consumer Health Information about Physical and Psychiatric Disabilities, Including Descriptions of Major Causes of Disability, Assistive and Adaptive Aids, Workplace Issues, and Accessibility Concerns

Along with Information about the Americans with Disabilities Act, a Glossary, and Resources for Additional Help and Information

Edited by Dawn D. Matthews. 616 pages. 2000. 0-7808-0389-2. $78.

"It is a must for libraries with a consumer health section." — *American Reference Books Annual 2002*

"A much needed addition to the Omnigraphics *Health Reference Series*. A current reference work to provide people with disabilities, their families, caregivers or those who work with them, a broad range of information in one volume, has not been available until now. . . . It is recommended for all public and academic library reference collections." — *E-Streams, May '01*

"An excellent source book in easy-to-read format covering many current topics; highly recommended for all libraries." — *Choice, Association of College and Research Libraries, Jan '01*

"Recommended reference source." —*Booklist, American Library Association, Jul '00*

■

Domestic Violence Sourcebook, 2nd Edition

Basic Consumer Health Information about the Causes and Consequences of Abusive Relationships, Including Physical Violence, Sexual Assault, Battery, Stalking, and Emotional Abuse, and Facts about the Effects of Violence on Women, Men, Young Adults, and the Elderly, with Reports about Domestic Violence in Selected Populations, and Featuring Facts about Medical Care, Victim Assistance and Protection, Prevention Strategies, Mental Health Services, and Legal Issues

Along with a Glossary of Related Terms and Resources for Additional Help and Information

Edited by Dawn D. Matthews. 628 pages. 2004. 0-7808-0669-7. $78.

ALSO AVAILABLE: Domestic Violence & Child Abuse Sourcebook, 1st Edition. Edited by Helene Henderson. 1,064 pages. 2001. 0-7808-0235-7. $78.

"Interested lay persons should find the book extremely beneficial. . . . A copy of *Domestic Violence and Child Abuse Sourcebook* should be in every public library in the United States." — *Social Science & Medicine, No. 56, 2003*

"This is important information. The Web has many resources but this sourcebook fills an important societal need. I am not aware of any other resources of this type." — *Doody's Review Service, Sep '01*

"Recommended for all libraries, scholars, and practitioners." — *Choice, Association of College & Research Libraries, Jul '01*

"Recommended reference source." —*Booklist, American Library Association, Apr '01*

"Important pick for college-level health reference libraries." — *The Bookwatch, Mar '01*

"Because this problem is so widespread and because this book includes a lot of issues within one volume, this work is recommended for all public libraries." — *American Reference Books Annual, 2001*

■

Drug Abuse Sourcebook, 2nd Edition

Basic Consumer Health Information about Illicit Substances of Abuse and the Misuse of Prescription and Over-the-Counter Medications, Including Depressants, Hallucinogens, Inhalants, Marijuana, Stimulants, and Anabolic Steroids

Along with Facts about Related Health Risks, Treatment Programs, Prevention Programs, a Glossary of Abuse and Addiction Terms, a Glossary of Drug-Related Street Terms, and a Directory of Resources for More Information

Edited by Catherine Ginther. 607 pages. 2004. 0-7808-0740-5. $78.

ALSO AVAILABLE: Drug Abuse Sourcebook, 1st Edition. Edited by Karen Bellenir. 629 pages. 2000. 0-7808-0242-X. $78.

"Containing a wealth of information . . . . This resource belongs in libraries that serve a lower-division undergraduate or community college clientele as well as the general public." — *Choice, Association of College and Research Libraries, Jun '01*

"Recommended reference source." —*Booklist, American Library Association, Feb '01*

"Highly recommended." — *The Bookwatch, Jan '01*

"Even though there is a plethora of books on drug abuse, this volume is recommended for school, public, and college libraries." —*American Reference Books Annual, 2001*

SEE ALSO Alcoholism Sourcebook, Substance Abuse Sourcebook

■

Ear, Nose & Throat Disorders Sourcebook

Basic Information about Disorders of the Ears, Nose, Sinus Cavities, Pharynx, and Larynx, Including Ear Infections, Tinnitus, Vestibular Disorders, Allergic and Non-Allergic Rhinitis, Sore Throats, Tonsillitis, and Cancers That Affect the Ears, Nose, Sinuses, and Throat

Along with Reports on Current Research Initiatives, a Glossary of Related Medical Terms, and a Directory of Sources for Further Help and Information

Edited by Karen Bellenir and Linda M. Shin. 576 pages. 1998. 0-7808-0206-3. $78.

■

Eating Disorders Sourcebook

Basic Consumer Health Information about Eating Disorders, Including Information about Anorexia Nervosa, Bulimia Nervosa, Binge Eating, Body Dysmorphic Disorder, Pica, Laxative Abuse, and Night Eating Syndrome

Along with Information about Causes, Adverse Effects, and Treatment and Prevention Issues, and Featuring a Section on Concerns Specific to Children and Adolescents, a Glossary, and Resources for Further Help and Information

Edited by Dawn D. Matthews. 322 pages. 2001. 0-7808-0335-3. $78.

SEE ALSO Diet & Nutrition Sourcebook, Digestive Diseases & Disorders Sourcebook, Gastrointestinal Diseases & Disorders Sourcebook

■

Emergency Medical Services Sourcebook

Basic Consumer Health Information about Preventing, Preparing for, and Managing Emergency Situations, When and Who to Call for Help, What to Expect in the Emergency Room, the Emergency Medical Team, Patient Issues, and Current Topics in Emergency Medicine

Along with Statistical Data, a Glossary, and Sources of Additional Help and Information

Edited by Jenni Lynn Colson. 494 pages. 2002. 0-7808-0420-1. $78.

Endocrine & Metabolic Disorders Sourcebook

Basic Information for the Layperson about Pancreatic and Insulin-Related Disorders Such as Pancreatitis, Diabetes, and Hypoglycemia; Adrenal Gland Disorders Such as Cushing's Syndrome, Addison's Disease, and Congenital Adrenal Hyperplasia; Pituitary Gland Disorders Such as Growth Hormone Deficiency, Acromegaly, and Pituitary Tumors; Thyroid Disorders Such as Hypothyroidism, Graves' Disease, Hashimoto's Disease, and Goiter; Hyperparathyroidism; and Other Diseases and Syndromes of Hormone Imbalance or Metabolic Dysfunction

Along with Reports on Current Research Initiatives

Edited by Linda M. Shin. 574 pages. 1998. 0-7808-0207-1. $78.

■

Environmental Health Sourcebook, 2nd Edition

Basic Consumer Health Information about the Environment and Its Effect on Human Health, Including the Effects of Air Pollution, Water Pollution, Hazardous Chemicals, Food Hazards, Radiation Hazards, Biological Agents, Household Hazards, Such as Radon, Asbestos, Carbon Monoxide, and Mold, and Information about Associated Diseases and Disorders, Including Cancer, Allergies, Respiratory Problems, and Skin Disorders

Along with Information about Environmental Concerns for Specific Populations, a Glossary of Related Terms, and Resources for Further Help and Information

Edited by Dawn D. Matthews. 673 pages. 2003. 0-7808-0632-8. $78.

ALSO AVAILABLE: Environmentally Induced Disorders Sourcebook, 1st Edition. Edited by Allan R. Cook. 620 pages. 1997. 0-7808-0083-4. $78.

Environmentally Induced Disorders Sourcebook, 1st Edition

SEE Environmental Health Sourcebook, 2nd Edition

Ethnic Diseases Sourcebook

Basic Consumer Health Information for Ethnic and Racial Minority Groups in the United States, Including General Health Indicators and Behaviors, Ethnic Diseases, Genetic Testing, the Impact of Chronic Diseases, Women's Health, Mental Health Issues, and Preventive Health Care Services

Along with a Glossary and a Listing of Additional Resources

Edited by Joyce Brennfleck Shannon. 664 pages. 2001. 0-7808-0336-1. $78.

"Recommended for health sciences libraries where public health programs are a priority."
— E-Streams, Jan '02

"Not many books have been written on this topic to date, and the Ethnic Diseases Sourcebook is a strong addition to the list. It will be an important introductory resource for health consumers, students, health care personnel, and social scientists. It is recommended for public, academic, and large hospital libraries."
— American Reference Books Annual 2002

"Recommended reference source."
— Booklist, American Library Association, Oct '01

"Will prove valuable to any library seeking to maintain a current, comprehensive reference collection of health resources. . . . An excellent source of health information about genetic disorders which affect particular ethnic and racial minorities in the U.S."
— The Bookwatch, Aug '01

■

Eye Care Sourcebook, 2nd Edition

Basic Consumer Health Information about Eye Care and Eye Disorders, Including Facts about the Diagnosis, Prevention, and Treatment of Common Refractive Problems Such as Myopia, Hyperopia, Astigmatism, and Presbyopia, and Eye Diseases, Including Glaucoma, Cataract, Age-Related Macular Degeneration, and Diabetic Retinopathy

Along with a Section on Vision Correction and Refractive Surgeries, Including LASIK and LASEK, a Glossary, and Directories of Resources for Additional Help and Information

Edited by Amy L. Sutton. 543 pages. 2003. 0-7808-0635-2. $78.

ALSO AVAILABLE: Ophthalmic Disorders Sourcebook, 1st Edition. Edited by Linda M. Ross. 631 pages. 1996. 0-7808-0081-8. $78.

". . . a solid reference tool for eye care and a valuable addition to a collection."
— American Reference Books Annual, 2004

Family Planning Sourcebook

Basic Consumer Health Information about Planning for Pregnancy and Contraception, Including Traditional Methods, Barrier Methods, Hormonal Methods, Permanent Methods, Future Methods, Emergency Contraception, and Birth Control Choices for Women at Each Stage of Life

Along with Statistics, a Glossary, and Sources of Additional Information

Edited by Amy Marcaccio Keyzer. 520 pages. 2001. 0-7808-0379-5. $78.

"Recommended for public, health, and undergraduate libraries as part of the circulating collection."
— E-Streams, Mar '02

"Information is presented in an unbiased, readable manner, and the sourcebook will certainly be a necessary addition to those public and high school libraries where Internet access is restricted or otherwise problematic." — American Reference Books Annual 2002

"Recommended reference source."
— Booklist, American Library Association, Oct '01

"Will prove valuable to any library seeking to maintain a current, comprehensive reference collection of health resources. . . . Excellent reference."
— The Bookwatch, Aug '01

SEE ALSO Pregnancy & Birth Sourcebook

■

Fitness & Exercise Sourcebook, 2nd Edition

Basic Consumer Health Information about the Fundamentals of Fitness and Exercise, Including How to Begin and Maintain a Fitness Program, Fitness as a Lifestyle, the Link between Fitness and Diet, Advice for Specific Groups of People, Exercise as It Relates to Specific Medical Conditions, and Recent Research in Fitness and Exercise

Along with a Glossary of Important Terms and Resources for Additional Help and Information

Edited by Kristen M. Gledhill. 646 pages. 2001. 0-7808-0334-5. $78.

ALSO AVAILABLE: Fitness & Exercise Sourcebook, 1st Edition. Edited by Dan R. Harris. 663 pages. 1996. 0-7808-0186-5. $78.

"This work is recommended for all general reference collections."
— American Reference Books Annual 2002

"Highly recommended for public, consumer, and school grades fourth through college."
— E-Streams, Nov '01

"Recommended reference source." — Booklist, American Library Association, Oct '01

"The information appears quite comprehensive and is considered reliable. . . . This second edition is a welcomed addition to the series."
— Doody's Review Service, Sep '01

"This reference is a valuable choice for those who desire a broad source of information on exercise, fitness, and chronic-disease prevention through a healthy lifestyle." —*American Medical Writers Association Journal, Fall '01*

"Will prove valuable to any library seeking to maintain a current, comprehensive reference collection of health resources. . . . Excellent reference."
— *The Bookwatch, Aug '01*

■

Food & Animal Borne Diseases Sourcebook

Basic Information about Diseases That Can Be Spread to Humans through the Ingestion of Contaminated Food or Water or by Contact with Infected Animals and Insects, Such as Botulism, E. Coli, Hepatitis A, Trichinosis, Lyme Disease, and Rabies

Along with Information Regarding Prevention and Treatment Methods, and Including a Special Section for International Travelers. Describing Diseases Such as Cholera, Malaria, Travelers' Diarrhea, and Yellow Fever, and Offering Recommendations for Avoiding Illness

Edited by Karen Bellenir and Peter D. Dresser. 535 pages. 1995. 0-7808-0033-8. $78.

"Targeting general readers and providing them with a single, comprehensive source of information on selected topics, this book continues, with the excellent caliber of its predecessors, to catalog topical information on health matters of general interest. Readable and thorough, this valuable resource is highly recommended for all libraries."
— *Academic Library Book Review, Summer '96*

"A comprehensive collection of authoritative information." — *Emergency Medical Services, Oct '95*

■

Food Safety Sourcebook

Basic Consumer Health Information about the Safe Handling of Meat, Poultry, Seafood, Eggs, Fruit Juices, and Other Food Items, and Facts about Pesticides, Drinking Water, Food Safety Overseas, and the Onset, Duration, and Symptoms of Foodborne Illnesses, Including Types of Pathogenic Bacteria, Parasitic Protozoa, Worms, Viruses, and Natural Toxins

Along with the Role of the Consumer, the Food Handler, and the Government in Food Safety; a Glossary, and Resources for Additional Help and Information

Edited by Dawn D. Matthews. 339 pages. 1999. 0-7808-0326-4. $78.

"This book is recommended for public libraries and universities with home economic and food science programs." — *E-Streams, Nov '00*

"Recommended reference source."
— *Booklist, American Library Association, May '00*

"This book takes the complex issues of food safety and foodborne pathogens and presents them in an easily understood manner. [It does] an excellent job of covering a large and often confusing topic."
— *American Reference Books Annual, 2000*

Forensic Medicine Sourcebook

Basic Consumer Information for the Layperson about Forensic Medicine, Including Crime Scene Investigation, Evidence Collection and Analysis, Expert Testimony, Computer-Aided Criminal Identification, Digital Imaging in the Courtroom, DNA Profiling, Accident Reconstruction, Autopsies, Ballistics, Drugs and Explosives Detection, Latent Fingerprints, Product Tampering, and Questioned Document Examination

Along with Statistical Data, a Glossary of Forensics Terminology, and Listings of Sources for Further Help and Information

Edited by Annemarie S. Muth. 574 pages. 1999. 0-7808-0232-2. $78.

"Given the expected widespread interest in its content and its easy to read style, this book is recommended for most public and all college and university libraries."
— *E-Streams, Feb '01*

"Recommended for public libraries."
— *Reference & User Services Quarterly, American Library Association, Spring 2000*

"Recommended reference source."
— *Booklist, American Library Association, Feb '00*

"A wealth of information, useful statistics, references are up-to-date and extremely complete. This wonderful collection of data will help students who are interested in a career in any type of forensic field. It is a great resource for attorneys who need information about types of expert witnesses needed in a particular case. It also offers useful information for fiction and nonfiction writers whose work involves a crime. A fascinating compilation. All levels." — *Choice, Association of College and Research Libraries, Jan 2000*

"There are several items that make this book attractive to consumers who are seeking certain forensic data. . . . This is a useful current source for those seeking general forensic medical answers."
— *American Reference Books Annual, 2000*

■

Gastrointestinal Diseases & Disorders Sourcebook

Basic Information about Gastroesophageal Reflux Disease (Heartburn), Ulcers, Diverticulosis, Irritable Bowel Syndrome, Crohn's Disease, Ulcerative Colitis, Diarrhea, Constipation, Lactose Intolerance, Hemorrhoids, Hepatitis, Cirrhosis, and Other Digestive Problems, Featuring Statistics, Descriptions of Symptoms, and Current Treatment Methods of Interest for Persons Living with Upper and Lower Gastrointestinal Maladies

Edited by Linda M. Ross. 413 pages. 1996. 0-7808-0078-8. $78.

". . . very readable form. The successful editorial work that brought this material together into a useful and understandable reference makes accessible to all readers information that can help them more effectively understand and obtain help for digestive tract problems."
— *Choice, Association of College & Research Libraries, Feb '97*

■

Genetic Disorders Sourcebook, 3rd Edition

Basic Consumer Health Information about Hereditary Diseases and Disorders, Including Facts about the Human Genome, Genetic Inheritance Patterns, Disorders Associated with Specific Genes, Such as Sickle Cell Disease, Hemophilia, and Cystic Fibrosis, Chromosome Disorders, Such as Down Syndrome, Fragile X Syndrome, and Turner Syndrome, and Complex Diseases and Disorders Resulting from the Interaction of Environmental and Genetic Factors, Such as Allergies, Cancer, and Obesity

Along with Facts about Genetic Testing, Suggestions for Parents of Children with Special Needs, Reports on Current Research Initiatives, a Glossary of Genetic Terminology, and Resources for Additional Help and Information

Edited by Karen Bellenir. 777 pages. 2004. 0-7808-0742-1. $78.

ALSO AVAILABLE: *Genetic Disorders Sourcebook, 1st Edition.* Edited by Karen Bellenir. 642 pages. 1996. 0-7808-0034-6. $78.

Genetic Disorders Sourcebook, 2nd Edition. Edited by Kathy Massimini. 768 pages. 2001. 0-7808-0241-1. $78.

"Recommended for public libraries and medical and hospital libraries with consumer health collections."
— *E-Streams, May '01*

"Recommended reference source."
— *Booklist, American Library Association, Apr '01*

"Important pick for college-level health reference libraries." — *The Bookwatch, Mar '01*

"Provides essential medical information to both the general public and those diagnosed with a serious or fatal genetic disease or disorder." —*Choice, Association of College and Research Libraries, Jan '97*

■

Head Trauma Sourcebook

Basic Information for the Layperson about Open-Head and Closed-Head Injuries, Treatment Advances, Recovery, and Rehabilitation

Along with Reports on Current Research Initiatives

Edited by Karen Bellenir. 414 pages. 1997. 0-7808-0208-X. $78.

■

Headache Sourcebook

Basic Consumer Health Information about Migraine, Tension, Cluster, Rebound and Other Types of Headaches, with Facts about the Cause and Prevention of Headaches, the Effects of Stress and the Environment, Headaches during Pregnancy and Menopause, and Childhood Headaches

Along with a Glossary and Other Resources for Additional Help and Information

Edited by Dawn D. Matthews. 362 pages. 2002. 0-7808-0337-X. $78.

"Highly recommended for academic and medical reference collections." — *Library Bookwatch, Sep '02*

■

Health Insurance Sourcebook

Basic Information about Managed Care Organizations, Traditional Fee-for-Service Insurance, Insurance Portability and Pre-Existing Conditions Clauses, Medicare, Medicaid, Social Security, and Military Health Care

Along with Information about Insurance Fraud

Edited by Wendy Wilcox. 530 pages. 1997. 0-7808-0222-5. $78.

"Particularly useful because it brings much of this information together in one volume. This book will be a handy reference source in the health sciences library, hospital library, college and university library, and medium to large public library."
— *Medical Reference Services Quarterly, Fall '98*

Awarded "Books of the Year Award"
— *American Journal of Nursing, 1997*

"The layout of the book is particularly helpful as it provides easy access to reference material. A most useful addition to the vast amount of information about health insurance. The use of data from U.S. government agencies is most commendable. Useful in a library or learning center for healthcare professional students."
— *Doody's Health Sciences Book Reviews, Nov '97*

■

Health Reference Series Cumulative Index 1999

A Comprehensive Index to the Individual Volumes of the Health Reference Series, Including a Subject Index, Name Index, Organization Index, and Publication Index

Along with a Master List of Acronyms and Abbreviations

Edited by Edward J. Prucha, Anne Holmes, and Robert Rudnick. 990 pages. 2000. 0-7808-0382-5. $78.

"This volume will be most helpful in libraries that have a relatively complete collection of the Health Reference Series." — *American Reference Books Annual, 2001*

"Essential for collections that hold any of the numerous *Health Reference Series* titles."
— *Choice, Association of College and Research Libraries, Nov '00*

■

Healthy Aging Sourcebook

Basic Consumer Health Information about Maintaining Health through the Aging Process, Including Advice on Nutrition, Exercise, and Sleep, Help in Making Decisions about Midlife Issues and Retirement, and

Guidance Concerning Practical and Informed Choices in Health Consumerism

Along with Data Concerning the Theories of Aging, Different Experiences in Aging by Minority Groups, and Facts about Aging Now and Aging in the Future; and Featuring a Glossary, a Guide to Consumer Help, Additional Suggested Reading, and Practical Resource Directory

Edited by Jenifer Swanson. 536 pages. 1999. 0-7808-0390-6. $78.

"Recommended reference source."
—*Booklist, American Library Association, Feb '00*

SEE ALSO *Physical & Mental Issues in Aging Sourcebook*

◼

Healthy Children Sourcebook

Basic Consumer Health Information about the Physical and Mental Development of Children between the Ages of 3 and 12, Including Routine Health Care, Preventative Health Services, Safety and First Aid, Healthy Sleep, Dental Care, Nutrition, and Fitness, and Featuring Parenting Tips on Such Topics as Bedwetting, Choosing Day Care, Monitoring TV and Other Media, and Establishing a Foundation for Substance Abuse Prevention

Along with a Glossary of Commonly Used Pediatric Terms and Resources for Additional Help and Information.

Edited by Chad T. Kimball. 647 pages. 2003. 0-7808-0247-0. $78.

"It is hard to imagine that any other single resource exists that would provide such a comprehensive guide of timely information on health promotion and disease prevention for children aged 3 to 12."
—*American Reference Books Annual, 2004*

"The strengths of this book are many. It is clearly written, presented and structured."
—*Journal of the National Medical Association, 2004*

◼

Healthy Heart Sourcebook for Women

Basic Consumer Health Information about Cardiac Issues Specific to Women, Including Facts about Major Risk Factors and Prevention, Treatment and Control Strategies, and Important Dietary Issues

Along with a Special Section Regarding the Pros and Cons of Hormone Replacement Therapy and Its Impact on Heart Health, and Additional Help, Including Recipes, a Glossary, and a Directory of Resources

Edited by Dawn D. Matthews. 336 pages. 2000. 0-7808-0329-9. $78.

"A good reference source and recommended for all public, academic, medical, and hospital libraries."
—*Medical Reference Services Quarterly, Summer '01*

"Because of the lack of information specific to women on this topic, this book is recommended for public libraries and consumer libraries."
—*American Reference Books Annual, 2001*

"Contains very important information about coronary artery disease that all women should know. The information is current and presented in an easy-to-read format. The book will make a good addition to any library."
—*American Medical Writers Association Journal, Summer '00*

"Important, basic reference."
—*Reviewer's Bookwatch, Jul '00*

SEE ALSO *Heart Diseases & Disorders Sourcebook, Women's Health Concerns Sourcebook*

◼

Heart Diseases & Disorders Sourcebook, 2nd Edition

SEE *Cardiovascular Diseases & Disorders Sourcebook, 3rd Edition*

◼

Hepatitis Sourcebook, 1st Edition

Basic Consumer Health Information about Hepatitis A, Hepatitis B, Hepatitis C, and Other Forms of Hepatitis, Including Autoimmune Hepatitis, Alcoholic Hepatitis, Nonalcoholic Steatohepatitis, and Toxic Hepatitis, with Facts about Risk Factors, Screening Methods, Diagnostic Tests, and Treatment Options

Along with Information on Liver Health, Tips for People Living with Chronic Hepatitis, Reports on Current Research Initiatives, a Glossary of Terms Related to Hepatitis, and a Directory of Sources for Further Help and Information

Edited by Sandra J. Judd. 575 pages. 2005. 0-7808-0749-9. $78.

◼

Household Safety Sourcebook

Basic Consumer Health Information about Household Safety, Including Information about Poisons, Chemicals, Fire, and Water Hazards in the Home

Along with Advice about the Safe Use of Home Maintenance Equipment, Choosing Toys and Nursery Furniture, Holiday and Recreation Safety, a Glossary, and Resources for Further Help and Information

Edited by Dawn D. Matthews. 606 pages. 2002. 0-7808-0338-8. $78.

"This work will be useful in public libraries with large consumer health and wellness departments."
—*American Reference Books Annual, 2003*

"As a sourcebook on household safety this book meets its mark. It is encyclopedic in scope and covers a wide range of safety issues that are commonly seen in the home."
—*E-Streams, Jul '02*

Hypertension Sourcebook

Basic Consumer Health Information about the Causes, Diagnosis, and Treatment of High Blood Pressure, with Facts about Consequences, Complications, and Co-Occurring Disorders, Such as Coronary Heart Disease, Diabetes, Stroke, Kidney Disease, and Hypertensive Retinopathy, and Issues in Blood Pressure Control, Including Dietary Choices, Stress Management, and Medications

Along with Reports on Current Research Initiatives and Clinical Trials, a Glossary, and Resources for Additional Help and Information

Edited by Dawn D. Matthews and Karen Bellenir. 613 pages. 2004. 0-7808-0674-3. $78.

■

Immune System Disorders Sourcebook, 2nd Edition

Basic Consumer Health Information about Disorders of the Immune System, Including Immune System Function and Response, Diagnosis of Immune Disorders, Information about Inherited Immune Disease, Acquired Immune Disease, and Autoimmune Diseases, Including Primary Immune Deficiency, Acquired Immunodeficiency Syndrome (AIDS), Lupus, Multiple Sclerosis, Type 1 Diabetes, Rheumatoid Arthritis, and Graves Disease

Along with Treatments, Tips for Coping with Immune Disorders, a Glossary, and a Directory of Additional Resources

Edited by Joyce Brennfleck Shannon. 671 pages. 2005. 0-7808-0748-0. $78.

ALSO AVAILABLE: Immune System Disorders Sourcebook. Edited by Allan R. Cook. 608 pages. 1997. 0-7808-0209-8. $78.

■

Infant & Toddler Health Sourcebook

Basic Consumer Health Information about the Physical and Mental Development of Newborns, Infants, and Toddlers, Including Neonatal Concerns, Nutrition Recommendations, Immunization Schedules, Common Pediatric Disorders, Assessments and Milestones, Safety Tips, and Advice for Parents and Other Caregivers

Along with a Glossary of Terms and Resource Listings for Additional Help

Edited by Jenifer Swanson. 585 pages. 2000. 0-7808-0246-2. $78.

"As a reference for the general public, this would be useful in any library." — *E-Streams, May '01*

"Recommended reference source." — *Booklist, American Library Association, Feb '01*

"This is a good source for general use." —*American Reference Books Annual, 2001*

Infectious Diseases Sourcebook

Basic Consumer Health Information about Non-Contagious Bacterial, Viral, Prion, Fungal, and Parasitic Diseases Spread by Food and Water, Insects and Animals, or Environmental Contact, Including Botulism, E. Coli, Encephalitis, Legionnaires' Disease, Lyme Disease, Malaria, Plague, Rabies, Salmonella, Tetanus, and Others, and Facts about Newly Emerging Diseases, Such as Hantavirus, Mad Cow Disease, Monkeypox, and West Nile Virus

Along with Information about Preventing Disease Transmission, the Threat of Bioterrorism, and Current Research Initiatives, with a Glossary and Directory of Resources for More Information

Edited by Karen Bellenir. 634 pages. 2004. 0-7808-0675-1. $78.

■

Injury & Trauma Sourcebook

Basic Consumer Health Information about the Impact of Injury, the Diagnosis and Treatment of Common and Traumatic Injuries, Emergency Care, and Specific Injuries Related to Home, Community, Workplace, Transportation, and Recreation

Along with Guidelines for Injury Prevention, a Glossary, and a Directory of Additional Resources

Edited by Joyce Brennfleck Shannon. 696 pages. 2002. 0-7808-0421-X. $78.

"This publication is the most comprehensive work of its kind about injury and trauma." — *American Reference Books Annual, 2003*

"This sourcebook provides concise, easily readable, basic health information about injuries. . . . This book is well organized and an easy to use reference resource suitable for hospital, health sciences and public libraries with consumer health collections." — *E-Streams, Nov '02*

"Practitioners should be aware of guides such as this in order to facilitate their use by patients and their families." — *Doody's Health Sciences Book Review Journal, Sep-Oct '02*

"Recommended reference source." — *Booklist, American Library Association, Sep '02*

"Highly recommended for academic and medical reference collections." — *Library Bookwatch, Sep '02*

■

Kidney & Urinary Tract Diseases & Disorders Sourcebook

Basic Information about Kidney Stones, Urinary Incontinence, Bladder Disease, End Stage Renal Disease, Dialysis, and More

Along with Statistical and Demographic Data and Reports on Current Research Initiatives

Edited by Linda M. Ross. 602 pages. 1997. 0-7808-0079-6. $78.

659

Learning Disabilities Sourcebook, 2nd Edition

Basic Consumer Health Information about Learning Disabilities, Including Dyslexia, Developmental Speech and Language Disabilities, Non-Verbal Learning Disorders, Developmental Arithmetic Disorder, Developmental Writing Disorder, and Other Conditions That Impede Learning Such as Attention Deficit/ Hyperactivity Disorder, Brain Injury, Hearing Impairment, Klinefelter Syndrome, Dyspraxia, and Tourette Syndrome

Along with Facts about Educational Issues and Assistive Technology, Coping Strategies, a Glossary of Related Terms, and Resources for Further Help and Information

Edited by Dawn D. Matthews. 621 pages. 2003. 0-7808-0626-3. $78.

ALSO AVAILABLE: Learning Disabilities Sourcebook, 1st Edition. Edited by Linda M. Shin. 579 pages. 1998. 0-7808-0210-1. $78.

"The second edition of *Learning Disabilities Sourcebook* far surpasses the earlier edition in that it is more focused on information that will be useful as a consumer health resource."
— *American Reference Books Annual, 2004*

"Teachers as well as consumers will find this an essential guide to understanding various syndromes and their latest treatments. [An] invaluable reference for public and school library collections alike."
— *Library Bookwatch, Apr '03*

Named "Outstanding Reference Book of 1999."
— *New York Public Library, Feb 2000*

"An excellent candidate for inclusion in a public library reference section. It's a great source of information. Teachers will also find the book useful. Definitely worth reading."
— *Journal of Adolescent & Adult Literacy, Feb 2000*

"Readable . . . provides a solid base of information regarding successful techniques used with individuals who have learning disabilities, as well as practical suggestions for educators and family members. Clear language, concise descriptions, and pertinent information for contacting multiple resources add to the strength of this book as a useful tool." — *Choice, Association of College and Research Libraries, Feb '99*

"Recommended reference source."
— *Booklist, American Library Association, Sep '98*

"A useful resource for libraries and for those who don't have the time to identify and locate the individual publications." — *Disability Resources Monthly, Sep '98*

Leukemia Sourcebook

Basic Consumer Health Information about Adult and Childhood Leukemias, Including Acute Lymphocytic Leukemia (ALL), Chronic Lymphocytic Leukemia (CLL), Acute Myelogenous Leukemia (AML), Chronic Myelogenous Leukemia (CML), and Hairy Cell Leukemia, and Treatments Such as Chemotherapy, Radiation Therapy, Peripheral Blood Stem Cell and Marrow Transplantation, and Immunotherapy

Along with Tips for Life During and After Treatment, a Glossary, and Directories of Additional Resources

Edited by Joyce Brennfleck Shannon. 587 pages. 2003. 0-7808-0627-1. $78.

"Unlike other medical books for the layperson, . . . the language does not talk down to the reader. . . . This volume is highly recommended for all libraries."
— *American Reference Books Annual, 2004*

Liver Disorders Sourcebook

Basic Consumer Health Information about the Liver and How It Works; Liver Diseases, Including Cancer, Cirrhosis, Hepatitis, and Toxic and Drug Related Diseases; Tips for Maintaining a Healthy Liver; Laboratory Tests, Radiology Tests, and Facts about Liver Transplantation

Along with a Section on Support Groups, a Glossary, and Resource Listings

Edited by Joyce Brennfleck Shannon. 591 pages. 2000. 0-7808-0383-3. $78.

"A valuable resource."
— *American Reference Books Annual, 2001*

"This title is recommended for health sciences and public libraries with consumer health collections."
— *E-Streams, Oct '00*

"Recommended reference source."
— *Booklist, American Library Association, Jun '00*

Lung Disorders Sourcebook

Basic Consumer Health Information about Emphysema, Pneumonia, Tuberculosis, Asthma, Cystic Fibrosis, and Other Lung Disorders, Including Facts about Diagnostic Procedures, Treatment Strategies, Disease Prevention Efforts, and Such Risk Factors as Smoking, Air Pollution, and Exposure to Asbestos, Radon, and Other Agents

Along with a Glossary and Resources for Additional Help and Information

Edited by Dawn D. Matthews. 678 pages. 2002. 0-7808-0339-6. $78.

"This title is a great addition for public and school libraries because it provides concise health information on the lungs."
— *American Reference Books Annual, 2003*

"Highly recommended for academic and medical reference collections." — *Library Bookwatch, Sep '02*

Medical Tests Sourcebook, 2nd Edition

Basic Consumer Health Information about Medical Tests, Including Age-Specific Health Tests, Important Health Screenings and Exams, Home-Use Tests, Blood and Specimen Tests, Electrical Tests, Scope Tests, Genetic Testing, and Imaging Tests, Such as X-Rays,

Ultrasound, Computed Tomography, Magnetic Resonance Imaging, Angiography, and Nuclear Medicine

Along with a Glossary and Directory of Additional Resources

Edited by Joyce Brennfleck Shannon. 654 pages. 2004. 0-7808-0670-0. $78.

ALSO AVAILABLE: Medical Tests, 1st Edition. Edited by Joyce Brennfleck Shannon. 691 pages. 1999. 0-7808-0243-8. $78.

"Recommended for hospital and health sciences libraries with consumer health collections."
—E-Streams, Mar '00

"This is an overall excellent reference with a wealth of general knowledge that may aid those who are reluctant to get vital tests performed."
—Today's Librarian, Jan 2000

"A valuable reference guide."
—American Reference Books Annual, 2000

■

Men's Health Concerns Sourcebook, 2nd Edition

Basic Consumer Health Information about the Medical and Mental Concerns of Men, Including Theories about the Shorter Male Lifespan, the Leading Causes of Death and Disability, Physical Concerns of Special Significance to Men, Reproductive and Sexual Concerns, Sexually Transmitted Diseases, Men's Mental and Emotional Health, and Lifestyle Choices That Affect Wellness, Such as Nutrition, Fitness, and Substance Use

Along with a Glossary of Related Terms and a Directory of Organizational Resources in Men's Health

Edited by Robert Aquinas McNally. 644 pages. 2004. 0-7808-0671-9. $78.

ALSO AVAILABLE: Men's Health Concerns Sourcebook, 1st Edition. Edited by Allan R. Cook. 738 pages. 1998. 0-7808-0212-8. $78.

"This comprehensive resource and the series are highly recommended."
—American Reference Books Annual, 2000

"Recommended reference source."
—Booklist, American Library Association, Dec '98

■

Mental Health Disorders Sourcebook, 3rd Edition

Basic Consumer Health Information about Mental and Emotional Health and Mental Illness, Including Facts about Depression, Bipolar Disorder, and Other Mood Disorders, Phobias, Post-Traumatic Stress Disorder (PTSD), Obsessive-Compulsive Disorder, and Other Anxiety Disorders, Impulse Control Disorders, Eating Disorders, Personality Disorders, and Psychotic Disorders, Including Schizophrenia and Dissociative Disorders

Along with Statistical Information, a Special Section Concerning Mental Health Issues in Children and

Adolescents, a Glossary, and Directories of Resources for Additional Help and Information

Edited by Karen Bellenir. 661 pages. 2005. 0-7808-0747-2. $78.

ALSO AVAILABLE: Mental Health Disorders Sourcebook, 1st Edition. Edited by Karen Bellenir. 548 pages. 1995. 0-7808-0040-0. $78.

ALSO AVAILABLE: Mental Health Disorders Sourcebook, 2nd Edition. Edited by Karen Bellenir. 605 pages. 2000. 0-7808-0240-3. $78.

"Well organized and well written."
—American Reference Books Annual, 2001

"Recommended reference source."
—Booklist, American Library Association, Jun '00

■

Mental Retardation Sourcebook

Basic Consumer Health Information about Mental Retardation and Its Causes, Including Down Syndrome, Fetal Alcohol Syndrome, Fragile X Syndrome, Genetic Conditions, Injury, and Environmental Sources

Along with Preventive Strategies, Parenting Issues, Educational Implications, Health Care Needs, Employment and Economic Matters, Legal Issues, a Glossary, and a Resource Listing for Additional Help and Information

Edited by Joyce Brennfleck Shannon. 642 pages. 2000. 0-7808-0377-9. $78.

"Public libraries will find the book useful for reference and as a beginning research point for students, parents, and caregivers."
—American Reference Books Annual, 2001

"The strength of this work is that it compiles many basic fact sheets and addresses for further information in one volume. It is intended and suitable for the general public. This sourcebook is relevant to any collection providing health information to the general public."
—E-Streams, Nov '00

"From preventing retardation to parenting and family challenges, this covers health, social and legal issues and will prove an invaluable overview."
—Reviewer's Bookwatch, Jul '00

■

Movement Disorders Sourcebook

Basic Consumer Health Information about Neurological Movement Disorders, Including Essential Tremor, Parkinson's Disease, Dystonia, Cerebral Palsy, Huntington's Disease, Myasthenia Gravis, Multiple Sclerosis, and Other Early-Onset and Adult-Onset Movement Disorders, Their Symptoms and Causes, Diagnostic Tests, and Treatments

Along with Mobility and Assistive Technology Information, a Glossary, and a Directory of Additional Resources

Edited by Joyce Brennfleck Shannon. 655 pages. 2003. 0-7808-0628-X. $78.

". . . a good resource for consumers and recommended for public, community college and undergraduate libraries."
—American Reference Books Annual, 2004

Muscular Dystrophy Sourcebook

Basic Consumer Health Information about Congenital, Childhood-Onset, and Adult-Onset Forms of Muscular Dystrophy, Such as Duchenne, Becker, Emery-Dreifuss, Distal, Limb-Girdle, Facioscapulohumeral (FSHD), Myotonic, and Ophthalmoplegic Muscular Dystrophies, Including Facts about Diagnostic Tests, Medical and Physical Therapies, Management of Co-Occurring Conditions, and Parenting Guidelines

Along with Practical Tips for Home Care, a Glossary, and Directories of Additional Resources

Edited by Joyce Brennfleck Shannon. 577 pages. 2004. 0-7808-0676-X. $78.

Obesity Sourcebook

Basic Consumer Health Information about Diseases and Other Problems Associated with Obesity, and Including Facts about Risk Factors, Prevention Issues, and Management Approaches

Along with Statistical and Demographic Data, Information about Special Populations, Research Updates, a Glossary, and Source Listings for Further Help and Information

Edited by Wilma Caldwell and Chad T. Kimball. 376 pages. 2001. 0-7808-0333-7. $78.

"The book synthesizes the reliable medical literature on obesity into one easy-to-read and useful resource for the general public."
— *American Reference Books Annual 2002*

"This is a very useful resource book for the lay public."
— *Doody's Review Service, Nov '01*

"Well suited for the health reference collection of a public library or an academic health science library that serves the general population." — *E-Streams, Sep '01*

"Recommended reference source."
— *Booklist, American Library Association, Apr '01*

" Recommended pick both for specialty health library collections and any general consumer health reference collection." — *The Bookwatch, Apr '01*

Ophthalmic Disorders Sourcebook, 1st Edition

SEE *Eye Care Sourcebook, 2nd Edition*

Oral Health Sourcebook

SEE *Dental Care & Oral Health Sourcebook, 2nd Ed.*

Osteoporosis Sourcebook

Basic Consumer Health Information about Primary and Secondary Osteoporosis and Juvenile Osteoporosis and Related Conditions, Including Fibrous Dysplasia, Gaucher Disease, Hyperthyroidism, Hypophosphatasia, Myeloma, Osteopetrosis, Osteogenesis Imperfecta, and Paget's Disease

Along with Information about Risk Factors, Treatments, Traditional and Non-Traditional Pain Management, a Glossary of Related Terms, and a Directory of Resources

Edited by Allan R. Cook. 584 pages. 2001. 0-7808-0239-X. $78.

"This would be a book to be kept in a staff or patient library. The targeted audience is the layperson, but the therapist who needs a quick bit of information on a particular topic will also find the book useful."
— *Physical Therapy, Jan '02*

"This resource is recommended as a great reference source for public, health, and academic libraries, and is another triumph for the editors of Omnigraphics."
— *American Reference Books Annual 2002*

"Recommended for all public libraries and general health collections, especially those supporting patient education or consumer health programs."
— *E-Streams, Nov '01*

"Will prove valuable to any library seeking to maintain a current, comprehensive reference collection of health resources. . . . From prevention to treatment and associated conditions, this provides an excellent survey."
— *The Bookwatch, Aug '01*

"Recommended reference source."
— *Booklist, American Library Association, July '01*

SEE ALSO *Women's Health Concerns Sourcebook*

Pain Sourcebook, 2nd Edition

Basic Consumer Health Information about Specific Forms of Acute and Chronic Pain, Including Muscle and Skeletal Pain, Nerve Pain, Cancer Pain, and Disorders Characterized by Pain, Such as Fibromyalgia, Shingles, Angina, Arthritis, and Headaches

Along with Information about Pain Medications and Management Techniques, Complementary and Alternative Pain Relief Options, Tips for People Living with Chronic Pain, a Glossary, and a Directory of Sources for Further Information

Edited by Karen Bellenir. 670 pages. 2002. 0-7808-0612-3. $78.

ALSO AVAILABLE: *Pain Sourcebook, 1st Edition.*
Edited by Allan R. Cook. 667 pages. 1997. 0-7808-0213-6. $78.

"A source of valuable information. . . . This book offers help to nonmedical people who need information about pain and pain management. It is also an excellent reference for those who participate in patient education."
— *Doody's Review Service, Sep '02*

"The text is readable, easily understood, and well indexed. This excellent volume belongs in all patient education libraries, consumer health sections of public libraries, and many personal collections."
— *American Reference Books Annual, 1999*

"A beneficial reference." — *Booklist Health Sciences Supplement, American Library Association, Oct '98*

"The information is basic in terms of scholarship and is appropriate for general readers. Written in journalistic style . . . intended for non-professionals. Quite thorough in its coverage of different pain conditions and summarizes the latest clinical information regarding pain treatment." — *Choice, Association of College and Research Libraries, Jun '98*

"Recommended reference source."
— *Booklist, American Library Association, Mar '98*

■

Pediatric Cancer Sourcebook

Basic Consumer Health Information about Leukemias, Brain Tumors, Sarcomas, Lymphomas, and Other Cancers in Infants, Children, and Adolescents, Including Descriptions of Cancers, Treatments, and Coping Strategies

Along with Suggestions for Parents, Caregivers, and Concerned Relatives, a Glossary of Cancer Terms, and Resource Listings

Edited by Edward J. Prucha. 587 pages. 1999. 0-7808-0245-4. $78.

"An excellent source of information. Recommended for public, hospital, and health science libraries with consumer health collections." — *E-Streams, Jun '00*

"Recommended reference source."
— *Booklist, American Library Association, Feb '00*

"A valuable addition to all libraries specializing in health services and many public libraries."
—*American Reference Books Annual, 2000*

■

Physical & Mental Issues in Aging Sourcebook

Basic Consumer Health Information on Physical and Mental Disorders Associated with the Aging Process, Including Concerns about Cardiovascular Disease, Pulmonary Disease, Oral Health, Digestive Disorders, Musculoskeletal and Skin Disorders, Metabolic Changes, Sexual and Reproductive Issues, and Changes in Vision, Hearing, and Other Senses

Along with Data about Longevity and Causes of Death, Information on Acute and Chronic Pain, Descriptions of Mental Concerns, a Glossary of Terms, and Resource Listings for Additional Help

Edited by Jenifer Swanson. 660 pages. 1999. 0-7808-0233-0. $78.

"This is a treasure of health information for the layperson." — *Choice Health Sciences Supplement, Association of College & Research Libraries, May 2000*

"Recommended for public libraries."
—*American Reference Books Annual, 2000*

"Recommended reference source."
— *Booklist, American Library Association, Oct '99*

SEE ALSO *Healthy Aging Sourcebook*

Podiatry Sourcebook

Basic Consumer Health Information about Foot Conditions, Diseases, and Injuries, Including Bunions, Corns, Calluses, Athlete's Foot, Plantar Warts, Hammertoes and Clawtoes, Clubfoot, Heel Pain, Gout, and More

Along with Facts about Foot Care, Disease Prevention, Foot Safety, Choosing a Foot Care Specialist, a Glossary of Terms, and Resource Listings for Additional Information

Edited by M. Lisa Weatherford. 380 pages. 2001. 0-7808-0215-2. $78.

"Recommended reference source."
— *Booklist, American Library Association, Feb '02*

"There is a lot of information presented here on a topic that is usually only covered sparingly in most larger comprehensive medical encyclopedias."
— *American Reference Books Annual 2002*

■

Pregnancy & Birth Sourcebook, 2nd Edition

Basic Consumer Health Information about Conception and Pregnancy, Including Facts about Fertility, Infertility, Pregnancy Symptoms and Complications, Fetal Growth and Development, Labor, Delivery, and the Postpartum Period, as Well as Information about Maintaining Health and Wellness during Pregnancy and Caring for a Newborn

Along with Information about Public Health Assistance for Low-Income Pregnant Women, a Glossary, and Directories of Agencies and Organizations Providing Help and Support

Edited by Amy L. Sutton. 626 pages. 2004. 0-7808-0672-7. $78.

ALSO AVAILABLE: *Pregnancy & Birth Sourcebook, 1st Edition.* Edited by Heather E. Aldred. 737 pages. 1997. 0-7808-0216-0. $78.

"A well-organized handbook. Recommended."
— *Choice, Association of College and Research Libraries, Apr '98*

"Recommended reference source."
— *Booklist, American Library Association, Mar '98*

"Recommended for public libraries."
— *American Reference Books Annual, 1998*

SEE ALSO *Congenital Disorders Sourcebook, Family Planning Sourcebook*

■

Prostate Cancer Sourcebook

Basic Consumer Health Information about Prostate Cancer, Including Information about the Associated Risk Factors, Detection, Diagnosis, and Treatment of Prostate Cancer

Along with Information on Non-Malignant Prostate Conditions, and Featuring a Section Listing Support and Treatment Centers and a Glossary of Related Terms

Edited by Dawn D. Matthews. 358 pages. 2001. 0-7808-0324-8. $78.

■

Public Health Sourcebook

Basic Information about Government Health Agencies, Including National Health Statistics and Trends, Healthy People 2000 Program Goals and Objectives, the Centers for Disease Control and Prevention, the Food and Drug Administration, and the National Institutes of Health

Along with Full Contact Information for Each Agency

Edited by Wendy Wilcox. 698 pages. 1998. 0-7808-0220-9. $78.

■

Reconstructive & Cosmetic Surgery Sourcebook

Basic Consumer Health Information on Cosmetic and Reconstructive Plastic Surgery, Including Statistical Information about Different Surgical Procedures, Things to Consider Prior to Surgery, Plastic Surgery Techniques and Tools, Emotional and Psychological Considerations, and Procedure-Specific Information

Along with a Glossary of Terms and a Listing of Resources for Additional Help and Information

Edited by M. Lisa Weatherford. 374 pages. 2001. 0-7808-0214-4. $78.

Rehabilitation Sourcebook

Basic Consumer Health Information about Rehabilitation for People Recovering from Heart Surgery, Spinal Cord Injury, Stroke, Orthopedic Impairments, Amputation, Pulmonary Impairments, Traumatic Injury, and More, Including Physical Therapy, Occupational Therapy, Speech/ Language Therapy, Massage Therapy, Dance Therapy, Art Therapy, and Recreational Therapy

Along with Information on Assistive and Adaptive Devices, a Glossary, and Resources for Additional Help and Information

Edited by Dawn D. Matthews. 531 pages. 1999. 0-7808-0236-5. $78.

■

Respiratory Diseases & Disorders Sourcebook

Basic Information about Respiratory Diseases and Disorders, Including Asthma, Cystic Fibrosis, Pneumonia, the Common Cold, Influenza, and Others, Featuring Facts about the Respiratory System, Statistical and Demographic Data, Treatments, Self-Help Management Suggestions, and Current Research Initiatives

Edited by Allan R. Cook and Peter D. Dresser. 771 pages. 1995. 0-7808-0037-0. $78.

SEE ALSO Lung Disorders Sourcebook

■

Sexually Transmitted Diseases Sourcebook, 2nd Edition

Basic Consumer Health Information about Sexually Transmitted Diseases, Including Information on the Diagnosis and Treatment of Chlamydia, Gonorrhea, Hepatitis, Herpes, HIV, Mononucleosis, Syphilis, and Others

Along with Information on Prevention, Such as Condom Use, Vaccines, and STD Education; And Featuring a Section on Issues Related to Youth and Adolescents, a Glossary, and Resources for Additional Help and Information

Edited by Dawn D. Matthews. 538 pages. 2001. 0-7808-0249-7. $78.

ALSO AVAILABLE: Sexually Transmitted Diseases Sourcebook, 1st Edition. Edited by Linda M. Ross. 550 pages. 1997. 0-7808-0217-9. $78.

"Recommended for consumer health collections in public libraries, and secondary school and community college libraries."
— *American Reference Books Annual 2002*

"Every school and public library should have a copy of this comprehensive and user-friendly reference book."
— *Choice, Association of College & Research Libraries, Sep '01*

"This is a highly recommended book. This is an especially important book for all school and public libraries." — *AIDS Book Review Journal, Jul-Aug '01*

"Recommended reference source."
— *Booklist, American Library Association, Apr '01*

"Recommended pick both for specialty health library collections and any general consumer health reference collection." — *The Bookwatch, Apr '01*

■

Skin Disorders Sourcebook

Basic Information about Common Skin and Scalp Conditions Caused by Aging, Allergies, Immune Reactions, Sun Exposure, Infectious Organisms, Parasites, Cosmetics, and Skin Traumas, Including Abrasions, Cuts, and Pressure Sores

Along with Information on Prevention and Treatment

Edited by Allan R. Cook. 647 pages. 1997. 0-7808-0080-X. $78.

"... comprehensive, easily read reference book."
— *Doody's Health Sciences Book Reviews, Oct '97*

SEE ALSO Burns Sourcebook

■

Sleep Disorders Sourcebook, 2nd Edition

Basic Consumer Health Information about Sleep and Sleep Disorders, Including Insomnia, Sleep Apnea, Restless Legs Syndrome, Narcolepsy, Parasomnias, and Other Health Problems That Affect Sleep, Plus Facts about Diagnostic Procedures, Treatment Strategies, Sleep Medications, and Tips for Improving Sleep Quality

Along with a Glossary of Related Terms and Resources for Additional Help and Information

Edited by Amy L. Sutton. 567 pages. 2005. 0-7808-0745-6. $78.

ALSO AVAILABLE: Sleep Disorders Sourcebook, 1st Edition. Edited by Jenifer Swanson. 439 pages. 1998. 0-7808-0234-9. $78.

"This text will complement any home or medical library. It is user-friendly and ideal for the adult reader."
— *American Reference Books Annual, 2000*

"A useful resource that provides accurate, relevant, and accessible information on sleep to the general public. Health care providers who deal with sleep disorders patients may also find it helpful in being prepared to answer some of the questions patients ask."
— *Respiratory Care, Jul '99*

"Recommended reference source."
— *Booklist, American Library Association, Feb '99*

■

Smoking Concerns Sourcebook

Basic Consumer Health Information about Nicotine Addiction and Smoking Cessation, Featuring Facts about the Health Effects of Tobacco Use, Including Lung and Other Cancers, Heart Disease, Stroke, and Respiratory Disorders, Such as Emphysema and Chronic Bronchitis

Along with Information about Smoking Prevention Programs, Suggestions for Achieving and Maintaining a Smoke-Free Lifestyle, Statistics about Tobacco Use, Reports on Current Research Initiatives, a Glossary of Related Terms, and Directories of Resources for Additional Help and Information

Edited by Karen Bellenir. 621 pages. 2004. 0-7808-0323-X. $78.

■

Sports Injuries Sourcebook, 2nd Edition

Basic Consumer Health Information about the Diagnosis, Treatment, and Rehabilitation of Common Sports-Related Injuries in Children and Adults

Along with Suggestions for Conditioning and Training, Information and Prevention Tips for Injuries Frequently Associated with Specific Sports and Special Populations, a Glossary, and a Directory of Additional Resources

Edited by Joyce Brennfleck Shannon. 614 pages. 2002. 0-7808-0604-2. $78.

ALSO AVAILABLE: Sports Injuries Sourcebook, 1st Edition. Edited by Heather E. Aldred. 624 pages. 1999. 0-7808-0218-7. $78.

"This is an excellent reference for consumers and it is recommended for public, community college, and undergraduate libraries."
— *American Reference Books Annual, 2003*

"Recommended reference source."
— *Booklist, American Library Association, Feb '03*

■

Stress-Related Disorders Sourcebook

Basic Consumer Health Information about Stress and Stress-Related Disorders, Including Stress Origins and Signals, Environmental Stress at Work and Home, Mental and Emotional Stress Associated with Depres-

sion, Post-Traumatic Stress Disorder, Panic Disorder, Suicide, and the Physical Effects of Stress on the Cardiovascular, Immune, and Nervous Systems

Along with Stress Management Techniques, a Glossary, and a Listing of Additional Resources

Edited by Joyce Brennfleck Shannon. 610 pages. 2002. 0-7808-0560-7. $78.

"Well written for a general readership, the *Stress-Related Disorders Sourcebook* is a useful addition to the health reference literature." — *American Reference Books Annual, 2003*

"I am impressed by the amount of information. It offers a thorough overview of the causes and consequences of stress to the layperson. . . . A well-done and thorough reference guide for professionals and nonprofessionals alike." — *Doody's Review Service, Dec '02*

■

Stroke Sourcebook

Basic Consumer Health Information about Stroke, Including Ischemic, Hemorrhagic, Transient Ischemic Attack (TIA), and Pediatric Stroke, Stroke Triggers and Risks, Diagnostic Tests, Treatments, and Rehabilitation Information

Along with Stroke Prevention Guidelines, Legal and Financial Information, a Glossary, and a Directory of Additional Resources

Edited by Joyce Brennfleck Shannon. 606 pages. 2003. 0-7808-0630-1. $78.

"This volume is highly recommended and should be in every medical, hospital, and public library." — *American Reference Books Annual, 2004*

■

Substance Abuse Sourcebook

Basic Health-Related Information about the Abuse of Legal and Illegal Substances Such as Alcohol, Tobacco, Prescription Drugs, Marijuana, Cocaine, and Heroin; and Including Facts about Substance Abuse Prevention Strategies, Intervention Methods, Treatment and Recovery Programs, and a Section Addressing the Special Problems Related to Substance Abuse during Pregnancy

Edited by Karen Bellenir. 573 pages. 1996. 0-7808-0038-9. $78.

"A valuable addition to any health reference section. Highly recommended." — *The Book Report, Mar/Apr '97*

". . . a comprehensive collection of substance abuse information that's both highly readable and compact. Families and caregivers of substance abusers will find the information enlightening and helpful, while teachers, social workers and journalists should benefit from the concise format. Recommended." — *Drug Abuse Update, Winter '96/'97*

SEE ALSO *Alcoholism Sourcebook, Drug Abuse Sourcebook*

Surgery Sourcebook

Basic Consumer Health Information about Inpatient and Outpatient Surgeries, Including Cardiac, Vascular, Orthopedic, Ocular, Reconstructive, Cosmetic, Gynecologic, and Ear, Nose, and Throat Procedures and More

Along with Information about Operating Room Policies and Instruments, Laser Surgery Techniques, Hospital Errors, Statistical Data, a Glossary, and Listings of Sources for Further Help and Information

Edited by Annemarie S. Muth and Karen Bellenir. 596 pages. 2002. 0-7808-0380-9. $78.

"Large public libraries and medical libraries would benefit from this material in their reference collections." — *American Reference Books Annual, 2004*

"Invaluable reference for public and school library collections alike." — *Library Bookwatch, Apr '03*

■

Thyroid Disorders Sourcebook

Basic Consumer Health Information about Disorders of the Thyroid and Parathyroid Glands, Including Hypothyroidism, Hyperthyroidism, Graves Disease, Hashimoto Thyroiditis, Thyroid Cancer, and Parathyroid Disorders, Featuring Facts about Symptoms, Risk Factors, Tests, and Treatments

Along with Information about the Effects of Thyroid Imbalance on Other Body Systems, Environmental Factors That Affect the Thyroid Gland, a Glossary, and a Directory of Additional Resources

Edited by Joyce Brennfleck Shannon. 599 pages. 2005. 0-7808-0745-6. $78.

■

Transplantation Sourcebook

Basic Consumer Health Information about Organ and Tissue Transplantation, Including Physical and Financial Preparations, Procedures and Issues Relating to Specific Solid Organ and Tissue Transplants, Rehabilitation, Pediatric Transplant Information, the Future of Transplantation, and Organ and Tissue Donation

Along with a Glossary and Listings of Additional Resources

Edited by Joyce Brennfleck Shannon. 628 pages. 2002. 0-7808-0322-1. $78.

"Along with these advances [in transplantation technology] have come a number of daunting questions for potential transplant patients, their families, and their health care providers. This reference text is the best single tool to address many of these questions. . . . It will be a much-needed addition to the reference collections in health care, academic, and large public libraries." — *American Reference Books Annual, 2003*

"Recommended for libraries with an interest in offering consumer health information." — *E-Streams, Jul '02*

"This is a unique and valuable resource for patients facing transplantation and their families." — *Doody's Review Service, Jun '02*

Traveler's Health Sourcebook

Basic Consumer Health Information for Travelers, Including Physical and Medical Preparations, Transportation Health and Safety, Essential Information about Food and Water, Sun Exposure, Insect and Snake Bites, Camping and Wilderness Medicine, and Travel with Physical or Medical Disabilities

Along with International Travel Tips, Vaccination Recommendations, Geographical Health Issues, Disease Risks, a Glossary, and a Listing of Additional Resources

Edited by Joyce Brennfleck Shannon. 613 pages. 2000. 0-7808-0384-1. $78.

"Recommended reference source."
— Booklist, American Library Association, Feb '01

"This book is recommended for any public library, any travel collection, and especially any collection for the physically disabled."
—American Reference Books Annual, 2001

■

Vegetarian Sourcebook

Basic Consumer Health Information about Vegetarian Diets, Lifestyle, and Philosophy, Including Definitions of Vegetarianism and Veganism, Tips about Adopting Vegetarianism, Creating a Vegetarian Pantry, and Meeting Nutritional Needs of Vegetarians, with Facts Regarding Vegetarianism's Effect on Pregnant and Lactating Women, Children, Athletes, and Senior Citizens

Along with a Glossary of Commonly Used Vegetarian Terms and Resources for Additional Help and Information

Edited by Chad T. Kimball. 360 pages. 2002. 0-7808-0439-2. $78.

"Organizes into one concise volume the answers to the most common questions concerning vegetarian diets and lifestyles. This title is recommended for public and secondary school libraries." — E-Streams, Apr '03

"Invaluable reference for public and school library collections alike." — Library Bookwatch, Apr '03

"The articles in this volume are easy to read and come from authoritative sources. The book does not necessarily support the vegetarian diet but instead provides the pros and cons of this important decision. The *Vegetarian Sourcebook* is recommended for public libraries and consumer health libraries."
— American Reference Books Annual, 2003

■

Women's Health Concerns Sourcebook, 2nd Edition

Basic Consumer Health Information about the Medical and Mental Concerns of Women, Including Maintaining Health and Wellness, Gynecological Concerns, Breast Health, Sexuality and Reproductive Issues, Menopause, Cancer in Women, the Leading Causes of Death and Disability among Women, Physical Concerns of Special Significance to Women, and Women's Mental and Emotional Health

Along with a Glossary of Related Terms and Directories of Resources for Additional Help and Information

Edited by Amy L. Sutton. 748 pages. 2004. 0-7808-0673-5. $78.

ALSO AVAILABLE: Women's Health Concerns Sourcebook, 1st Edition. Edited by Heather E. Aldred. 567 pages. 1997. 0-7808-0219-5. $78.

"Handy compilation. There is an impressive range of diseases, devices, disorders, procedures, and other physical and emotional issues covered . . . well organized, illustrated, and indexed." —Choice, Association of College and Research Libraries, Jan '98

SEE ALSO Breast Cancer Sourcebook, Cancer Sourcebook for Women, Healthy Heart Sourcebook for Women, Osteoporosis Sourcebook

■

Workplace Health & Safety Sourcebook

Basic Consumer Health Information about Workplace Health and Safety, Including the Effect of Workplace Hazards on the Lungs, Skin, Heart, Ears, Eyes, Brain, Reproductive Organs, Musculoskeletal System, and Other Organs and Body Parts

Along with Information about Occupational Cancer, Personal Protective Equipment, Toxic and Hazardous Chemicals, Child Labor, Stress, and Workplace Violence

Edited by Chad T. Kimball. 626 pages. 2000. 0-7808-0231-4. $78.

"As a reference for the general public, this would be useful in any library." —E-Streams, Jun '01

"Provides helpful information for primary care physicians and other caregivers interested in occupational medicine. . . . General readers; professionals."
— Choice, Association of College & Research Libraries, May '01

"Recommended reference source."
— Booklist, American Library Association, Feb '01

"Highly recommended." —The Bookwatch, Jan '01

■

Worldwide Health Sourcebook

Basic Information about Global Health Issues, Including Malnutrition, Reproductive Health, Disease Dispersion and Prevention, Emerging Diseases, Risky Health Behaviors, and the Leading Causes of Death

Along with Global Health Concerns for Children, Women, and the Elderly, Mental Health Issues, Research and Technology Advancements, and Economic, Environmental, and Political Health Implications, a Glossary, and a Resource Listing for Additional Help and Information

Edited by Joyce Brennfleck Shannon. 614 pages. 2001. 0-7808-0330-2. $78.

"Named an Outstanding Academic Title." —Choice, Association of College & Research Libraries, Jan '02

"Yet another handy but also unique compilation in the extensive Health Reference Series, this is a useful work because many of the international publications reprinted or excerpted are not readily available. Highly recommended."
— *Choice, Association of College & Research Libraries, Nov '01*

"Recommended reference source."
— *Booklist, American Library Association, Oct '01*

Teen Health Series

Helping Young Adults Understand, Manage, and Avoid Serious Illness

Alcohol Information for Teens
Health Tips About Alcohol And Alcoholism

Including Facts about Underage Drinking, Preventing Teen Alcohol Use, Alcohol's Effects on the Brain and the Body, Alcohol Abuse Treatment, Help for Children of Alcoholics, and More

Edited by Joyce Brennfleck Shannon. 370 pages. 2005. 0-7808-0741-3. $58.

Asthma Information for Teens
Health Tips about Managing Asthma and Related Concerns

Including Facts about Asthma Causes, Triggers, Symptoms, Diagnosis, and Treatment

Edited by Karen Bellenir. 386 pages. 2005. 0-7808-0770-7. $58.

Cancer Information for Teens
Health Tips about Cancer Awareness, Prevention, Diagnosis, and Treatment

Including Facts about Frequently Occurring Cancers, Cancer Risk Factors, and Coping Strategies for Teens Fighting Cancer or Dealing with Cancer in Friends or Family Members

Edited by Wilma R. Caldwell. 428 pages. 2004. 0-7808-0678-6. $58.

"Recommended for school libraries, or consumer libraries that see a lot of use by teens."
— *E-Streams, May 2005*

"A valuable educational tool."
— *American Reference Books Annual, 2005*

"Young adults and their parents alike will find this new addition to the *Teen Health Series* an important reference to cancer in teens."
— *Children's Bookwatch, February 2005*

Diet Information for Teens
Health Tips about Diet and Nutrition

Including Facts about Nutrients, Dietary Guidelines, Breakfasts, School Lunches, Snacks, Party Food, Weight Control, Eating Disorders, and More

Edited by Karen Bellenir. 399 pages. 2001. 0-7808-0441-4. $58.

"Full of helpful insights and facts throughout the book. . . . An excellent resource to be placed in public libraries or even in personal collections."
— *American Reference Books Annual 2002*

"Recommended for middle and high school libraries and media centers as well as academic libraries that educate future teachers of teenagers. It is also a suitable addition to health science libraries that serve patrons who are interested in teen health promotion and education."
— *E-Streams, Oct '01*

"This comprehensive book would be beneficial to collections that need information about nutrition, dietary guidelines, meal planning, and weight control. . . . This reference is so easy to use that its purchase is recommended."
— *The Book Report, Sep-Oct '01*

"This book is written in an easy to understand format describing issues that many teens face every day, and then provides thoughtful explanations so that teens can make informed decisions. This is an interesting book that provides important facts and information for today's teens."
— *Doody's Health Sciences Book Review Journal, Jul-Aug '01*

"A comprehensive compendium of diet and nutrition. The information is presented in a straightforward, plain-spoken manner. This title will be useful to those working on reports on a variety of topics, as well as to general readers concerned about their dietary health."
— *School Library Journal, Jun '01*

Drug Information for Teens
Health Tips about the Physical and Mental Effects of Substance Abuse

Including Facts about Alcohol, Anabolic Steroids, Club Drugs, Cocaine, Depressants, Hallucinogens, Herbal Products, Inhalants, Marijuana, Narcotics, Stimulants, Tobacco, and More

Edited by Karen Bellenir. 452 pages. 2002. 0-7808-0444-9. $58.

"A clearly written resource for general readers and researchers alike."
— *School Library Journal*

"The chapters are quick to make a connection to their teenage reading audience. The prose is straightforward and the book lends itself to spot reading. It should be useful both for practical information and for research, and it is suitable for public and school libraries."
— *American Reference Books Annual, 2003*

"Recommended reference source."
— *Booklist, American Library Association, Feb '03*

"This is an excellent resource for teens and their parents. Education about drugs and substances is key to discouraging teen drug abuse and this book provides this much needed information in a way that is interesting and factual." —*Doody's Review Service, Dec '02*

■

Eating Disorders Information for Teens

Health Tips about Anorexia, Bulimia, Binge Eating, and Other Eating Disorders

Including Information on the Causes, Prevention, and Treatment of Eating Disorders, and Such Other Issues as Maintaining Healthy Eating and Exercise Habits

Edited by Sandra Augustyn Lawton. 337 pages. 2005. 0-7808-0783-9. $58.

■

Fitness Information for Teens

Health Tips about Exercise, Physical Well-Being, and Health Maintenance

Including Facts about Aerobic and Anaerobic Conditioning, Stretching, Body Shape and Body Image, Sports Training, Nutrition, and Activities for Non-Athletes

Edited by Karen Bellenir. 425 pages. 2004. 0-7808-0679-4. $58.

"This book will be a great addition to any public, junior high, senior high, or secondary school library."
—*American Reference Books Annual, 2005*

■

Mental Health Information for Teens

Health Tips about Mental Health and Mental Illness

Including Facts about Anxiety, Depression, Suicide, Eating Disorders, Obsessive-Compulsive Disorders, Panic Attacks, Phobias, Schizophrenia, and More

Edited by Karen Bellenir. 406 pages. 2001. 0-7808-0442-2. $58.

"In both language and approach, this user-friendly entry in the *Teen Health Series* is on target for teens needing information on mental health concerns." —*Booklist, American Library Association, Jan '02*

"Readers will find the material accessible and informative, with the shaded notes, facts, and embedded glossary insets adding appropriately to the already interesting and succinct presentation."
—*School Library Journal, Jan '02*

"This title is highly recommended for any library that serves adolescents and parents/caregivers of adolescents." —*E-Streams, Jan '02*

"Recommended for high school libraries and young adult collections in public libraries. Both health professionals and teenagers will find this book useful."
—*American Reference Books Annual 2002*

"This is a nice book written to enlighten the society, primarily teenagers, about common teen mental health

issues. It is highly recommended to teachers and parents as well as adolescents."
—*Doody's Review Service, Dec '01*

■

Sexual Health Information for Teens

Health Tips about Sexual Development, Human Reproduction, and Sexually Transmitted Diseases

Including Facts about Puberty, Reproductive Health, Chlamydia, Human Papillomavirus, Pelvic Inflammatory Disease, Herpes, AIDS, Contraception, Pregnancy, and More

Edited by Deborah A. Stanley. 391 pages. 2003. 0-7808-0445-7. $58.

"This work should be included in all high school libraries and many larger public libraries. . . . highly recommended."
—*American Reference Books Annual 2004*

"Sexual Health approaches its subject with appropriate seriousness and offers easily accessible advice and information." —*School Library Journal, Feb. 2004*

■

Skin Health Information For Teens

Health Tips about Dermatological Concerns and Skin Cancer Risks

Including Facts about Acne, Warts, Hives, and Other Conditions and Lifestyle Choices, Such as Tanning, Tattooing, and Piercing, That Affect the Skin, Nails, Scalp, and Hair

Edited by Robert Aquinas McNally. 429 pages. 2003. 0-7808-0446-5. $58.

"This volume, as with others in the series, will be a useful addition to school and public library collections."
—*American Reference Books Annual 2004*

"This volume serves as a one-stop source and should be a necessity for any health collection."
—*Library Media Connection*

■

Sports Injuries Information For Teens

Health Tips about Sports Injuries and Injury Protection

Including Facts about Specific Injuries, Emergency Treatment, Rehabilitation, Sports Safety, Competition Stress, Fitness, Sports Nutrition, Steroid Risks, and More

Edited by Joyce Brennfleck Shannon. 405 pages. 2003. 0-7808-0447-3. $58.

Suicide Information for Teens

Health Tips about Suicide Causes and Prevention

Including Facts about Depression, Risk Factors, Getting Help, Survivor Support, and More

Edited by Joyce Brennfleck Shannon. 368 pages. 2005. 0-7808-0737-5. $58.